Cardiopulmonary Rehabilitation: Basic Theory and Application

Second Edition

Contemporary Perspectives in Rehabilitation

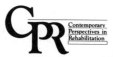

Steven L. Wolf, PhD, FAPTA
Editor-in-Chief

PUBLISHED VOLUMES

The Biomechanics of the Foot and Ankle
Robert Donatelli, MA, PT

Pharmacology in Rehabilitation
Charles D. Ciccone, PhD, PT

Wound Healing: Alternatives in Management
Luther C. Kloth, MS, PT, Joseph M. McCulloch, PhD, PT, and
Jeffrey A. Feedar, BS, PT

Thermal Agents in Rehabilitation, 2nd Edition
Susan L. Michlovitz, MS, PT

Electrotherapy in Rehabilitation
Meryl R. Gersh, MS, PT

Dynamics of Human Biologic Tissues
Dean P. Currier, PhD, PT and Roger M. Nelson, PhD, PT

Concepts in Hand Rehabilitation
Barbara G. Stanley, BS, PT and Susan M. Tribuzi, BS, OTR

Cardiopulmonary Rehabilitation: Basic Theory and Application

Second Edition

Frances J. Brannon, PhD
Professor, Assistant Chairperson, Coordinator of
    Graduate Studies, and Coordinator of Exercise
Physiology Laboratory
Department of Physical Education
Slippery Rock University
Slippery Rock, Pennsylvania

Margaret W. Foley, MN
St. Josephs's Hospital of Atlanta
Atlanta, Georgia

Julie Ann Starr, MS, PT
Clinical Assistant Professor
Department of Physical Therapy
Sargent College of Allied Health Professions
Boston University
Boston, Massachusetts

Mary Geyer Black, MS, PT
Director of Rehabilitative Services
Butler Memorial Hospital
Butler, Pennsylvania

 F. A. DAVIS COMPANY • Philadelphia

Printed in the United States of America

Last digit indicates print number: 10 9 8 7 6 5 4 3 2 1

acquisitions editor: Jean-François Vilain
developmental editor: Ralph Zickgraf
production editor: Crystal S. McNichol

As new scientific information becomes available through basic and clinical research, recommended treatments and drug therapies undergo changes. The author(s) and publisher have done everything possible to make this book accurate, up to date, and in accord with accepted standards at the time of publication. The authors, editors, and publisher are not responsible for errors or omissions or for consequences from application of the book, and make no warranty, expressed or implied, in regard to the contents of the book. Any practice described in this book should be applied by the reader in accordance with professional standards of care used in regard to the unique circumstances that may apply in each situation. The reader is advised always to check product information (package inserts) for changes and new information regarding dose and contraindications before administering any drug. Caution is especially urged when using new or infrequently ordered drugs.

Library of Congress Cataloging-in-Publication Data

Cardiopulmonary rehabilitation : basic theory and application /
   Frances J. Brannon . . . [et al.].—2nd ed.
      p. cm.—(Contemporary perspectives in rehabilitation : v. 10)
      Rev. ed. of: Cardiac rehabilitation / Frances J. Brannon, Mary J. Geyer, Margaret W. Foley.
c1988.
      Includes bibliographical references and index.
      ISBN 0-8036-1126-6 (hardbound: alk. paper);
      1. Heart—Diseases—Exercise therapy.   2. Heart—Diseases-
-Patients—Rehabilitation.   3. Cardiopulmonary system—Diseases-
-Patients—Rehabilitation.   I. Brannon, Frances J., 1935–
II. Brannon, Frances J., 1935–   Cardiac rehabilitation.
III. Series.
   [DNLM: 1. Exercise Therapy.   2. Heart Diseases—rehabilitation.
3. Lung Diseases—rehabilitation.   W1 CO769NS v. 10]
RC684.E9.C39   1992
616.1′2062—dc20
DNLM/DLC   92-18329
for Library of Congress   CIP

To my sister, Marjorie B. Stephens, and to my brother, Jennings Brannon, who have done for me what few people would.

Frances J. Brannon

To Terry—whose patience, support, and editorial assistance made my contribution possible —and to our families, whose encouragement and hours of babysitting allowed me to "get it done!"

Margaret W. Foley

To my family—George, Jillian, Jana, and Adam—and to my Mom and Dad who taught me to finish what I start.

Julie Ann Starr

Foreword

In 1988, *Cardiac Rehabilitation: Basic Theory and Application* became the second book in our *Contemporary Perspectives in Rehabilitation* series. At the time we prided ourselves on the fact that, like the volume's predecessor, *Thermal Agents in Rehabilitation*, this book would emphasize a problem-solving format designed to complement the way in which clinicians gather data for the primary purpose of reaching logical decisions for the optimal care of the cardiac patient. The authors sought to integrate basic theory from multiple resources so that the text would also serve as a condensed and valued resource. In retrospect the first edition met another objective; namely to facilitate the acquisition and development of information about cardiac rehabilitation that would be useful in the classroom, clinic, or laboratory. Furthermore the content was designed to (1) meet the needs of undergraduate students in physical therapy, health sciences nursing, sports medicine, athletic training, and physical education; (2) serve as a concise yet comprehensive review for physical therapists studying for cardiopulmonary specialization examinations; and (3) stimulate clinicians responsible for monitoring, generating, or evaluating the status of patients within a cardiopulmonary treatment program.

Based on the performance of the first edition, it is fair to say that these goals were met very successfully. The question then arose as to how a second edition could be better than the first. Based on the belief that clinicians who are engaged in cardiopulmonary rehabilitation treatment are even more eager and qualified to make important clinical decisions than they were 5 years ago and that students of cardiopulmonary pathologies are more astute and inquisitive, the authors have expanded problem solving chapters as well as the scope of this text. Four chapters have been added and an *increased emphasis placed on the pulmonary system*. The existing chapters have been extensively revised, and references have been made contemporary for all chapters. Elaborate and sophisticated case studies to challenge the reader are included.

Added to this edition are comprehensive chapters on the anatomy and function of the respiratory system and on chronic lung diseases. A detailed discussion on assessment of pulmonary patients emphasizes the interview and physical examination process, including the incorporation of laboratory findings into the assessment, and the development of exercise prescriptions. The case studies included in this chapter will be thought provoking for student and clinician alike. One of the most popular chapters in the first edition, "The Exercise Prescription," has been revised, and a totally new chapter on additional components for the pulmonary rehabilitation program has been developed. The comprehensive chapters on ECGs and their interpretations remain intact and serve as an excellent resource to challenge the analytic skills of the reader.

For those clinicians who enjoyed the first edition of *Cardiac Rehabilitation: Basic Theory and Application*, we hope that our expansion into pulmonary treatment and our updating of cardiac rehabilitation approaches will prove enlightening. To those clinicians and students who are experiencing this text for the first time, we hope that you will appreciate the comprehensive yet concise treatment given to the rehabilitative management of patients with cardiopulmonary deficits, and we trust that your thinking and clinical acumen will greatly benefit.

Steven L. Wolf, PhD, FAPTA
Series Editor

Preface to the Second Edition

The first edition of this text, *Cardiac Rehabilitation: Basic Theory and Application*, was an attempt to give students and practicing clinicians information necessary to develop their decision-making skills so as to provide comprehensive and quality rehabilitation programs for cardiac patients. Practical application of theoretical concepts based on current research was emphasized, with a particular strength of the text being the presentation of case studies to reinforce and illustrate problem-solving techniques.

The second edition follows the practical approach of the first, but the scope of the second edition has been broadened to include knowledges, and applications of those knowledges, necessary to provide quality rehabilitation programs for the pulmonary patient. The title of the text has, therefore, been changed to *Cardiopulmonary Rehabilitation: Basic Theory and Application*.

All chapters have been updated, and four new chapters have been added that specifically address the rehabilitation of the pulmonary patient. Chapter 3 presents the anatomy and physiology of respiration; Chapter 6 discusses the pathophysiology of COPD; Chapter 10 addresses the assessment of the pulmonary patient; and Chapter 14, "Additional Components of Pulmonary Rehabilitation," presents skills and techniques of pulmonary rehabilitation that are not commonly encountered in programs designed primarily for the cardiac patient.

Extensive revisions have been made in Chapters 11, 12, and 13 to reflect the current theories, practices, and procedures used in exercise prescription and programming for cardiopulmonary patients.

We hope that the practical nature of this text will continue to serve those educators responsible for disseminating information to future clinicians. The text was also written to assist practicing clinicians who are responsible for providing quality care in the rehabilitation of the cardiopulmonary patient.

FJB
MWF
JAS

Acknowledgments

In addition to the acknowledgments cited in the first edition of our text, we would like to thank the following:

My family and friends (especially those at the "Round Table" at Slippery Rock University) who have given me encouragement and support and have helped me keep my sense of humor so that this edition of *Cardiopulmonary Rehabilitation* was "not so painful." My appreciation goes also to our helpful reviewers: Nancy Blackshaw, Linda Crane, and Walter Erickson. I would also like to express my gratitude to my co-authors, Peggy Foley and Julie Starr, with whom I have had countless conversations, and who were always willing to do what had to be done to accomplish the writing of this edition, which I believe is an even better text than the first. Finally, and again, a special thanks to Jean-François Vilain—for being Jean-François!

FJB

A very special thank you to my husband Terry for his love, understanding, and support when I agreed to undertake this project and for his many hours of assistance as it ensued.

To our children, Allison and Sean, who always *tried* to wait until one more sentence was written, and to our parents Peggy and Jim Wiley and Alice and John Foley, who "vacationed in Atlanta" to babysit their grandchildren to allow me time for research and writing—I am forever grateful.

My thanks also go to Eddie Smith, my typist, and to those friends and colleagues who enthusiastically encouraged me.

Finally, to Dr. Frances Brannon who, after talking me into working on this second edition, could not ever have been a more helpful resource and supportive co-author and friend.

MWF

First and foremost, I would like to thank George Coggeshall, Jr. for his support, guidance, expertise, and constructive editing and willingness to support this project to the end and to endure life with a woman glued to a computer. I want to acknowledge my dynamic trio, Jillian, Jana, and Adam, for their ability to make me smile and enjoy life in spite of all the writing. To them, I promise, "Just a minute, I'm almost done" will not be uttered again (at least for a little while). I would also like to thank Elizabeth Eagan-Bengston for her knowledge, willingness to help, bright enthusiasm, and soaring optimism that saw me through many difficult hours. I would like to acknowledge Ms. Barbara O'Brien for keeping my life and my children's lives in beautiful harmony, which only she could have provided during these past months while this book was in progress. I would like to thank Marj Levy for her willingness to lend a hand when I really needed one. Finally, I would like to thank Dr. Frances Brannon. Her faith in this book and in me and her always gentle prodding made this all come true.

JAS

Preface to the First Edition

Recent innovations in health care delivery systems and a more informed public have contributed to an unprecedented interest in health, wellness, fitness, and nutrition; in the prevention of degenerative diseases, such as cardiac disease; and in the rehabilitation of individuals with such diseases. This timely text fills a void for many allied health professionals involved in providing scientifically-based exercise programs for healthy populations as well as those with cardiac disease. The specialized field of cardiac rehabilitation attracts many health professionals, including physical therapists, exercise physiologists, respiratory therapists, nurses, psychologists, nutritionists, and certainly physicians. Although each specialist brings unique skills to the field, the knowledge that an individual clinician possesses regarding cardiac rehabilitation programming is often incomplete. Therefore, we have written this book to enhance the allied health professionals' understanding of the basic scientific theory and principles associated with outpatient (Phases II, III) cardiac rehabilitation. Specific innovations in instrumentation, surgical procedures, pharmacology, and behavioral medicine techniques are presented. Every effort has been made to include the most current references and research available regarding the information presented.

Our goal is to offer a comprehensive description (which integrates information from a variety of disciplines) of the current state of knowledge and clinical practices in the field of cardiopulmonary rehabilitation for both the student and the experienced clinician. The text begins with an overview of cardiac rehabilitation; Chapters 2 and 3 present cardiac and circulatory anatomy and physiology; Chapter 4 discusses the pathophysiology of coronary heart disease (CHD); Chapter 5 explores surgical and pharmacologic management of the CHD patient; Chapter 6, on ECG interpretation, includes sample rhythm strips illustrating arrhythymias that the clinician must be able to readily identify as either benign or life-threatening. A self-test is included, which is valuable as a review of the material and considerably enhances the identification process. We then discuss physiologic assessment in Chapter 7, the exercise prescription in Chapter 8, and the exercise training session in Chapter 9. The last chapter is devoted to risk factor modification. The Appendix contains a variety of sample forms for patient, physician, and cardiopulmonary rehabilitation staff, along with health risk appraisals, stress inventories, and dietary information.

Another major goal of our book is to facilitate the acquisition and development of decision-making skills. The depth and breadth of the content provide the means for acquiring these skills. We also have provided nine case studies to which we refer in the later chapters in order to integrate the information from chapter to chapter and to foster the development of problem-solving skills. In this way, the learner may follow the course of treatment described for a specific individual beginning with physiologic assessment and criteria for test termination, followed by the writing of the exercise prescription, and ending with the progression through the training program. This method of presentation is unique to this book and has not been so used in any text in this field.

Throughout the text, illustrations are provided to clarify complex technical data such as formulae, physiologic processes, and algorithms. Photographs of specific procedures have been included as needed, and anatomic illustrations have been chosen for their simplicity and their pedagogic value.

It should be emphasized that the concepts presented are to be used as guidelines to assist the clinician in the evaluation and treatment process since no one method applies to all situations. We hope that the practical nature of the text will aid the decision-making process of the clinician who is responsible for conducting the outpatient cardiac rehabilitation program and is, therefore, responsible for making the ultimate decisions regarding patient care.

ACKNOWLEDGMENTS

The task of completing a major text of this nature was made easier by the support and encouragement of our families and friends. We would especially like to thank the following:

Dr. Kathleen Byrne
Elise and Clovis Faltot
Joan Faltot
Lt. Terry Foley
Claudia Hickly
Marjorie Stephens
Peggy and Jim Wiley

A special thanks also goes to all the patients, program directors, and medical directors (Dr. Herbert Gray, Dr. Wilfredo Rubio, Dr. Surendra Sethi, Dr. Michael Wusylko) of the Bio-Energetiks Rehabilitation Clinics.

We wish to offer our gratitude to the following reviewers who read various drafts of the manuscript: Carolyn Burnett, Jane Golden, Thomas W. Hare, Thomas Hon, Nancy Humberstone, Althea Jones, Steven L. Wolf, and Lana K. Woods. Finally, our thanks go to the staff at F. A. Davis who contributed to make the book a reality: Susan Ferragino, Mary Helen Bond, Herbert Powell, Jr., Philip Ashley, and Jean-François Vilain.

FJB
MJG
MWF

Contents

CHAPTER 1

Cardiopulmonary Rehabilitation: Overview

HISTORIC PERSPECTIVE OF CORONARY HEART DISEASE

Thirty years ago, persons with cardiovascular disease were given little hope of leading normal lives.[1] Cardiac patients were treated as invalids, and the prospects of returning to full-time work were dismal. Perhaps the Framingham Study[2] provided the impetus to change the direction for treatment and hence prognosis for the cardiac patient. With the examination of 5200 men and women at regular intervals, a pattern of the etiology of cardiovascular disease began to appear. Of course, very little can be done to change family history, but other risk factors indicated that lifestyle might exacerbate the incidence of coronary heart disease (CHD). Elevated blood pressure, blood fats and blood sugar, cigarette smoking, and lack of exercise seem to be interrelated and to lead to an increased risk of developing CHD.[2] Could CHD be prevented or the age of CHD onset be delayed if the risk factors that seem to be responsible could be modified? The answer to that question remains to be found, but current research[3] indicates that regular exercise of the appropriate type and intensity and modification of other risk factors contribute to longevity in a normal population,[4-10] as well as to the secondary prevention of cardiac events in CHD populations.[11-14]

Exercise has become an integral part of medicine by assisting in the diagnosis of cardiovascular disease and by serving as an adjunct to traditional medical practice in the treatment of persons with CHD.[15-18]

Despite the recent declines in CHD mortality, cardiovascular disease remains the single most prevalent cause of death in the United States today.[19] Although research and advances in surgical and medical treatment have most likely contributed to the declining CHD death rates, modifications of factors related to coronary risk also are important. However, behavioral approaches to induce individuals to modify negative health habits have only recently been given appropriate attention.[19,20]

Current trends in cardiac rehabilitation indicate that programs are changing to include a multispecialty approach in which emphasis on exercise therapy is followed by intervention that addresses various risk factors. Risk factor modification is becoming

1

increasingly scientific, and the specialized skills of many health professionals working as a team are required to provide effective rehabilitative services. This multispecialty approach is not new to inpatient rehabilitation programs, and both free-standing and hospital-based outpatient cardiac rehabilitation programs also are increasing their specialized services to include the expertise of the physical therapist, the respiratory therapist, the exercise physiologist, the psychologist, the registered dietitian or nutritionist, the nurse cardiac specialist, and various exercise specialists and health educators. Regardless of the specialization of the health professionals who, under the supervision of the physician medical director(s), provide the rehabilitative services in a specific setting, current trends in cardiac rehabilitation emphasize more professional approaches to stress management, nutritional counseling, and smoking cessation. Unfortunately, insurance reimbursement for largely "educational" approaches to risk factor modification is virtually nonexistent. In many cases, the cost of utilizing the skills of all the aforementioned professionals thus becomes prohibitive. Overlap in the educational backgrounds of these professionals and education of existing staff may, however, provide quality programming in many areas of specialization. For example, a nurse cardiac specialist can be trained in the theory and practice of cardiac exercise physiology. It is for that purpose that this text was written: to provide the basic theory of outpatient cardiac rehabilitation and the practical application of the theory so that allied health professionals at various educational levels might gain sufficient information to function optimally as cardiac rehabilitation specialists.

INPATIENT CARDIAC REHABILITATION

The inpatient exercise program (Phase I) is begun in the hospital, usually in the coronary care unit (CCU). Persons with uncomplicated myocardial infarctions (MI), coronary artery bypass grafts (CABG), pulmonary disease, or peripheral vascular disease (PVD) may begin their programs early during their hospital stays. The once routine therapy of bed rest has been replaced by allowing patients to sit in chairs by the third postinfarction or postsurgical day. Early mobilization in this form has resulted in improved cardiac function and has benefited patients psychologically.[22] Goals of inpatient cardiac rehabilitation include (1) preventing the deleterious effects of bed rest, (2) assessing the hemodynamic response to exercise, (3) managing the psychosocial issues of cardiac disease, and (4) educating the patient and family.[23-25]

The inpatient exercise program usually begins in the intensive care unit (ICU). Once a patient is medically stable following a cardiac event and an initial assessment has been completed, exercise sessions can begin. Activities are prescribed at low intensities, 1 to 2 METs, and they include active assistive range-of-motion exercises in the supine position.[26] Exercise intensity gradually progresses to 2 and 3 METs and includes sitting and standing exercises and progressive ambulation. Stair climbing is performed prior to discharge from the hospital.[25] Table 1–1 illustrates activities and progressions that have been used in inpatient rehabilitation programs to help patients achieve functional capacities that permit self-care.

Monitoring patients during Phase I cardiac rehabilitation usually requires the use of the ICU or the ward's electrocardiography (ECG) equipment (telemetry or hard-wire monitors), as well as periodic pulse checks for heart rate evaluations. A maximum heart rate increase of 20 beats per minute above resting (in the absence of arrhythmias, displaced ST segment, or angina) is a fairly safe guideline for exercise intensity during

Phase I cardiac rehabilitation.[27] Blood pressures are easily measured prior to and after exercise. If there is reason for concern, blood pressures should be monitored every few minutes. Systolic blood pressures should not rise more than 20 mm Hg or fall more than 10 to 15 mm Hg. Pulse pressures should not be less than 20 mm Hg between systolic and diastolic pressures.[28]

Education for a healthier lifestyle is an integral part of each phase of rehabilitation. Patient education begins in Phase I cardiac rehabilitation with individual or group instructions. Emphasis is placed on identification and modification of reversible risk factors in order to prevent further cardiac events.

Prior to discharge from the hospital, a low-level symptom-limited graded exercise test (LL-GXT) should be performed.[24,29-31] The purpose of this test is to evaluate the patient's functional capacity. A symptom-limited heart rate is established by the LL-GXT, and it can be used to prescribe a safe and effective exercise program for the next phase of cardiac rehabilitation.

OUTPATIENT CARDIAC EXERCISE TRAINING PROGRAMS

Supervised Programs

Outpatient (Phase II) exercise training ideally should be provided in a facility that offers continuous ECG monitoring, emergency equipment, and medically supervised exercise.[10] Outpatient treatment is usually initiated within a few weeks following hospital discharge. However, to qualify for insurance reimbursement, rehabilitation should begin sometime within the first year following a diagnosis of coronary artery disease, coronary artery bypass surgery, myocardial infarction, coronary angioplasty, or other cardiac event that warrants rehabilitative services. Unsupervised programs are not recommended for the majority of cardiac patients, because the safety of unsupervised exercise programs is yet to be determined.[21] Patients with the following characteristics should be trained in a medically supervised setting:

1. Low maximal functional capacity
2. Severely depressed left ventricular function
3. Complex ventricular arrhythmias
4. Exercise-induced hypotension
5. Exertional angina
6. Inability to self-monitor exercise heart rate

Patients with the characteristics listed are at increased risk for adverse cardiac events during exercise.[32]

Most increases in cardiopulmonary functional capacity occur in outpatient exercise programs. Because Phase I (inpatient) patients are discharged from the hospital as soon as they are stable, there is insufficient time for significant physiologic adaptation to occur.

Patients are generally referred to supervised outpatient cardiac rehabilitation programs by their cardiologists or primary physicians. The medical director of the outpatient program must supervise all laboratory assessment and exercise therapy sessions. The medical director is responsible for the medical management of the patient's rehabil-

TABLE 1-1 Inpatient Rehabilitation: Seven-Step Myocardial Infarction Program
(Grady Memorial Hospital and the Emory University School of Medicine)

Step	Date	MD Initials	Nurse/PT Notes	Supervised Exercise	CCU/Ward Activity	Educational-Recreational Activity
CCU						
1				Active and passive ROM all extremities, in bed Teach patient ankle plantar and dorsiflexion—repeat hourly when awake	Partial self-care Feed self Dangle legs on side of bed Use bedside commode Sit in chair 15 min 1–2 times/day	Orientation to CCU Personal emergencies, social service aid as needed
2				Active ROM all extremities, sitting on side of bed	Sit in chair 15–30 min 2–3 times/day Complete self-care in bed	Orientation to rehabilitation team, program Smoking cessation Educational literature if requested Planning transfer from CCU
Ward						
3				Warm-up exercises, 2 METs: Stretching Calisthenics Walking 50 ft and back at slow pace	Sit in chair ad lib To ward class in wheelchair Walk in room	Normal cardiac anatomy and function Development of atherosclerosis What happens with myocardial infarction 1–2 METs craft activity
4				ROM and calisthenics, 2.5 METs	OOB as tolerated Walk to bathroom	Coronary risk factors and their control

4

Step	Exercise	Ward Activity	Educational, Craft, and Diversional Activity
5	Walk length of hall (75 ft) and back, average pace Teach pulse counting ROM and calisthenics, 3 METs Check pulse counting Practice walking few stairsteps Walk 300 ft bid	Walk to ward class, with supervision Walk to waiting room or telephone Walk in ward corridor prn	Diet Energy conservation Work simplification techniques (as needed) 2–3 METs craft activity
6	Continue above activities Walk down flight of steps (return by elevator) Walk 500 ft bid Instruct on home exercise	Tepid shower or tub bath, with supervision To OT, cardiac clinic teaching room, with supervision	Heart attack management: Medications Exercise Surgery Response to symptoms Family, community adjustments on return home Craft activity prn
7	Continue above activities Walk up flight of steps Walk 500 ft bid Continue home exercise instruction; present information regarding outpatient exercise program	Continue all previous ward activities	Discharge planning: Medications, diet, activity Return appointments Scheduled tests Return to work Community resources Educational literature Medication cards Craft activity prn

Source: From NK Wenger and GF Fletcher: Rehabilitation of the patient with symptomatic atherosclerotic coronary heart disease. In JW Hurst, et al (eds): The Heart, ed 6. McGraw-Hill, New York, 1986. Used by permission.

itation program. Physicians conduct and interpret routine ECG monitoring and interpret laboratory assessment results, and they are responsible for administering emergency medical care with the assistance of trained, qualified staff.

Generally, the program director (exercise physiologist, physical therapist, or nurse cardiac specialist) is responsible for administering stress tests and other laboratory evaluations (under the direct supervision of a physician), writing exercise prescriptions, revising exercise prescriptions (after physician review), and discharging most adminis- trative and managerial functions. The program director, in addition to management/ administrative experience, must have a thorough understanding of human anatomy and the physiology of exercise, as well as a knowledge of basic ECG interpretation, patho- physiology, and pharmacology, so that exercise prescriptions and patient progression can proceed as safely as possible.

A consulting nutritionist may counsel patients about proper diet, and a consulting psychologist may work with patients on management of stress and other risk factor modifications such as cessation of smoking. These tasks may also be assigned to health educators or specialists in the field who have been trained to provide such services.

In most cases, the outpatient program is begun soon after the patient is discharged from a hospital. Continuous monitoring of the patient during the early stages of the rehabilitation program is standard procedure. In the course of the exercise therapy program, stable patients are gradually weaned from continuous monitoring in order to effect self-regulation of the recognition of their exercise limitations in preparation for Phase III or home exercise programs. Stable patients learn to count their own pulse rates and to rate their perceived exertions in order to modify their exercise intensities (Chap- ters 11 and 12) and to reinforce knowledge of the contraindications to exercise.

Generally, exercise therapy is conducted three times per week over a minimum period of 3 months. At the end of the 3 months, a re-evaluation, including a stress test, is administered. The re-evaluation provides valuable information about the improve- ment in cardiopulmonary function, allows for exercise prescription revisions, and serves as an important motivator for the patient.

Decisions as to when the patient may progress to a medically unsupervised (less intensely monitored Phase III or community program) or home program are based on (1) the patient's functional classification at re-evaluation (an aerobic capacity of at least 5 METs as determined by the stress test[10]); (2) the patient's ability to self-monitor his or her exercise program; (3) the stability (or absence of contraindications to exercise) of the patient; and (4) the psychologic and emotional status of the patient. The decision to recommend a patient for home or Phase III exercise is usually made by the rehabilitation team as a whole after a careful consideration of the patient's safety and functional and medical status and the likelihood of his or her compliance. Many patients develop a dependency on the rehabilitation staff and must be slowly phased from the supervised program by decreasing the frequency of supervised visits over a period of time and encouraging unsupervised exercise at home. In this way, the more dependent patients can build confidence in their own abilities to make decisions regarding their exercise programs as the staff provides feedback regarding their conduct during unsupervised exercise. This process helps to eliminate the feeling of abandonment that many patients report following the sudden cessation of a formal supervised program.

Even though a patient may no longer be actively involved in the supervised exercise therapy program, periodic re-evaluations should be scheduled to ensure that the exer- cise program and cardiopulmonary function are being maintained. Re-evaluations also help in the early detection of conditions for which further medical evaluations are indicated.

PHASE III (COMMUNITY) PROGRAMS

Persons with CHD who are exercising without medical supervision should probably do so only after "graduating" from a medically supervised program. With the current increase in knowledge and continued research into the science of exercise, it is inappropriate for patients to be advised "to do what you feel like doing" without exercise evaluations and concrete guidelines for their exercise target heart rates. Once patients have completed programs in which they learn what is necessary to maintain their cardiopulmonary function, they should be able to engage in unsupervised programs fairly safely. At the Phase III level, maintenance of cardiopulmonary function is the primary goal; therefore, many such programs are ineligible for third-party reimbursement.

A criticism of unsupervised programs is that they often lack personnel with the ability to give sound advice about exercise prescriptions and progression. To improve compliance, these centers often employ recreational games as a part of the rehabilitation process. That procedure is discouraged by those who seek closer controls over exercise heart rates and emphasize avoidance of emotional responses to exercise and similar competitive situations that may affect the safety of CHD patients. Physicians should decide whether the unsupervised program in their area meets the standards necessary for patient safety. The decision should be made on an individual basis in accordance with the guidelines previously discussed.

HISTORIC PERSPECTIVE OF PULMONARY DISEASE

A few decades ago, patients with pulmonary disease were given a standard prescription for rest and avoidance of exercise.[33] Well into the 1960s, the stress imposed by exercise was considered deleterious to such people.[34] They were treated as invalids and sometimes referred to as respiratory cripples.[35] The impetus to change direction in the treatment of pulmonary dysfunction came in 1964 as a result of a study by Pierce and his co-workers.[34] Patients with severe chronic obstructive pulmonary disease (COPD) were pre-tested for their exercise abilities and trained via treadmill walking programs. By using post-test data, decreases in exercising heart rate, respiratory rate, minute ventilation, oxygen consumption, and carbon dioxide production at similar exercise intensities were noted. An increase in exercise tolerance also was reported. Reconditioning of patients with COPD was found to be possible. Much research has since reported the positive effects of exercise training on patients with COPD.[36-42] Indeed, the view taken by Barach in 1951—that there might be a physiologic response to exercise training in patients with COPD based on the "progressive improvement in ability to talk without dyspnea,"—was supported.[43]

Exercise testing and training are now integral parts of the rehabilitation of the patient with COPD. There is little doubt that pulmonary rehabilitation enhances a patient's sense of well-being, improves exercise capacity, decreases the need for hospitalization, lowers overall health costs, and prolongs the survival in this patient population.[44,45]

Research has largely been focused on the exercise training of the patient population with COPD. Other types of chronic pulmonary diseases also are debilitating, and, until recently, their rehabilitation potential had been questioned. In one study, the results of a pre-training and post-training 6-minute walk test revealed that patients with pulmonary diseases other than COPD (primarily with restrictive pulmonary diseases) could significantly increase their walking distances.[46] The authors concluded that both COPD patients and "non-COPD" pulmonary patients appear to benefit from monitored exercise programs.

The second major emphasis in pulmonary rehabilitation is education. The education sessions are best provided by a variety of health care professionals. Topics such as the pulmonary disease process, available treatment modalities, smoking cessation, and energy-saving techniques give patients information they need to be better participants and managers in their own care.

Chronic pulmonary disease has been steadily increasing in incidence, and it is now estimated to afflict as many as 18.5 million Americans.[47] Since it is a leading cause of chronic disability,[48] pulmonary rehabilitation programs are more necessary now than ever before. Therefore, a major purpose of this text is to provide the basic theory of pulmonary rehabilitation and the practical application of the theory so that allied health professionals at all educational levels might gain sufficient information to function optimally in their roles as pulmonary rehabilitation specialists.

ACUTE PULMONARY CARE (INPATIENT)

Acute respiratory tract infections are the most frequently occurring infections; they range in severity from the common cold to pneumonia.[49] Acute pulmonary disease may result in decreased oxygen delivered to the body and decreased carbon dioxide eliminated from the body. The goals of acute pulmonary care are to improve ventilation and gas exchange, improve secretion clearance, and maintain functional capacity.[50] The role of the clinician involved in acute pulmonary care is to (1) instruct patients in breathing exercises in order to promote greater lung volumes and more efficient breathing patterns, (2) perform secretion removal techniques to enhance gas exchange, and (3) prescribe general conditioning exercises to maintain present levels of functioning. Because of the limitations on length of hospital stay, there is insufficient time to gain the physiologic adaptations of exercise training. Achievement of premorbid activity level is more compatible within the time frame of acute care. At this time, it is not within the scope of this text to provide detailed information on acute pulmonary care.

CHRONIC PULMONARY CARE (OUTPATIENT)

Chronic pulmonary disease and its associated dysfunction have a slow and insidious onset. Activities that result in the uncomfortable sensation of dyspnea are avoided by persons with pulmonary dysfunction. Family and friends often discourage these patients from exerting themselves for fear of untoward effects.[51] A slow but steady decrease in activity levels will soon follow. It is not uncommon for persons to lose many functional abilities before ever seeking medical help. One goal of pulmonary rehabilitation is to interrupt this downward spiraling of physical ability.[52]

A rehabilitation program can be initiated on inpatient admission or on an outpatient basis. Because of the confines of hospital admission, however, most increases in functional capacity will occur during outpatient rehabilitation. Candidates for outpatient pulmonary rehabilitation come from a variety of sources. In some cases, the outpatient program begins after hospitalization for an acute exacerbation of the disease. Other patients are diagnosed with chronic pulmonary disease as outpatients and are then referred for pulmonary rehabilitation. Finally, patients can be referred to pulmonary rehabilitation when their dyspnea interferes with their ability to maintain appropriate levels of physical activity. Enrollment in an outpatient pulmonary rehabilitation program is usually by physician referral.

An exercise test is often performed prior to admission to a pulmonary rehabilitation program. The results of this exercise test help to quantify patient symptoms, determine causes of dyspnea, assess functional abilities, determine potentials for work, and prescribe appropriate exercise programs.[53-55] Clinicians monitor patients by using rates of perceived shortness of breath, heart rates, respiratory rates, and oximetry (a photoelectric apparatus used to determine the amount of O_2 in the blood). During the course of the exercise therapy program, patients are gradually weaned to self-monitoring.

Generally, conditioning exercises are conducted three times per week for 6 to 8 weeks, although it often takes 6 to 12 months of exercise training for patients with COPD to show physiologic change. At the end of the rehabilitation program, patients are re-evaluated. A second exercise test is performed to assess the exercise prescription for continuation of care. An unfortunate reality is that pulmonary patients will often have respiratory setbacks. Continued contact and encouragement in the form of periodic evaluation is essential to maintain new levels of physical activity. However, insurance reimbursement for such care (maintenance) is difficult to obtain.[56] Patients are advised to join community-based groups that encourage compliance with their medical care. One such group is the Better Breathing Club, which is sponsored by the American Lung Association. Patients are also encouraged to subscribe to support groups such as Emphysema Anonymous.

HOME EXERCISE PROGRAMS

For both cardiac and pulmonary patients, a home exercise program is usually begun in conjunction with the outpatient program. When on the basis of exercise performance and laboratory data the rehabilitation staff deems it feasible, patients can be assigned exercises to be performed at home. They periodically return to the outpatient clinic with exercise logs of heart rates, perceived exertion rates, exercise parameters, and any problems that may have occurred during the home program. The staff members analyze the data, adjust the home program as necessary, and suggest methods for self-monitoring the changes in the home program. If no contraindications occur, the patient is advised to continue as before. Progression of patients to home programs is an ultimate goal of both the cardiac and pulmonary rehabilitation program. Once patients reach the level of functional capacity at which maintenance becomes the primary goal, they should be encouraged to continue exercising at home, with periodic evaluations, so that adequate cardiopulmonary functional capacity can be maintained.

MULTISPECIALTY APPROACH TO CARDIAC AND PULMONARY REHABILITATION

The primary goals of cardiac and pulmonary rehabilitation programs should be to increase the functional capacity of patients and to assist patients in attaining normal function, insofar as possible, in their daily lives. Throughout the many aspects of cardiopulmonary care, input from a diversity of health professionals is essential to provide the knowledge required to meet the medical, physical, social, and psychologic needs of the patient with cardiac and pulmonary disease. The team may include nurses, physicians, physical therapists, occupational therapists, respiratory therapists, exercise physiologists, vocational counselors, sex therapists, dietitians, psychiatrists, psychologists, social workers, recreational therapists, clergy, and, most important, the patient and the patient's family. It appears that hospitals and geographic regions differ in the extent of participation by the various allied health professionals. A comprehensive program dedicated to fulfilling the various needs of the patients that it serves should avail itself of these disciplines.[57]

SUMMARY

This chapter has presented a basic overview of cardiac and pulmonary rehabilitation programs. Cardiac rehabilitation programs are divided into three phases. Phase I programs begin during a patient's hospitalization and are of insufficient length and intensity to allow dramatic physiologic change. Most of the increases in cardiopulmonary functional capacity occur during the outpatient (Phase II) rehabilitation program. Phase II programs are physician-supervised, and they may employ specialists from several allied health disciplines. The outpatient program is usually conducted three times a week for a period of 12 weeks. Patients are gradually weaned from the outpatient program and encouraged to begin home exercise or unsupervised (Phase III) programs that include periodic re-evaluations by the outpatient cardiac rehabilitation staff.

Pulmonary rehabilitation programs are divided into inpatient acute and outpatient chronic phases. Inpatient care is usually of insufficient duration to allow dramatic physiologic training effects. Outpatient programs are usually conducted three times a week for a period of 6 to 8 weeks. As in cardiac rehabilitation, patients are gradually weaned from the structured programs and encouraged to begin home exercise programs. Follow-up evaluations by the outpatient pulmonary rehabilitation staff are important to ensure the highest level of patient compliance.

REFERENCES

1. Hellerstein, HK and Moir, TW: Distance running in the 1980's: Cardiovascular risks and benefits. In NK Wenger (ed): Exercise and the Heart, ed 2. FA Davis, Philadelphia, 1985, pp 75–86.
2. Dawber, TR: The Framingham Study: The Epidemiology of Atherosclerotic Disease. Harvard University Press, Cambridge, MA, 1980.
3. Mockeen, PC, et al: A thirteen year follow-up of a coronary heart disease risk factor screening and exercise program for 40–59 year-old men: Exercise habit maintenance and physiologic status. J Cardiopulmonary Rehabil 5:510–525, 1985.
4. Paffenbarger, RS Jr, et al: A natural history of athleticism and cardiovascular health. JAMA 252:491–495, 1984.
5. Eichner, ER: Exercise and heart disease: Epidemiology of the "exercise hypothesis." Am J Med 75:1008–1023, 1983.
6. Kannel, WB and Sorlic, P: Some health benefits of physical activity: The Framingham Study. Arch Intern Med 139:857–861, 1979.
7. Costas, R, et al: Relation of lipids, weight, and physical activity to incidence of coronary heart disease: The Puerto Rican Heart Study. Am J Cardiol 42:653–658, 1978.
8. Smith, EL, Reddan, W and Smith, PE: Physical activity and calcium modalities for bone mineral increase in aged women. Med Sci Sports Exerc 13:60–64, 1981.

9. Wallace, JP: Physical conditioning. In W. Regelson and FM Sinex (eds): Intervention in the Aging Process, Part A. Alan R Liss, New York, 1983, pp 307–323.
10. American College of Sports Medicine: Guidelines for Exercise Testing and Prescription. Lea & Febiger, Philadelphia, 1986, p 58.
11. Sparrow, D, et al: The influence of cigarette smoking on prognosis after a first myocardial infarction. J Chronic Dis 31:425–532, 1977.
12. Mulcahy, R, et al: Factors affecting the five-year survival rate of men following acute coronary heart disease. Am Heart J 93:556–559, 1977.
13. Coronary Drug Project Research Group: Influence of adherence to treatment and response of cholesterol on mortality in the coronary drug project. N Eng J Med 303:1038–1041, 1980.
14. Dyer, AR and Stamler, PJ: Alcoholic consumption and 17 year mortality in the Chicago Western Electric Study. Prev Med 9:78–90, 1980.
15. Fletcher, GF and Cantwell, JD: Exercise and Coronary Heart Disease. Charles C Thomas, Springfield, IL, 1979.
16. Blocker, WP and Cardus, D: Rehabilitation in Ischemic Heart Disease. Spectrum Publications, New York, 1983.
17. Fardy, PS, Yanowitz, FG and Wilson, PK: Cardiac Rehabilitation, Adult Fitness and Exercise Testing, ed 2. Lea & Febiger, Philadelphia, 1988, pp 3–16.
18. Froelicher, VF: Exercise Testing and Training. Le Jacq Publishing, New York, 1983.
19. Garrison, RJ, et al: Epidemiology of CHD: New Trends. Department of Epidemiology, National Heart, Lung and Blood Institute, NIH, Bethesda, MD.
20. Blumenthal, JA, et al: Continuing medical educator: Cardiac rehab: A new frontier for behavioral medicine. J Cardiac Rehabil 3:637–656, 1983.
21. Wenger, NK and Fletcher, GF: Rehabilitation of the patient with symptomatic atherosclerotic coronary heart disease. In J Hurst et al (eds): The Heart, ed 6. McGraw-Hill, New York, 1986.
22. Levine, S and Lown, B: "Armchair" treatment of acute coronary thrombosis. JAMA 148:1365, 1952.
23. Cahalin, LP, Ice, RG and Irwin, S: Program planning and implementation. In S Irwin and J Tecklin (eds): Cardiopulmonary Physical Therapy, ed 2. CV Mosby, St. Louis, 1990, p 149.
24. Graf, R: Rehabilitation during the acute and convalescent stages following myocardial infarction. In L Amundsen (ed): Cardiac Rehabilitation. Churchill Livingstone, New York, 1981, pp 101–105.
25. Brammel, H: Early rehabilitation of the post infarction patient. In C Long (ed): Prevention and Rehabilitation in Ischemic Heart Disease. Williams & Wilkins, Baltimore, 1980, pp 160–170.
26. Alpern, H and Mickle, E: Functional testing in the cardiac patient. In J Vyden (ed): Postmyocardial Infarction Management and Rehabilitation. Marcel Dekker, New York, pp 330–340.
27. Pollack, M, et al: Exercise prescription for rehabilitation of the cardiac patient. In M Pollock and D Schmidt (eds): Heart Disease and Rehabilitation. John Wiley & Sons, New York, 1986, p 495.
28. Freireich, R: Medical management of acute myocardial infarction. In S Irwin and J Tecklin (eds): Cardiopulmonary Physical Therapy, ed 2. CV Mosby, St. Louis, 1990, p. 95.
29. Fardy, P, Yanowitz, F and Wilson, P: Cardiac Rehabilitation, Adult Fitness and Exercise Testing, ed 2. Lea & Febiger, Philadelphia, 1988, pp 153–156.
30. Sivarajan, E, et al: Low level treadmill testing of 41 patients with acute myocardial infarction prior to discharge from the hospital. Heart Lung 6:975–980, 1977.
31. Madsen, E and Fraelicher, V: The use of exercise testing to evaluate patients after myocardial infarction. In M Pollack and D Schmidt (eds): Heart Disease and Rehabilitation. John Wiley & Sons, New York, 1986, p 465.
32. Williams, RS, et al: Guidelines for unsupervised exercise in patients with ischemic heart disease. J Cardiac Rehabil 1:213, 1981.
33. Hughes, R and Davison, R: Limitation of exercise reconditioning in cold. Chest 83(2):241–249, 1983.
34. Pierce, A, et al: Responses to exercise training in patients with emphysema. Arch Int Med 114:28–36, 1964.
35. Hale, T, Cumming, G and Spriggs, J: The effects of physical training in chronic obstructive pulmonary disease. Bull Europ Physiopath Resp 14:593–608, 1978.
36. Miller, W: Rehabilitation of patients with chronic obstructive pulmonary disease. Med Clin North Am 51:349–361, 1967.
37. Paez, P, et al: The physiological basis of training patients with emphysema. Am Rev Respir Dis 95:944–953, 1967.
38. Bass, H, Whitcomb, J and Forman, R: Exercise training: Therapy for patients with chronic obstructive pulmonary disease. Chest 57:116–121, 1970.
39. Vyas, M, et al: Response to exercise in patients with chronic airway obstruction. I. Effects of exercise training. Am Rev Respir Dis 103:390–400, 1971.
40. Woolf, C: A rehabilitation program for improving exercise tolerance in patients with chronic lung disease. Can Med Assoc J 106:1289–1292, 1972.
41. Bedout, D, et al: Clinical and physiological outcomes of a university hospital pulmonary rehabilitation program. Respir Care 28(11):1468–1471, 1983.
42. Carter, R, et al: Exercise conditioning in the rehabilitation of patients with chronic obstructive pulmonary disease. Arch Phys Med Rehabil 69:118–121, 1988.

43. Barach, A, Bickerman, H and Beck, G: Advances in the treatment of nontuberculous pulmonary disease. Bull NY Acad Med 28:353–384, 1952.
44. Belman, M and Wasserman, K: Exercise training and testing in patients with chronic obstructive pulmonary disease. Basics Respir Dis 10:1–6, 1981.
45. Sneider, R, O'Malley, J and Kahn, M: Trends in pulmonary rehabilitation at Eisenhower Medical Center: An 11-years' experience (1976–1987). J Cardiopulmonary Rehabil 11:453–461, 1988.
46. Foster, S and Thomas, H: Pulmonary rehabilitation in lung disease other than chronic obstructive pulmonary disease. Am Rev Respir Dis 141:601–604, 1990.
47. Hammon, W: Pathophysiology of chronic pulmonary disease. In D Frownfelter: Chest Physical Therapy and Pulmonary Rehabilitation: An Interdisciplinary Approach, ed 2. Year Book Medical Publishers, Chicago, 1987, p 91.
48. Feinleib, M, et al: Trends in COPD morbidity and mortality in the United States. Am Rev Respir Dis (Suppl)140:9–18, 1989.
49. Price, S and Wilson, L: Pathophysiology: Clinical Concepts of Disease Processes, ed 2. McGraw-Hill, New York, 1982, p 393.
50. Humberstone, N: Respiratory assessment and treatment. In S Irwin and J Tecklin: Cardiopulmonary Physical Therapy, ed 2. CV Mosby, St. Louis, 1990, p 303.
51. Moser, K, Archibald, C and Hansen, P: Better Living and Breathing: A Manual for Patients, ed 2. CV Mosby, St. Louis, 1980, p 46.
52. Frownfelter, D: Pulmonary rehabilitation. In D Frownfelter: Chest Physical Therapy and Rehabilitation. Year Book Medical Publishers, Chicago, 1987, p 295.
53. Zadai, C: Rehabilitation of the patient with chronic obstructive pulmonary disease. In S Irwin and J Tecklin: Cardiopulmonary Physical Therapy, ed 2. CV Mosby, St. Louis, 1990, p 496.
54. Hodgkin, J: Exercise testing and training. In J Hodgkin and T Petty: Chronic Obstructive Pulmonary Disease: Current Concepts, WB Saunders, Philadelphia, 1987, p 121.
55. American Thoracic Society Position Statement: Evaluation of impairment/disability secondary to respiratory disease. Am Rev Respir Dis 126:945–951, 1982.
56. Elkousy, N, et al: Outpatient pulmonary rehabilitation: A Medicare fiscal intermediary's viewpoint. J Cardiopulmonary Rehabil 11:492–497, 1988.
57. Miller, NH, et al: Position paper of the American Association of Cardiovascular and Pulmonary Rehabilitation. J Cardiopulmonary Rehabil 10(6):198–209, 1990.

CHAPTER 2

The Heart and Circulation

THE HEART

The heart is a hollow organ weighing approximately 250 to 300 g. It is not positioned in the center of the chest cavity; most of it lies to the left of center. The base of the heart is broad and is located superiorly, and the apex is at the inferior end and points anteriorly and approximately 45° to the left. The heart is enclosed in a fibrous protective sac called the pericardium. The major portion of the heart itself is composed of muscle referred to as the myocardium. The inner surface of the myocardium is lined with a smooth epithelial tissue called the endocardium, which allows the blood to pass through the chambers of the heart without damage to the blood cells.[1]

The outer, external surface of the myocardium is covered with a fibrous membrane, the epicardium, which merges at the base of the heart with the pericardium. The muscular tissue of the myocardium is arranged in layers that run in indefinite, circular, and oblique directions.[1]

The four chambers of the heart are the right and left atria and the right and left ventricles. The apex of the heart is formed by the tip of the left ventricle.[2]

The surfaces of the heart are the sternocostal, the diaphragmatic, and the posterior. The sternocostal surface (anterior) is formed primarily by the right atrium and the right ventricle. The diaphragmatic (inferior) surface of the heart is formed by the right and left ventricles. The posterior (base) surface of the heart is formed primarily by the left atrium, although the right atrium forms a small part of the posterior surface.[2]

The four borders of the heart are the right, left, superior, and inferior. The right border is formed by the right atrium; the left border is formed mainly by the left ventricle, but a small part is formed by the left atrium. The superior border is formed by both atria and is located in the area where the great vessels unite with the heart. The inferior border is formed primarily by the right ventricle and to a lesser extent by the left ventricle (Fig. 2–1).

Heart Chambers

The heart has four chambers that are arranged in pairs. The two atria are thin-walled cavities designed to receive blood into the heart. The right atrium receives blood from the systemic circulation through two openings: the superior and inferior venae

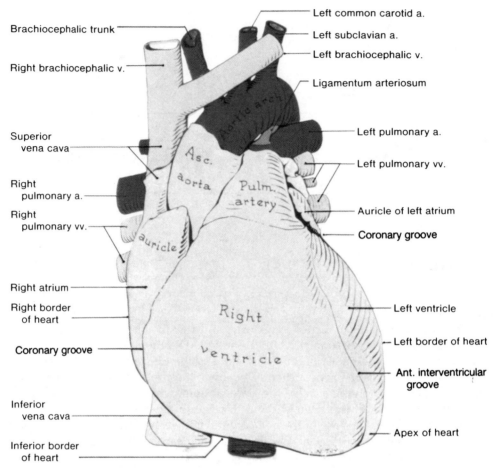

Brachiocephalic trunk

Right brachiocephalic v.

Superior
    vena cava

Right
    pulmonary a.

Right
    pulmonary vv.

Right atrium

Right border
    of heart

Coronary groove

Inferior
    vena cava

Inferior border
    of heart

Left common carotid a.

Left subclavian a.

Left brachiocephalic v.

Ligamentum arteriosum

Left pulmonary a.

Left pulmonary vv.

Auricle of left atrium

Coronary groove

Left ventricle

Left border of heart

Ant. interventricular
    groove

Apex of heart

FIGURE 2–1. The sternocostal aspect of the heart. (From Moore, KL: *Clinically Oriented Anatomy*, ed. 2, 1985, Williams & Wilkins Company, Baltimore, with permission.)

cavae. During systole of the atria, blood from the right atrium is sent through the right atrioventricular orifice to the right ventricle. This orifice contains the tricuspid valve, which opens to allow the blood to pass into the ventricle during atrial systole.[3] During ventricular systole, the tricuspid valve closes so that blood will not be pumped back into the atrium (Fig. 2–2).

The left atrium also is thin-walled. It has four openings at its superior and posterior wall (Fig. 2–3). These openings accommodate the four pulmonary veins that carry oxygenated blood from the lungs to the left atrium. Blood passes from the left atrium through the left atrioventricular orifice, which is controlled by the bicuspid or mitral valve. During ventricular contraction, the mitral valve is tightly closed to prevent blood surging back to the atrium.[4]

The walls of the ventricles are much thicker and stronger than those of the atria and are well suited to pump the blood greater distances. The right ventricle forms most of the front of the heart; it pumps the blood through the pulmonary orifice into the pulmonary artery (Fig. 2–4). The blood flow to the pulmonary artery is controlled by the semilunar or pulmonary valve, which prevents the flow of blood back to the right ventricle during systole. The right ventricle contracts to send the blood via the pulmo-

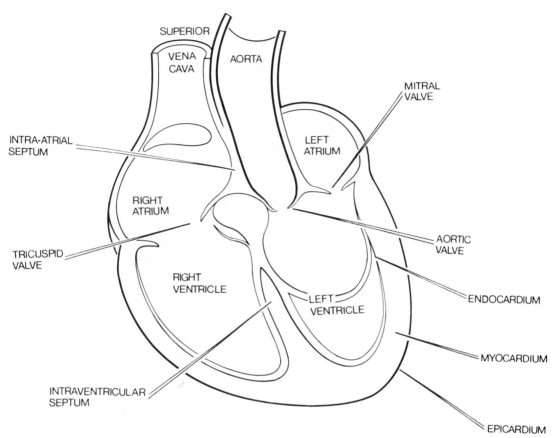

FIGURE 2–2. The heart and its chambers. (From Phillips and Feeney,[9] p. 11, with permission.)

nary artery through the pulmonary circulation to be oxygenated; hence, the right ventricle is referred to as the pulmonary pump.[4,5]

The walls of the left ventricle are thicker and stronger than the walls of the right ventricle. The left ventricle forms most of the left margin and the apex of the heart, and it is responsible for pumping blood throughout the entire systemic circulation: it is the systemic pump. Blood enters the systemic circulation from the left ventricle through the aortic orifice, guarded by the aortic valve, and into the aorta. The aorta is the largest artery in the body.[4,5]

THE CORONARY ARTERIES

The two major arteries that supply the heart with blood arise directly from the aorta at a point near the aortic valve (Fig. 2–5). Although there is considerable variation, the right coronary artery branches to send blood to the right atrium, the right ventricle, and, in most persons, the inferior wall of the left ventricle, the atrioventricular (AV) node, and the bundle of His. The sinoatrial (SA) node receives its blood supply from the right coronary artery in about 60 percent of human beings.[6]

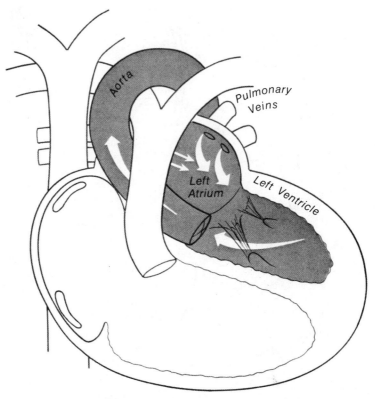

FIGURE 2–3. The left atrium and the pulmonary veins. (From Phillips and Feeney,[9] p. 9, with permission.)

The left coronary artery branches into two main divisions within approximately 2 cm from its point of origin. The left anterior descending (LAD) artery supplies the left ventricle, the interventricular septum, the right ventricle, and, in most persons, the inferior areas of the apex and both ventricles.[4,6]

The second main division of the left coronary artery, the left circumflex, supplies blood to the inferior walls of the left ventricle and to the left atrium. In about 40 percent of humans, the left circumflex supplies the SA node with blood.[4,6]

Circulation to the Heart

Blood circulating to the heart muscle itself via the coronary arteries must do so while the muscle fibers are relaxed, during diastole of the heart. To prevent the occurrence of an ischemic state, this is an important fact to remember when considering whether the heart muscle has adequate blood flow during exercise. Although blood is forced into the coronary arteries from the heart during systole, that blood cannot enter the cardiac muscle fibers to supply oxygen to the tissue until the heart is in diastole and the fibers are relaxed.[1] Perhaps that is the greatest single reason for keeping the exercising heart rate low in a coronary patient.

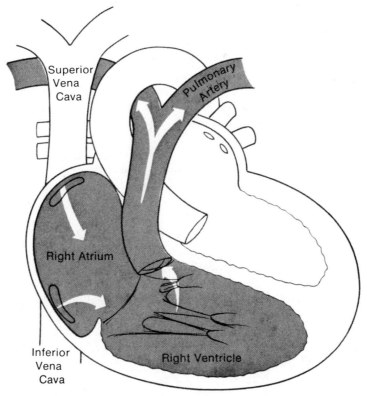

FIGURE 2–4. Blood flow from the right ventricle to the lungs. (From Phillips and Feeney,[9] p. 9, with permission.)

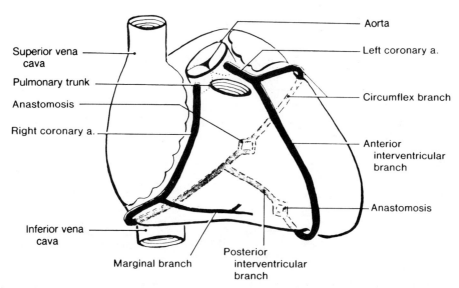

FIGURE 2–5. The coronary arteries. (From Moore, KL: *Clinically Oriented Anatomy*, ed. 2, 1985, Williams & Wilkins Company, Baltimore, with permission.)

METABOLISM OF CARDIAC TISSUE

Cardiac tissue contains large amounts of myoglobin, the enzymes of the Krebs cycle, and the electron transport system, and it is thus well suited for aerobic metabolism. For it to function properly, the heart must receive a constant supply of oxygen to support its almost exclusively aerobic metabolism. The principal source of energy production for cardiac muscle is the oxidation of free fatty acids. Although acetoacetic acid and lactic acid can be metabolized to produce energy, the energy of preference of the heart is supplied by fatty acid metabolism.[6,7] Examples of the anaerobic and aerobic pathways for adenosine 5'-triphosphate (ATP) production are given in Table 2–1.

The most common fatty acids have chains of 16 and 18 carbons. Through β-oxidation (oxidizing 2 carbons at one time), a 16-carbon-chain fatty acid could produce approximately 128 ATP when completely metabolized (16 ATP $\times$ 16 carbon/β-oxidation) = 16 ATP $\times$ 8 = 128 ATP.[6]

The importance of continuous O_2 delivery to the cardiac muscle can be seen in the relative contributions of anaerobic and aerobic metabolism to the production of ATP. During rest, cardiac tissue extracts approximately 70 percent of the O_2 that is delivered to it via the coronary arteries. This leaves a very limited reserve for increasing oxygen extraction during increased myocardial work. The increased demand for more oxygen during work is met by increasing the blood flow to the cardiac tissue. Consequently, the rate and force of cardiac contraction, and therefore cardiac output, increases in response to increased activity. Increased coronary blood flow is also achieved through a reduction in the resistance (dilation) of the coronary vessels.[6]

CONDUCTION

Although there are structural and functional similarities between cardiac and skeletal muscle, there are also major differences.[8] In addition to ordinary muscle tissue, cardiac muscle has two other major types of tissue: nodal and Purkinje. The nodal tissue is located at the junction of the superior vena cava and the right atrium (sinoatrial node)

TABLE 2–1 Anaerobic and Aerobic Metabolic Pathways for Production of ATP

Anaerobic Metabolism

1. Coronary circulation delivers glucose to cardiac tissue
2. Glucose via glycolysis (in cytoplasm) $\longrightarrow$ Pyruvate + 2 ATP

or

3. Lactate delivered by coronary circulation to cardiac tissue
4. Lactate (in cytoplasm) $\longrightarrow$ Pyruvate + 2 ATP

Aerobic Metabolism

1. Coronary circulation delivers free fatty acids to cardiac tissue
2. Free fatty acids undergo β-oxidation $\longrightarrow$ ~ 4 ATP + Acetyl Co A (Mitochondria)
3. Acetyl Co A enters Krebs cycle + O_2 $\longrightarrow$ ~ 12 ATP (approximately 6 total ATP with *each* 2-carbon oxidation) + H_2O + CO_2

or

4. Pyruvate (from cytoplasm) $\longrightarrow$ Acetyl Co A (Mitochondria)
5. Acetyl Co A $\longrightarrow$ Krebs cycle + O_2 $\longrightarrow$ 36 ATP + H_2O + CO_2

and at the junction of the right atrium and the right ventricle (atrioventricular node). The Purkinje fibers are the specialized conducting tissues of both ventricles.

Sinoatrial Node

The sinoatrial (SA) node (Fig. 2–6) is composed of small, slender, spindle-shaped cells that contain very few myofibrils but large amounts of thick connective tissue. The SA node, called the pacemaker of the heart, has sympathetic and parasympathetic innervation, although at rest the SA node is under continuous parasympathetic control via the vagus nerve. Small strands of fibers extend out from the main region of the SA node and are continuous with the ordinary muscle fibers of the atrium. Through this arrangement, once the SA node initiates an impulse (sinus rhythm), that impulse can spread from muscle fiber to muscle fiber throughout both atria (functional syncytium).[1,9]

Atrioventricular Node

The atrioventricular (AV) node is a band of fibers located at the lower end of the interatrial septum of the right atrium (Fig. 2–7). The AV nodal tissue merges with the atrioventricular bundle of His near the origin of the ventricles. The AV node normally functions to receive the impulse that originates from the SA node and conducts it to the bundle of His. In cases of impaired SA node function, the AV node can become the pacemaker of the heart and send out its own impulses to keep the heart beating (nodal rhythms). The AV node is also supplied with nerves from the sympathetic and parasympathetic systems.[1,9]

Purkinje Tissue

The AV bundle of His has two branches, the right and the left, located along either side of the intraventricular septum (Fig. 2–7). These branches terminate in the Purkinje fibers, which are the specialized conducting tissues of both ventricles. The fibers that comprise the Purkinje system have sarcoplasm that contains large amounts of glycogen but few myofibrils. The fibers of the Purkinje system terminate in twigs that penetrate the ventricles and are intimately associated with the contractile fibers of the ventricle muscles.[1,9]

Origin and Conduction of Heart Beat

The origin of the electric impulse that precedes the contraction of the heart is in the SA node (myogenic). This impulse spreads quickly through both atria, which then contract simultaneously. This wave of electrical activity next stimulates the AV node, which transmits the impulse down the bundle of His to the Purkinje fibers. Because the Purkinje fibers merge with the walls of the ventricles, the impulse spreads through the Purkinje system to the cells of the ventricles, and the ventricles contract together (Fig. 2–8). This rhythmic sequence of events occurs, on the average, 72 times per minute.[1]

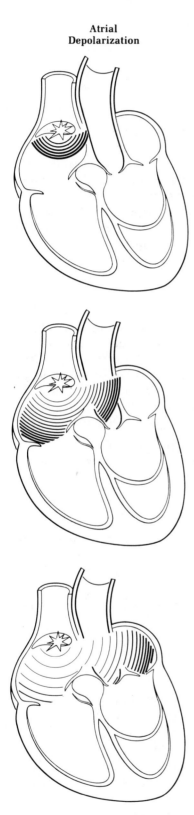

**Atrial
Depolarization**

FIGURE 2–6. Atrial impulse conduction. (From Phillips and Feeney,[9] p. 21, with permission.)

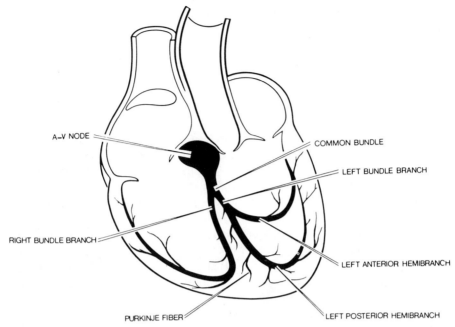

FIGURE 2–7. Ventricular conduction. (From Phillips and Feeney,[9] p. 23, with permission.)

Myocardial Fibers

The microscopic appearance of cardiac muscle fibers is similar to that of skeletal muscle fibers. Both types of muscle appear to be striated; their myofibrils have well-identified A, I, and Z bands.[8] Compared to skeletal muscle, cardiac tissue has numerous mitochondria and its T-tubules are larger, but the sarcoplasmic reticulum (SR) is not well developed.[8] A major functional difference between skeletal and cardiac muscle is that cardiac muscle exhibits a rhythmicity (myogenicity) of contraction whereas skeletal

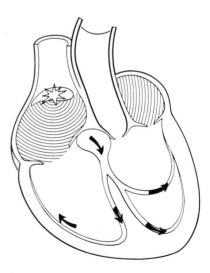

FIGURE 2–8. Schematic illustration of the conduction system of cardiac muscle. (From Phillips and Feeney,[9] p. 23, with permission.)

muscle contracts in response to direct neural stimulation. This inherent rhythmicity of cardiac tissue originates in the SA node.

GENERAL MYOLOGY

Muscle Tissue

The protoplasm of muscle cells has the ability to contract, and because most muscle cells are elongated, individual cells are called fibers. There are three types of muscle tissue in the body: smooth, skeletal, and cardiac. (Skeletal or striated muscle is sometimes further divided into skeletal and cardiac.[5])

Smooth muscle is closely associated with connective tissue structures and is found in the walls of the digestive tract, urinary tract, and blood vessels. Contraction of smooth muscle in those areas causes the structures to change in size and volume. Smooth muscle is also called involuntary or visceral, and the terms are used interchangeably. Each individual muscle fiber (cell) of smooth muscle tissue has a single oval nucleus. Unlike cardiac and skeletal muscle, smooth muscle can regenerate quite well following injury.[3]

The basic cellular structure of skeletal muscle can be described as a multinucleated cylinder that varies in length and may be longer than 30 cm. Skeletal muscle cells are striped and have light (isotropic) and dark (anisotropic) bands throughout. Synonymous terms for skeletal muscle are somatic, voluntary, and striated muscle. Skeletal muscles are responsible for moving the various parts of the skeleton.[3]

The individual cells of cardiac muscle are irregular in shape, contain a single oval nucleus, and seem to have incomplete cell membranes. Like skeletal muscle, cardiac muscle is striated. Unlike skeletal muscle, individual cardiac cells are joined through intercalated disks. Because cardiac cells have branches that appear to connect with adjacent fibers, the cells contract as a unit to act as a syncytium (a functional rather than an anatomic syncytium). The heart has two such functional syncytia: the atria and the ventricles.[1,3,8]

Although the muscles of the body are composed of three different types of contractile tissues, they are similar in that all are affected by the same kinds of stimuli: They will atrophy in response to inadequate activity, and they will hypertrophy as a result of increased work. Current theory regarding muscle contraction indicates that skeletal and cardiac muscle contractions are similar physiologic processes.

MUSCLE PROTEINS

Chemical study of muscle tissue indicates that a large portion of the solid material in muscle is protein. For instance, skeletal muscle is 75 percent water and 25 percent solid material. Of that solid material, 20 percent is protein and the remaining 5 percent is other material.[1]

Classification of Proteins

Considerable variation exists in classifying proteins, but a convenient classification method is according to protein function. The majority of proteins found in muscle tissue are either enzymatic (approximately 40 percent) or structural (almost 60 percent).[10,11] The remaining muscle proteins are the stroma proteins, which function to hold various structures intact.[11-13]

Enzymes. The protein enzymes are located primarily in the sarcoplasm and in the membranes of intracellular organoids. They control muscle metabolism. Thus, glycolysis (which occurs in the sarcoplasm) and the Krebs cycle (which occurs in the mitochondria) are controlled by protein enzymes.

Structural Proteins. The structural proteins, which constitute almost 60 percent of total muscle proteins, are abundant in the myofibrils.[13] The major proteins of the contractile process are myosin, actin, tropomysin, and troponin.[14] Minor proteins of uncertain function that may influence contraction are A-actinin, B-actinin, C-protein, M-protein, and desmin.[15] Desmin is particularly abundant in cardiac muscle. Myoglobin (muscle hemoglobin) is a protein found in the sarcoplasm.[14,16]

THE MUSCLE FIBER

The membrane of a muscle cell is the sarcolemma. Each muscle cell has at least one nucleus. It is surrounded by the cytoplasm, which, in muscle cells, is called the sarcoplasm. The myofibrils are the structures in the sarcoplasm of muscle cells that provide stability, and they are directly responsible for muscle contraction (Fig. 2–9). The function of the mitochondria found in muscle cells is the same as that for other cells of the body: energy production. There are abundantly more mitochondria in cardiac fibers than there are in skeletal muscle fibers. Skeletal muscle fibers respond to aerobic training by increasing the number and size of mitochondria in their cells, a response that apparently does not occur in cardiac tissue.[17]

The two important tubular systems found in muscle fibers are the transverse tubules (T-tubules) and the sarcoplasmic reticulum (Fig. 2–10). The T-tubules occur at

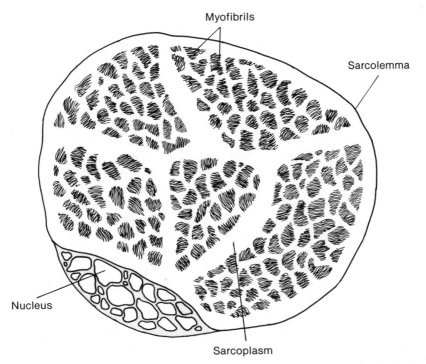

FIGURE 2–9. Cross section of a muscle fiber. (Reprinted with permission of the Macmillan Publishing Company from Grollman, S: The Human Body. Copyright © 1978 by Sigmund Grollman).

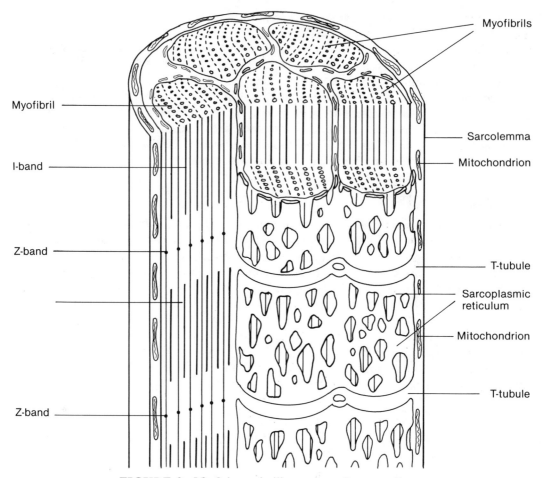

Myofibrils

Myofibril

I-band

Z-band

Z-band

Sarcolemma

Mitochondrion

T-tubule

Sarcoplasmic reticulum

Mitochondrion

T-tubule

FIGURE 2–10. Schematic illustration of myocardium.

regular intervals along the fibers; their function is to conduct waves of depolarization from the sarcolemma to deeper regions of the fiber. The numerous saclike structures that comprise the sarcoplasmic reticulum (SR) are located next to the T-tubules.[18] The SR seems to be a storage place for the calcium (Ca^{2+}) that is necessary for muscle contraction to occur. The T-tubules in cardiac tissue are significantly larger than those in skeletal muscle. Conversely, SRs are not as abundant in cardiac muscle as in skeletal muscle. The amount of Ca^{2+} released into the fiber during the contractile process seems to relate to the force of contraction that is generated by that fiber.[19]

The Myofibril

Muscle fibers contain numerous myofibrils, the filaments directly responsible for the contractile process. The smallest functional unit of the myofibril is the sarcomere, which is characterized by alternating light (I-band) and dark (A-band) bands. The A-band contains mainly the protein myosin, a thick, dark filament. The I-band is composed primarily of the protein actin, a much thinner filament than myosin (Fig. 2–10). During muscle contraction, cross-bridges located on myosin connect to the actin filaments. The thin actin filaments slide inward toward the center of the sarcomere, and the sarcomere shortens.[12,17,18,20,21]

Myosin. Chemical studies of myosin indicate that there are several forms and several large components. The fundamental unit of myosin is a protein with an average molecular weight of 470,000.[22] The ATPase (ability to split ATP) activity of the myofibril is confined to myosin; this ATPase ability is activated by CA^{2+} and inhibited by Mg^{2+}.[23,24]

Actin. Actin has been found to exist as G-actin (globular) and as F-actin (fibrous). It has a molecular weight of approximately 42,000. The conversion of F-actin to G-actin, and vice versa, involves a process of polymerization, which is necessary for muscle contraction. ATP has been found to bind to actin, and this binding is stronger to F-actin than to G-actin.[13,21,22]

The Regulatory Proteins. The two major proteins in the myofibril that exert a regulatory effect on contraction are tropomyosin and troponin.[12] In the resting state, tropomyosin seems to prevent actin and myosin from interacting. Once calcium enters the cell, it binds with troponin to remove the inhibiting effect of tropomyosin. At this point, actin and myosin can interact and muscle contraction occurs (Fig. 2–11).

Ca^{2+} plays a role in the contraction of skeletal and cardiac muscle. In the resting state, the regulatory protein tropomyosin prevents actin and myosin from interacting. When muscle cells are stimulated, Ca^{2+} is released from the SR and binds to the regulatory protein troponin, which removes the inhibiting effect of tropomyosin. Actin and myosin are now free to interact to cause contraction.[8]

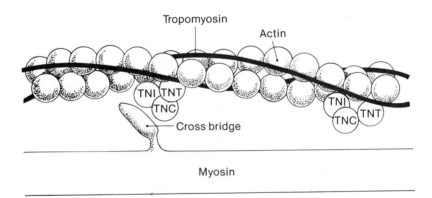

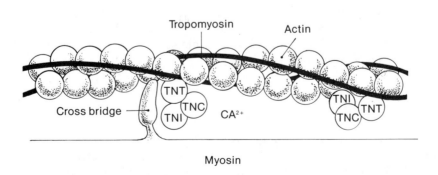

FIGURE 2–11. Schematic illustration of the regulatory proteins. TNI (troponin); TNT (tropomyosin, troponin); TNC (calcium-binding troponin). (Reprinted with permission of the Macmillan Publishing Company from Grollman, S: The Human Body. Copyright © 1978 by Sigmund Grollman.)

TABLE 2-2 Energy Formation in Muscle Cells

1. ATP-F-actomyosin $\xrightarrow[\text{Ca}^{2+}]{\text{nerve impulse}}$ G-actomyosin + ATP

2. ATP $\rightleftharpoons$ ADP + Pi (H_3PO_4) + E (energy used for contraction)
3. Phosphocreatine $\rightleftharpoons$ creatine + Pi (H_3PO_4) + E (energy used for resynthesis of ATP)
4. Glycogen (glycolysis) $\rightleftharpoons$ Lactic acid + E (energy used for resynthesis of phosphocreatine)
5. ⅕ Lactic acid + O_2 (Krebs cycle) $\longrightarrow$ CO_2 + H_2O + E (energy to drive reaction 6)
6. ⅘ Lactic acid + E $\longrightarrow$ Glycogen

Contraction Theory

Once a nerve impulse enters the muscle fiber, Ca^{2+} is released by the SR. Some of the Ca^{2+} combines with myosin to form an "activated myosin," which now has the property of the enzyme ATPase. This activated ATPase is able to react with ATP to remove its energy. This energy, in turn, is used to "pull" the actin filaments in among the myosin filaments. This is the sliding-filament theory of contraction.[8]

In the resting muscle cell, the myofibril is composed of F-actomyosin with ATP strongly attached to it to form an ATP-F-actomyosin complex. As a result of the ionic events that occur in response to nerve impulses, the ATP-F-actomyosin linkage is broken and G-actomyosin is formed. Table 2-2 summarizes the energy-forming events.

NEURAL CONTROL OF HEART RATE AND BLOOD VESSELS

The heart is regulated by the autonomic nervous system, which has two major divisions: the parasympathetic and the sympathetic (Fig. 2-12).

Parasympathetic Center

The parasympathetic system innervates the heart via the vagus nerve (X cranial). The center for this system, located in the medulla, is considered a cardioinhibitory center. Stimulation of the parasympathetic nerves (Fig. 2-13) causes a release of acetylcholine (cholinergic), which in turn both slows the heart from its normal intrinsic rate and decreases the force of its contraction. Vagal stimulation also causes the coronary arteries to dilate, which enhances coronary blood flow. At rest, the normal heart is under continual vagal control.[1,9]

Sympathetic Center

The sympathetic center (adrenergic) is located in the medulla oblongata. Stimulation of this center causes an increase in the rate and the force of contraction of the cardiac muscle. The chemical mediator for sympathetic stimulation is primarily norepinephrine, although epinephrine also is released (Fig. 2-13). The sympathetic system has two types of receptors that respond to stimulation: the alpha and beta (β_1 and β_2) receptors. When stimulated, the majority of alpha receptors cause coronary arteriolar

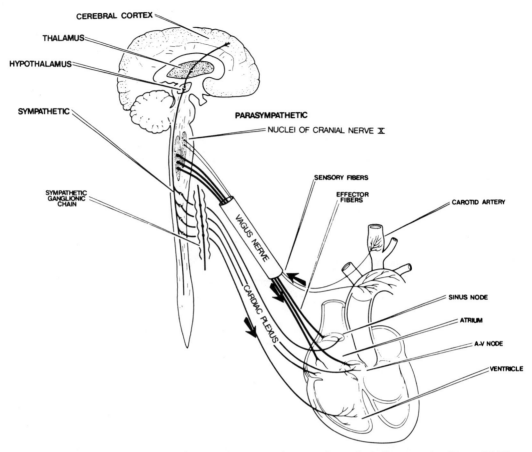

FIGURE 2–12. The autonomic nervous system innervation of cardiac muscle. (From Phillips and Feeney,[9] p. 63, with permission.)

vasoconstriction. In contrast, beta receptors when stimulated cause coronary arteriolar vasodilation. In cardiac tissue, however, norepinephrine binding to the beta receptors has a stimulating effect that causes the rate and force of contraction to increase. A balance between the alpha and beta receptors is necessary for the heart to function properly.[1,9,25]

Additional Mechanisms of Control of Heart Beat

Although neural regulation seems to be the heart's main mode of control, other factors influence heart action. The pressoreceptors (baroreceptors) located in the aorta and carotid sinus are sensitive to changes in blood pressure. When blood pressure is increased, the pressoreceptors send this information to the medulla oblongata and stimulate the parasympathetic system to decrease the rate and force of the cardiac contraction.

The chemoreceptors located in the carotid body are sensitive to changes in such blood chemicals as O_2, CO_2, and lactic acid. For instance, either an increase in CO_2 (and

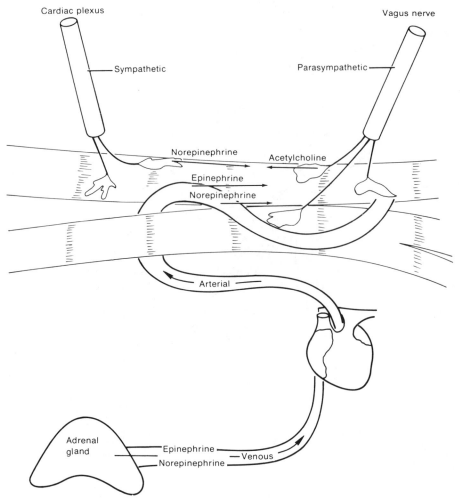

FIGURE 2–13. The influence of the sympathetic and parasympathetic nervous systems on heart rate. (From Phillips and Feeney,[9] p. 66, with permission.)

a decrease in O_2) or lactic acid concentration (causing decreased pH) will cause the heart rate to increase. Increased levels of O_2 will cause the heart action to decrease.[25]

Body temperature plays an important role in controlling the rate of heart action. Increased body temperature causes the heart rate to increase, whereas a decrease in body temperature causes the heart rate to decrease.[8]

The concentration of ions in the blood is important in proper heart action. Increased concentration of potassium (hyperkalemia) widens the PR interval and the QRS complex, produces tall T waves, and decreases the rate and force of contraction. Hypokalemia, if not treated, may cause the T waves to flatten, prolong the PR and QT intervals, and cause arrhythmias that may progress to ventricular fibrillation.[8,25]

Excessive calcium concentration (hypercalcemia) increases the action of the heart and produces prolonged contractions.[26] Hypocalcemia depresses heart action. All these factors govern heart action, and proper balance among them is necessary for normal cardiac function.[8]

PERIPHERAL CIRCULATION

Blood circulates when the pressure in one area or structure of the body is higher than in another. Blood flows from an area of higher pressure to one of lower pressure. Blood pressure can be defined as the pressure exerted by the blood against the walls of the vessels.[27] During systole (contraction) of the ventricles, the pressure exerted against the walls of the vessels is greater than during diastole (relaxation) of the ventricles. Systolic and diastolic arterial blood pressure are usually determined indirectly by the auscultatory method with the bell of the stethoscope applied to the brachial artery. Average systolic arterial blood pressures usually range from 90 to 120 mm Hg (millimeters of mercury), and the average diastolic arterial pressure range is from 60 to 90 mm Hg. Resting arterial systolic blood pressures consistently above 140 mm Hg and resting diastolic arterial blood pressures in excess of 100 mm Hg are considered to be abnormal.[27] Although blood pressures vary with such factors as age, emotional states, and exercise, a primary determinant of blood pressure is the volume of blood in the arteries. Thus, an increase in the blood volume in the arteries tends to cause an increase in arterial pressures; conversely, a decrease in volume tends to cause a decrease in arterial pressure. Two important factors that affect blood volume, and thus blood pressure, are cardiac output and peripheral resistance.[4,28]

Cardiac Output

An increase in cardiac output (amount of blood ejected from the heart per minute) tends to increase arterial blood volume and therefore increase blood pressure. The volume of blood pumped per minute depends on the number of contractions (heart beats) per minute and the amount of blood pumped with each contraction. The amount of blood pumped per beat (stroke volume) depends on the force of ventricular contraction. The greater the force of contraction, the greater the stroke volume and the systolic pressure tend to be.[4,28]

Increases in heart rate result in increases in cardiac output. This causes arterial blood volume and therefore arterial blood pressure to increase. Conversely, when the heart beats more slowly and/or with less force, there are decreases in cardiac output, arterial volume, and arterial blood pressure.[4,28]

REGULATION OF CARDIAC OUTPUT

Stroke volume is directly related to contractility and, consequently, to the strength of the heart beat. The main regulator for stroke volume is the ratio of sympathetic to parasympathetic impulses innervating the heart. An increase in sympathetic impulses causes a more forceful contraction of the heart. This increases the stroke volume. Blood concentrations of epinephrine also affect stroke volume in that increases in blood epinephrine increase stroke volume.[4,28]

The pressoreceptors (baroreceptors) in the aortic arch and carotid sinus are the main mechanisms responsible for controlling heart rate. If the blood pressure within those areas increases, impulses are sent to the cardioinhibitory center in the medulla oblongata, which causes the heart rate to slow. A decrease in the blood pressure in the aortic arch or carotid sinus causes a reflex acceleration of the heart.[4,28]

Pressoreceptors in the right atrium of the heart also affect heart rate. Increases in the right atrial blood pressure cause a reflex acceleration, and decreases in that pressure cause a reflex slowing of the heart beat.[4,28,29]

Other factors affecting heart rate, and therefore cardiac output, include emotions, exercise, blood temperature, and hormones. Anxiety, fear, and anger tend to increase heart rate and cardiac output, whereas grief tends to decrease heart rate and cardiac output. Increases in heart rate are observed during exercise, along with increases in the temperature of the blood and levels of epinephrine.[4,28,29]

Peripheral Resistance

A change in peripheral resistance (resistance to blood flow) tends to cause the volume of blood within the arteries to change and thus change blood pressure. An increase in peripheral resistance tends to increase arterial blood volume and therefore increase arterial blood pressure. A decrease in peripheral resistance tends to cause decreased blood volume and therefore decreased arterial blood pressure. Peripheral resistance is influenced by the viscosity of the blood and the diameter of the arterioles and capillaries. When the amount of blood flowing from the arteries to the arterioles decreases, more blood is left in the arteries. This increases blood volume and tends to cause an increase in arterial blood pressure.[4,28]

REGULATION OF PERIPHERAL RESISTANCE

The amount of resistance encountered by the peripheral circulation depends primarily on the viscosity of the blood and the diameter of the arterioles. To a large extent, the viscosity (thickness) of the blood determines the ease with which the blood flows. The hematocrit, or the ratio of the formed elements (red blood cells, white blood cells, and platelets) to the plasma content of whole blood, exerts a great influence on viscosity, as does the number of plasma proteins circulating in the blood. If the formed elements (mainly red blood cells) increase, then viscosity increases and so does peripheral resistance. Normally, blood viscosity changes very little. In cases such as hemorrhage, viscosity decreases (as does total blood volume) and thereby lowers peripheral resistance and arterial blood pressure. When the hematocrit rises above 50 percent (as in polycythemia), the corresponding increase in blood viscosity causes decreased blood flow and also increases the work of the heart.[28]

Arteriole diameter (vasoconstriction and vasodilation) is influenced by many factors, among which are arterial blood pressure, oxygen and carbon dioxide content of the blood, pH of the blood, and substances such as hormones (epinephrine, norepinephrine), histamines, and lactic acid. Decreases in arteriole diameters (vasoconstriction) increase the peripheral resistance and therefore increase blood pressure. Increases in arterial blood pressure stimulate the aortic and carotid baroreceptors and thereby cause parasympathetic impulses to be sent to the cardioinhibitory system in the medulla oblongata, which inhibits the vasoconstriction center. As a result, impulses are sent to the heart and blood vessels, thereby causing the heart rate to decrease and the arterioles to dilate and reduce arterial blood pressure. Decreases in arterial blood pressure have the opposite effect.[4,28]

SUMMARY

This chapter has dealt with the basic structure and function of the heart, the proteins and protein enzymes responsible for cardiac contraction, and similarities between skeletal muscle and cardiac tissue.

A discussion of muscle fiber structure included the comments that more mitochondria are found in cardiac fibers than in skeletal fibers and that aerobic training does not appear to increase the number and size of mitochondria in cardiac muscle cells. The T-tubules in cardiac tissue are larger than those in skeletal muscle, but the sarcoplasmic reticulum is not as abundant in cardiac tissue.

The ultrastructure of the myofibril and the A-bands and I-bands and the relation of the three to actin and myosin were presented. Muscle contraction theory, including the role of tropomyosin and troponin as regulatory proteins, was discussed.

In presenting the function of the heart, particular attention was given to the fact that the heart has three kinds of tissue: nodal, Purkinje, and ordinary muscle. The origin and conduction of the heart beat are functions of the coordination of those three tissues.

A discussion of the anatomy of the heart included the four chambers (two atria and two ventricles), the three surfaces (sternocostal, diaphragmatic, and posterior), and the four borders (right, left, superior, and inferior). Circulation to the heart is provided by two major arteries: the right and left coronary arteries.

Metabolism of the heart was described as primarily aerobic, with the preferred substrate being fatty acids. The importance of a continuous O_2 delivery to cardiac muscle was emphasized.

Factors controlling the rate and force of cardiac contraction were shown to be primarily neural (cholinergic or adrenergic). Other factors influencing heart action are the pressoreceptors, chemoreceptors, body temperature, and the concentration of ions (potassium and calcium) in the blood.

A primary determinant of peripheral blood pressure is the volume of blood in the arteries. Increases in arterial blood volume tend to increase blood pressure. Factors affecting blood volume and thus blood pressure are cardiac output and peripheral resistance. Increases in heart rate and stroke volume increase cardiac output, which tends to increase arterial blood pressure. Increases in peripheral resistance tend to increase arterial blood volume and therefore to increase arterial blood pressure. Peripheral resistance is influenced by the viscosity of the blood and the diameter of the arterioles and capillaries. Blood viscosity is determined largely by the hematocrit, and arteriole diameter is influenced by blood pressure, pH, and blood concentrations of oxygen, carbon dioxide, hormones, lactic acid, and histamines.

REFERENCES

1. Grollman, S: The Human Body, ed 4. Macmillan, New York, 1978, pp 85–262.
2. Moore, L: Clinically Oriented Anatomy, ed 2. Williams & Wilkins, Baltimore, 1985.
3. Sinclair, D: An Introduction to Functional Anatomy, ed 5. JB Lippincott, Philadelphia, 1975, pp 50–53.
4. Anthony, CP and Thibodeau, GA: Textbook of Anatomy and Physiology, ed 12. CV Mosby, St. Louis, 1987, pp 416–477.
5. Vick, RL: Contemporary Medical Physiology. Addison-Wesley, Menlo Park, CA, 1984, pp 160–195.
6. Amsterdam, EA and Mason, DT: Coronary artery disease: Pathology and clinical correlations. In EA Amsterdam et al (eds): Exercise in Cardiovascular Health and Disease. Yorke, New York, 1977, pp 13–18.

7. Devlin, TM (ed): Textbook of Biochemistry with Clinical Correlations, ed 12. John Wiley & Sons, New York, 1986, p 817.
8. Guyton, AC: Textbook of Medical Physiology, ed 7. WB Saunders, Philadelphia, 1986, pp 121–162.
9. Phillips, RE and Feeney, MK: The Cardiac Rhythms, ed 2. WB Saunders, Philadelphia; 1980, pp 21–68.
10. Dowhen, RM: In VB Mountcastle (ed): Medical Physiology, ed 14. CV Mosby, St. Louis, 1980, p 83.
11. Orten, JM and Neuhaus, OW: Human Biochemistry, ed 10. CV Mosby, St. Louis, 1982, pp 27–59.
12. Bell, GH, Emslie-Smith, D and Paterson, CR: Textbook of Physiology and Biochemistry, ed 9. Longman Group, London, 1976, pp 10–329.
13. Keele, CA, et al: Samson Wrights' Applied Physiology, ed 13. Oxford University Press, New York, 1982, p 249.
14. Schottelius, BA and Schottelius, DD: Textbook of Physiology. CV Mosby, St. Louis, 1978, pp 87–1097.
15. Gordon, AM: Muscle. In T Ruch and HD Patton (eds): Physiology and Biophysics. WB Saunders, Philadelphia, 1982, p 182.
16. Mannberg, HG and Goody, RS: Proteins of contractile systems. Ann Rev Biochem 45:427, 1976.
17. Amsterdam, EA, Wilmore, JH and DeMaria, AN: Exercise in Cardiovascular Health and Disease. Yorke, New York, 1977, pp 70–94.
18. Edington, DW and Edgerton, VR: The Biology of Physical Activity. Houghton Mifflin, Boston, 1976, pp 23–26.
19. Jensen, D: The Principles of Physiology, ed 2. Appleton-Century-Crofts, New York, 1980, p 75.
20. Buchthal, F, Svensmark, O and Falck, PR: Mechanical and chemical events in muscle contraction. Physiol Rev 36:503–538, 1956.
21. Harrington, WF: Contractile proteins of muscle. In H Neurath et al (eds): The Proteins, ed 3, vol. 4. Academic Press, New York, 1979, pp 246–393.
22. White, A, et al: Principles of Biochemistry, ed 6. McGraw-Hill, New York, 1978, pp 1085–1103.
23. Taylor, EW: Mechanism of actomyosin ATPase and the problem of muscle contraction. Curr Topics Bioenerg 5:201, 1973.
24. Taylor, EW: Chemistry of muscle contraction. Ann Rev Biochem 42:577, 1972.
25. Smith, JJ and Kampine, JP: Circulatory Physiology, ed 3. Williams & Wilkins, Baltimore, 1990, pp 25–172.
26. Bigger, JT: A Primer on Calcium Ion Antagonists. Knoll Pharmaceutical, 1980.
27. Thomas, CL (ed): Taber's Cyclopedic Medical Dictionary, ed 6. FA Davis, Philadelphia, 1989, p 226.
28. West, JB (ed): Best and Taylor's Physiological Basis of Medical Practice, ed 12. Williams & Wilkins, Baltimore, 1991, pp 276–330.
29. Tortora, GJ: Principles of Human Anatomy, ed 4. Harper & Row, New York, 1989, pp 356–357.

CHAPTER 3

Anatomy and Physiology of Respiration

This chapter presents a brief review of respiratory anatomy and physiology. Respiratory anatomy includes the bony structure of the thorax, the musculature of ventilation and the composition of the lungs, the conducting airways, and the distal respiratory unit. Respiratory physiology includes an overview of lung volumes and capacities, flow rates, external and internal respiration, the regulation of respiration, the respiratory system's contribution to the acid-base balance within the body, and arterial oxygenation.

BONY STRUCTURES

The bony thorax has three major functions: It protects the vital organs of the cardiopulmonary system and upper abdominal viscera; it supports the shoulder girdle; and it provides skeletal attachment for the muscles of the upper limbs, chest, neck, and back.[1] The bony structures of the thorax include the sternum anteriorly, the ribs laterally, the thoracic vertebrae posteriorly, and the shoulder girdle including the clavicle, humerus, and scapula (Figs. 3–1 and 3–2).

The sternum is the anterior border of the thorax, which comprises the manubrium, the body, and the xiphoid process. A palpable landmark of the sternum is the sternal angle, which is the bony ridge of fibrocartilage at the union of the manubrium and the body. The sternum provides articulating surfaces for the ribs and the clavicle.

Twelve pairs of ribs form the lateral borders of the thorax. The first seven pairs are called true ribs because they attach by a single costocartilage to the sternal body. Ribs 8 to 12 are called false ribs because they lack direct anterior attachment to the sternum. Ribs 8 to 10 attach anteriorly to the cartilage of the rib above them, and not directly to the sternum. The last two pairs of ribs, 11 and 12, are also called floating ribs because they have no anterior attachment.

The thoracic vertebrae (T-1 through T-12) constitute the posterior aspect of the thorax. A synovial gliding joint is present between the head of a rib and the facets of the

33

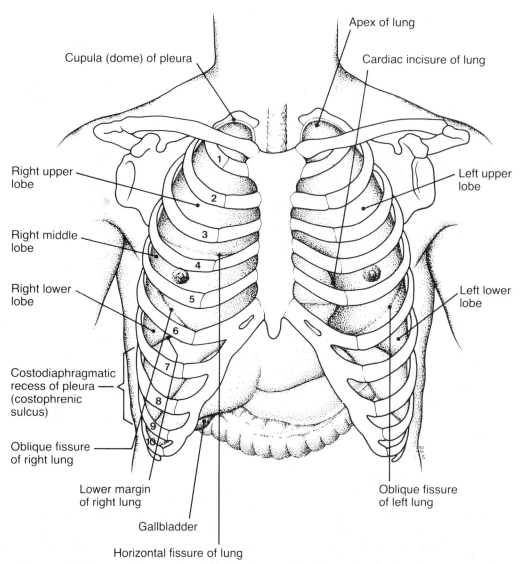

FIGURE 3–1. The bony thorax, anterior view. (From Rothstein, JM, Roy, SH, and Wolf, SL: The Rehabilitation Specialist's Handbook. FA Davis, Philadelphia, 1991, p. 586, with permission.)

vertebral bodies, superiorly and inferiorly to each rib. (Ribs 1, 10, 11, and 12 articulate with only one vertebral body.) Additional articulations exist between the neck and tubercle of the rib and the adjacent transverse process of the vertebrae.

The shoulder girdle can affect the motion of the thorax. The sternal end of the clavicle articulates with the superior border of the manubrium. The acromiom of the scapula attaches to the distal end of the clavicle. The glenoid fossa of the scapula articulates with the head of the humerus. The muscular attachments from the shoulder girdle to the thorax, head, and cervical spine can potentially be used to assist ventilation.

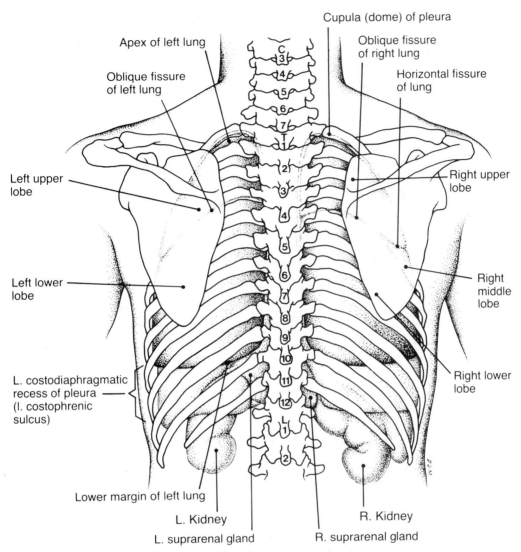

FIGURE 3-2. The bony thorax, posterior view. (From Rothstein, JM, Roy, SH, and Wolf, SL: The Rehabilitation Specialist's Handbook. FA Davis, Philadelphia, 1991, p. 587, with permission.)

MUSCULATURE

The musculature about the thorax can be divided into muscles of inspiration and those of expiration.

Inspiration

The principal inspiratory muscle is the diaphragm.[2] This dome-shaped muscle originates from the sternum, the ribs, and lumbar vertebrae, and lumbocostal arches; it forms the inferior border of the thorax. The muscle fibers insert into a central tendon. A right leaf (or right hemidiaphragm) is innervated by the right phrenic nerve, and a left leaf is innervated by the left phrenic nerve (Fig. 3–3).

When stimulated, the muscle fibers of the diaphragm contract; in doing so, they pull the central tendon and therefore the dome caudally. Thus, the descending diaphragm increases the volume of the thorax. Boyle's law states that, at a constant temperature, the volume to which a given quantity of gas is compressed is inversely proportional to the pressure ($V \propto 1/P$).[3] Therefore, according to Boyle's law, by increasing the volume within the thorax, the pressure within the thorax is reduced. The pressure inside the thorax (intrathoracic) during a diaphragmatic contraction becomes less than the pressure outside the thorax (atmospheric). Air then enters the lungs to equalize the two pressures.

During quiet inspiration, muscles of ventilation other than the diaphragm also are active.[4-6] Both the internal and external intercostals contract to keep the ribs aligned rather than to actually raise the rib cage.[7,8] The scaleni muscles are used to stabilize and may help to elevate the rib cage.[9,10]

Deep inspiration requires that the accessory muscles of inspiration contract more fully and thereby further increase the volume (by decreasing the pressure) within the thorax. The external intercostals contract to lift the ribs; the sternocleidomastoids elevate the sternum; and the levatores costarum and serratus posterior superior raise the ribs. The trapezius, rhomboid major, rhomboid minor, and levator scapulae elevate and fix

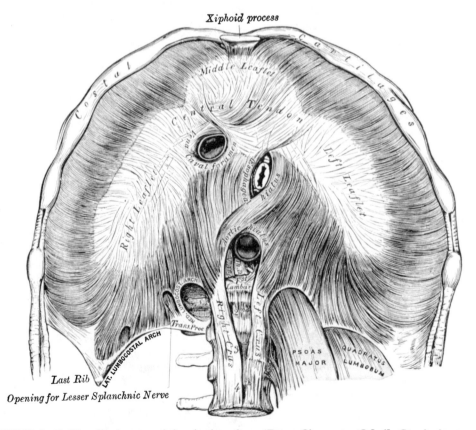

FIGURE 3–3. The diaphragm, abdominal surface. (From Clemente, C [ed]: Gray's Anatomy, ed 30. Lea & Febiger, Philadelphia, 1985. Reproduced with permission.)

the scapulae when the head and neck are fixed. With stabilization of the shoulder girdle, the pectoralis minor, the pectoralis major, and the serratus anterior also will elevate the ribs. The sacrospinalis can further assist in raising the ribs and increasing the volume within the thorax by extending the vertebral column.[4]

Expiration

Quiet expiration is mainly a passive process involving relaxation of the inspiratory muscles. With relaxation of the muscles of inspiration, the elastic properties of lung tissue recoil and pull the chest wall inward, which returns the thorax to its resting position.[11] By Boyle's law, as the thorax decreases in volume, there is an increase in the intrathoracic pressure. Air is passively exhaled to preserve a pressure equilibrium between intrathoracic and atmospheric pressures. In the standing position, the abdominal muscles have been shown to actively generate some tension during quiet expiration.[12]

The elastic properties of the lung parenchyma, with its inward recoiling force, are opposed by the tendency of the force within the thoracic cage to spring outward and upward. These two forces are at equilibrium at the end of a quiet exhalation. This state of equilibrium is referred to as resting end-expiratory pressure (REEP).

Forced expiration is an active process. The abdominal muscles (rectus abdominis, external and internal obliques, and the transverse abdominis) contract to compress the abdominal viscera. Since the viscera are prevented from moving posteriorly by the vertebral column and caudally by the pelvis, the abdominal contents are forced cephally, which pushes the diaphragm upward. The ribs are pulled downward by the action of the quadratus lumborum, internal intercostals, and the serratus posterior inferiores.[4] By flexing the vertebral column[13] and by exerting pressure with the arms on the chest wall,[14] forced expiration can be enhanced. As the thorax decreases in volume, intrathoracic pressure is increased and air is forced out of the lungs.

LUNGS

The lungs are the primary organs of external respiration. Each lung has an apex, a base, a costal, and a mediastinal surface. The apex may reach as high as 1.5 to 2.5 cm above the clavicle.[11] The base of the lung is concave, and it rests on the diaphragm. The dome of the right hemidiaphragm is higher than that of the left because of the size of the underlying liver. The costal surface is large and convex; it conforms to the inner contour of the rib cage. The mediastinal surface is concave, which accommodates the heart. Since the heart is situated more within the left hemithorax than the right, the cardiac impression is larger and deeper on the left lung than on the right lung (Figs. 3–4 and 3–5). As a result, the left lung is narrower and longer and the right lung is larger, shorter, and wider.[11]

The inner surfaces of the thorax, sternum, ribs, vertebrae, and diaphragm are covered by a thin serous membrane called the parietal pleurae. Each lung is enveloped by a thin membrane called the visceral pleura. Both the visceral and the parietal pleurae actually are continuous with each other around the root of the lung; in the healthy individual, they are in actual contact with each other. The potential space between them, called the intrapleural space, has a slightly negative pressure. Within this potential space, there is a small amount of serous fluid that reduces friction and allows the

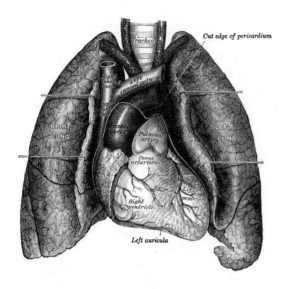

FIGURE 3–4. The lungs. (From Clemente, C [ed]: Gray's Anatomy, ed 30. Lea & Febiger, Philadelphia, 1985. Reproduced with permission.)

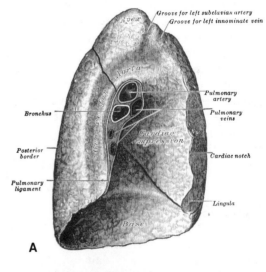

A

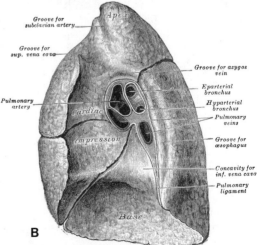

B

FIGURE 3–5. Mediastinal surfaces of the right and left lungs. (From Clemente, C [ed]: Gray's Anatomy, ed 30. Lea & Febiger, Philadelphia, 1985. Reproduced with permission.)

pleurae to glide over each other during ventilation. The right and left pleural sacs are completely separated from each other by the mediastinum, which comprises the thoracic viscera (a mass of organs and tissues separating the lungs).[4]

The left lung has one fissure line, the oblique fissure, that separates the upper and the lower lobes. The right lung also has an oblique fissure; it separates the upper lobe from the lower lobe posteriorly. The right lung contains a horizontal or transverse fissure that divides the upper and the middle lobes anteriorly. The visceral pleurae are continuous along the fissure lines.

Each lobe of the lung is divided into segments. The right lung has three lobes and ten segments and the left lung has two lobes and eight segments (Fig. 3–6).

CONDUCTING AIRWAYS

Air must be delivered from the atmosphere to the distal respiratory unit, where the actual gas exchange takes place. The conducting airways provide this transportation route.

Upper Conducting Airways

The upper airways of the respiratory system contain the nose, mouth, pharynx, and larynx (Fig. 3–7). The function of the nose is to filter, humidify, and warm the air prior to its delivery to the pharynx. The nose provides a large surface area that is lined with a respiratory mucous membrane. This membrane is comprised of ciliated epithelium, goblet cells, and mucous and serous glands. The mucous membrane filters the inhaled air by trapping foreign material in the mucus. The cilia sweep the mucus layer to the nasopharynx, where it is either swallowed or expectorated. The nose also contains sensory receptors that can initiate a sneeze: a forceful clearing mechanism.[1]

The pharynx includes the tonsils and adenoids. It is divided into three sections: the nasopharynx, oropharynx, and laryngeopharynx. The nasopharynx contains a ciliated mucus membrane and continues to filter and humidify the inspired air. The oropharynx and laryngeopharynx do not have cilia and mucous membranes. They conduct inspired air from the oral cavity into the trachea, but they are unable to humidify and filter the air. The oropharynx and the laryngeopharynx also provide the passageway from the oral cavity to the esophagus, so they are part of the digestive system as well.

The larynx connects the pharynx with the trachea. The entrance into the larynx is called the glottis. The epiglottis is a leaf-shaped elastic cartilage that covers and protects the glottis during swallowing. The larynx also has sensory fibers that can stimulate a cough: a forceful clearing mechanism of the lower airways. The larynx ensures that only air is inspired into the trachea and that solids and liquids pass only into the esophagus. Only a portion of the larynx contains a mucous membrane. Finally, the larynx contains the vocal cords that provide the mechanism for phonation. The larynx is the narrowest structure of the upper airway.[12]

Lower Conducting Airways

The lower conducting airways begin with the trachea, which branches into the right and left main stem bronchus. The bronchi further branch into lobar bronchi and

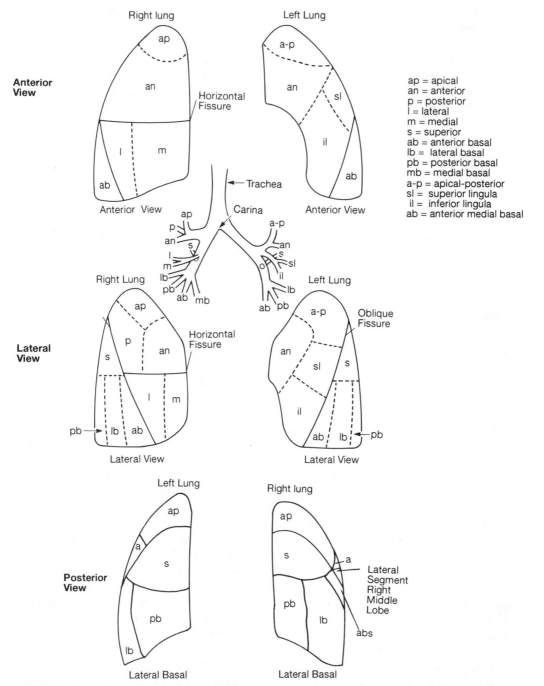

FIGURE 3–6. The segments of the lobes of the lungs. (From Rothstein, JM, Roy, SH, and Wolf, SL: The Rehabilitation Specialist's Handbook. FA Davis, Philadelphia, 1991, p. 589, with permission.)

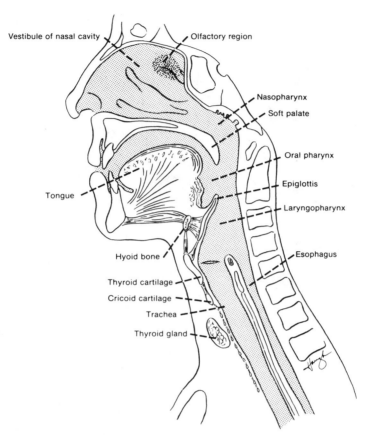

Vestibule of nasal cavity

Olfactory region

Nasopharynx

Soft palate

Oral pharynx

Epiglottis

Laryngopharynx

Esophagus

Tongue

Hyoid bone

Thyroid cartilage

Cricoid cartilage

Trachea

Thyroid gland

FIGURE 3–7. The upper airways. (From Frownfelter, D: Chest Physical Therapy and Pulmonary Rehabilitation: An Interdisciplinary Approach, ed 2. Mosby-Year Book, Inc., Chicago, 1987, p. 18, with permission.)

segmental bronchi for generations until they terminate in the bronchioles. The most distal conducting airway is called the terminal bronchiole (Fig. 3–8).

The trachea is considered to be the first-generation ventilatory passageway; it is the continuation of the airway inferior to the larynx. It originates at the lower border of the cricoid cartilage at the level of the sixth cervical vertebra and terminates at the level of the sternal angle. It is about 12 cm in length and has a cylindrical 2-cm lumen. Support and protection are provided anteriorly and laterally by C-shaped cartilage. The posterior wall of the trachea, which is shared with the anterior wall of the esophagus, is made up of fibrous tissue and the smooth muscle of the trachealis.

The mucous membrane of the trachea contains both goblet cells (which provide a mucus layer lining the trachea) and ciliated epithelial cells (which beat and move the mucus layer upward to the pharynx). Once the mucus layer reaches the level of the pharynx, it is either swallowed or expectorated. A number of reserve cells that lie beneath the ciliated and goblet cells can become either goblet cells or ciliated cells as needed. Below the reserve cells is a layer of gland cells that also help to produce mucus.

At the level of the sternal angle, the trachea bifurcates and creates the right and left main stem bronchi, which are the second generation of ventilatory passageway. This point of bifurcation is called the carina.

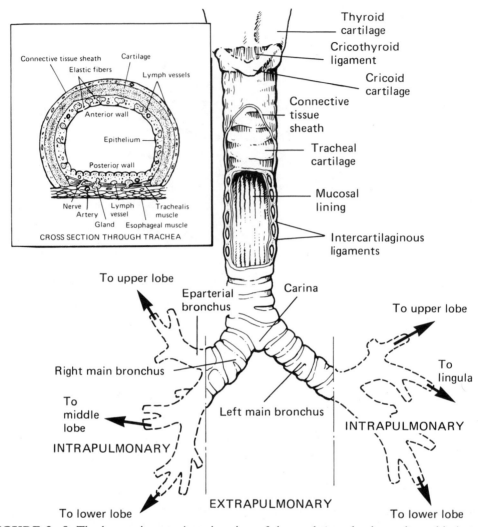

FIGURE 3–8. The lower airways. Anterior view of the trachea and primary bronchi. A cross-section through a part of the trachea shows the anterior and lateral support of the C-shaped cartilage. The trachealis muscle provides the necessary protective support posteriorly. (From Martin and Youtsey,[20] p. 27, with permission.)

Cartilage continues to support the smooth muscle and other tissues of the bronchial walls, although at this point it is shaped as flat plates rather than as rings.[14] The right main stem bronchus is shorter, less angular, and wider than the left main stem bronchus. It extends caudally into the right lung at the hilum. The left main stem bronchus angles more laterally at the tracheal bifurcation because of the presence of the heart. It enters caudally and laterally into the left lung at the hilum.

The main stem bronchi divide, on entering the lungs, into lobar bronchi (third-generation ventilatory passage). Each branch of the bronchi corresponds to a lobe of the lung. Branching continues into segmental bronchi (fourth generation), subsegmental bronchi (fifth generation), and so on. The cartilagenous support within the smooth muscle of the airway decreases with each generation, as does the number of cilia.[15] The term ''bronchiole'' is used when there is no longer any cartilage or any cilia in the smooth muscle of the airway. The bronchioles continue to divide until they become the final generation of the conducting airways, the terminal bronchioles. A terminal bronchiole is 0.5 to 1.0 mm in diameter.[16] There are 20 to 25 generations of conducting passages in all.

THE RESPIRATORY UNIT

The inspired air travels from the conducting airways to the distal respiratory unit, which contains the respiratory bronchioles, alveolar ducts, alveolar sacs, and the alveoli and pulmonary capillary bed (Fig. 3–9). In an adult, there are an estimated 300 million alveoli available for gas exchange.[17] The alveolar membrane, the pulmonary capillary membrane, and the interstitial space are all that separate the alveolar air from the pulmonary capillary red blood cells (Fig. 3–10).

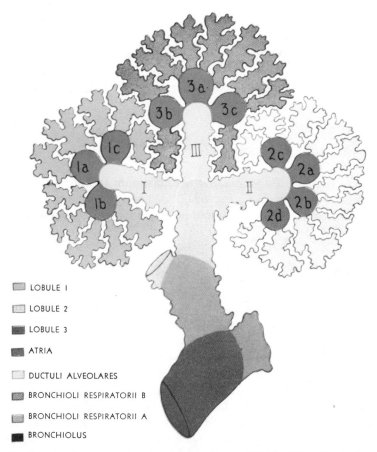

LOBULE 1
LOBULE 2
LOBULE 3
ATRIA
DUCTULI ALVEOLARES
BRONCHIOLI RESPIRATORII B
BRONCHIOLI RESPIRATORII A
BRONCHIOLUS

FIGURE 3–9. The respiratory unit, the acinus. (From Miller, WS: The Lung. Courtesy of Charles C Thomas, Publisher, Springfield, Illinois, 1950, p. 42.)

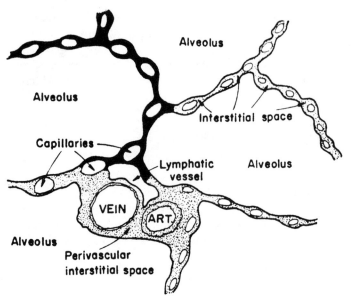

FIGURE 3-10. The alveolar capillary network. (From Guyton,[3] p. 487, with permission.)

Ventilation

Air is inspired through the nose or mouth and through all of the conducting airways until it reaches the acinus. The act of moving air in and out of the lungs is termed "ventilation." The terminology surrounding the amount of air involved in ventilation is the topic of the next section.

Lung Volumes and Capacities

At full inspiration, the lungs contain their maximum amount of gas. This volume of air, called total lung capacity (TLC), can be divided into four separate volumes of air: (1) tidal volume, (2) inspiratory reserve volume, (3) expiratory reserve volume, and (4) residual volume (Fig. 3-11).

TIDAL VOLUME

The amount of air that is inspired and expired during normal resting ventilation is called the tidal volume (V_T). For a young, healthy male the V_T is approximately 500 milliters (Fig. 3-11).[18] REEP, or the point during ventilation at which all forces about the rib cage are at equilibrium, occurs at the end of a tidal exhalation.

As the V_T (500 milliliters) enters the respiratory system, it travels through the conducting airways to reach the respiratory units. The amount of inspired air that actually reaches the respiratory unit and takes part in gas exchange is about 350 milliliters. The remaining 150 milliliters of the inhaled tidal breath remains in the conducting airways. This 150 milliliters of air is considered to be within the anatomical dead space of the lungs, since it does not take part in gas exchange. There is a numerical relation between the amount of air contained in the anatomical dead space V_{DS} and the total amount of air inhaled V_T. The normal dead space to tidal volume ratio V_{DS}/V_T in

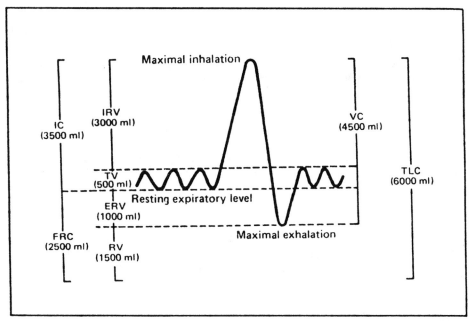

FIGURE 3–11. Lung volumes and capacities of a 23-year-old, 166-cm, healthy male. IRV = inspiratory reserve volume; TV = tidal volume; ERV = expiratory reserve volume; RV = residual volume; IC = inspiratory capacity; FRC = functional residual capacity; VC = vital capacity; TLC = total lung capacity. (From Youtsey,[18] p. 377, with permission.)

the example (Fig. 3–11) of a 23-year-old healthy man is 150 milliliters per 500 milliliters, or 30 percent.[18]

INSPIRATORY RESERVE VOLUME

When only a tidal breath occupies the lungs, there is "room" for additional air that can be further inhaled. This inspiratory volume, in excess of tidal breathing, is the inspiratory reserve volume (IRV). Aptly named, it is the volume of air that can be inspired when needed, but it is usually kept in reserve. Again referring to Figure 3–11, the IRV is approximately 3000 milliliters.[18]

EXPIRATORY RESERVE VOLUME

There is a quantity of air that can potentially be exhaled beyond the end of a tidal exhalation, or below REEP. Usually kept in reserve, this volume of air, called the expiratory reserve volume (ERV), is about 1000 milliliters in the example of a young male[18] (Fig. 3–11).

RESIDUAL VOLUME

The lungs are not completely emptied of air after maximal exhalation of the ERV. The external forces of the rib cage do not allow the lungs to fully collapse. The volume of air that remains within the lungs when the ERV has been exhaled is called the residual volume (RV). The normal value of the RV in a young, healthy male is approximately 1500 milliliters.[18]

As previously stated, the total of the four lung volumes is the TLC; that is, TLC = IRV + V_T + ERV + RV. Combinations of two or more lung volumes are termed "capacities."

INSPIRATORY CAPACITY

The sum of TV and IRV is called the inspiratory capacity (IC). In the young, healthy male (Fig. 3–11), the IC would be V_T + IRV, or 500 + 3000 = 3500 milliliters of air.

FUNCTIONAL RESIDUAL CAPACITY

The functional residual capacity (FRC) is the combined RV and ERV. Physiologically, it is the amount of air that is left in the lungs after a resting tidal exhalation. Thus, FRC = ERV + RV, or 1000 + 1500 = 2500 milliliters of air in the example (Fig. 3–11).

VITAL CAPACITY

Vital capacity (VC) comprises the three volumes that are under volitional control; that is, VC = IRV + V_T + ERV. The common method of measuring VC is to achieve maximal inspiration and then forcibly exhale all of the air as hard and as fast as possible until the ERV has been exhausted. Because the exhalation is forced, it is called the forced vital capacity (FVC). In our example, the maximum amount of air that could be exhaled after a maximal inhalation would be 4500 milliliters (3000 + 500 + 1000 milliliters).

Figures 3–12 and 3–13 are nomograms used for calculating lung volumes and capacities in healthy, nonsmoking men and women.

Volumes and capacities are dependent on the age, height, race, gender, and body position of a subject.[20] With increasing age, the lungs gradually lose their elastic properties and the thorax becomes stiffer.[21] Lung volumes will reflect those changes with an increase in the FRC.[21] The increase in FRC is due primarily to an increase in residual volume. With increasing age, there are also decreases in the IRV and VC.[12] Expiratory flow rates also are found to decrease as a result of the aging process.[22]

There is a direct relationship between a person's height and that person's measured lung volumes and capacities.[23] Arm span can be used to predict lung volumes in patients with spinal deformities that alter their heights.[24] Black males have smaller lung volumes than white males of equal height and age.[23,25,26] Smaller lung volumes are found in women than in men when age and height are the same for both.[27] A quantitative measurement of thoracic size may be a more reliable predictor of lung volumes and capacities than height, race, or gender.

Body position also can alter lung volumes and capacities. Both FRC and VC decrease when a subject moves from the erect posture of sitting or standing to the supine.[28] The effects of gravity on the thorax, diaphragm, and abdominal contents, as well as restriction of the supporting surface, are at least in part responsible for the changes. During conventional measurement of lung volumes and flow rates, the body position is erect, usually sitting.[29]

Any alteration in the properties of the lungs or chest wall will change lung volumes and capacities. A loss of the elastic properties of the lung parenchyma allows an

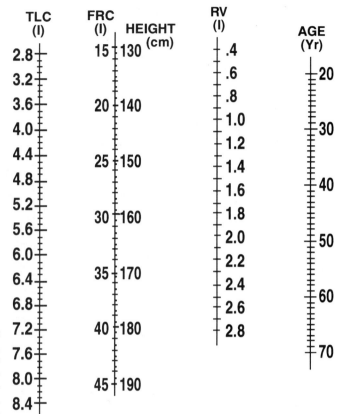

FIGURE 3–12. Nomograms for calculating lung volumes and capacities in healthy, nonsmoking males. TLC = total lung capacity; FRC = functional residual capacity; RV = residual volume. (From Cherniak, R: Pulmonary Function Testing. WB Saunders, Philadelphia, 1977, p. 247, with permission.)

MALES

unrestrained expansion of the chest. The result is an increase in RV, FRC, TLC; vital capacity will be decreased.[30] This can occur in certain obstructive disease states such as emphysema.

Fibrosis of the lung parenchyma increases the elastic properties of the lungs, which results in the characteristic pattern observed in restrictive pulmonary disease: a decrease in vital capacity and TLC.[31] Pleural fibrosis and restriction of the chest wall that are due to disease or deformity also can restrict the lungs' ability to expand and structurally reduce VC and TLC.[32,33] Figure 3–14 shows the normal lung volumes and capacities as well as the changes that occur with obstructive and restrictive pulmonary disease.

FLOW RATES AND MECHANICS

Flow rates are the measurements of gas volumes moved in a period of time. Expiratory flow rates, therefore, are measurements of exhaled gas volume divided by the amount of time of the exhalation. Flow rates reflect the ease with which the lungs can be ventilated, and they are related to the resistance to airflow, or the elasticity of the

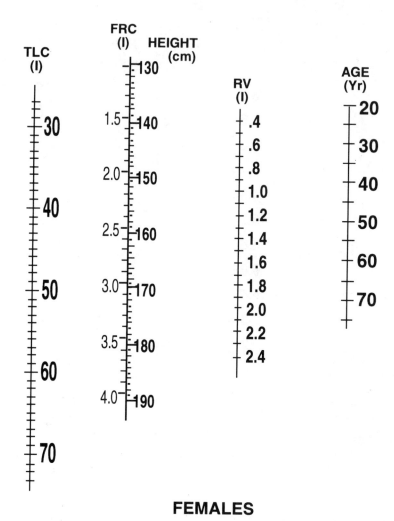

FEMALES

FIGURE 3–13. Nomograms for calculating lung volumes and capacities in healthy, nonsmoking females. TLC = total lung capacity; FRC = functional residual capacity; RV = residual volume. (From Cherniak, R: Pulmonary Function Testing. WB Saunders, Philadelphia, 1977, p. 248, with permission.)

lung parenchyma.[19] An important airflow measurement is the volume of air that can be forcefully exhaled during the first second of a forced vital capacity maneuver. This is called the forced expiratory volume in one second, or FEV_1. In a healthy individual, the FEV_1 is greater than 75 percent of the total FVC. For the example of the 70-kg male (Fig. 3–11), a normal value of FEV_1 should be 3.4 liters per second or greater (4500 liters $\times$ 0.75). (Nomograms for forced expiratory flow rates are given in Chapter 10.) Inspiratory flow rates can also be determined by measuring the amount of air inspired and the amount of time necessary for the inhalation.

Any alteration in the properties of the lungs or chest wall will also alter flow rates. Patients who present with obstructive pulmonary disease will have a VC that takes longer to exhale because of the loss of the elastic recoil of the lungs: the FEV_1 will be decreased. Patients who present with restrictive pulmonary disease may also have a

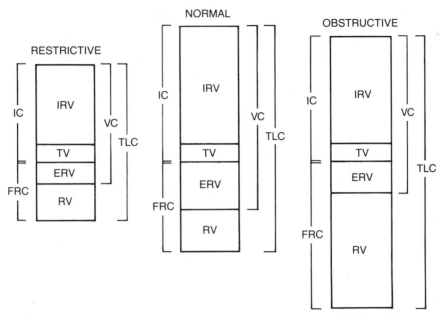

FIGURE 3–14. Lung volumes and capacities in normal as well as obstructive and restrictive pulmonary diseases. (From Rothstein, JM, Roy, SH, and Wolf, SL: The Rehabilitation Specialist's Handbook. FA Davis, Philadelphia, 1991, p. 604, with permission.)

volume of air exhaled in the first second that is less than would be predicted by their height, age, race, and gender. However, in the case of the patient with restrictive pulmonary disease, the decrease in FEV_1 is due to the overall lack of volume, not the ability to exhale it. Therefore, when corrected for vital capacity, FEV_1/FVC_1 the resulting percent is normal or greater than 75.

Measurement and interpretation of spirometric values are covered in greater detail in Chapter 6, Pulmonary Diseases, and Chapter 10, Pulmonary Assessment.

RESPIRATION

"Respiration" is a term used to describe the gaseous exchange that occurs between the atmospheric air and pulmonary capillaries or between the tissues and the surrounding capillaries. It should not be confused with ventilation, which describes only the movement of air. External respiration is the gaseous exchange that occurs at the alveolar/capillary membrane; internal respiration takes place at the tissue/capillary level. The following discussion describes the course of gas exchange, specifically, oxygen and carbon dioxide, during both external and internal respiration.

For external respiration to take place, there must first be an inhalation of air from the ambient environment, through the conducting airways, and into the alveoli. Oxygen diffuses through the alveolar wall, through the interstitial space, and through the pulmonary capillary wall. Most of the oxygen (98.5 percent) then travels through the blood plasma into the red blood cells and onto one of the gas-carrying sites of hemoglobin.[20] A small portion of oxygen (1.5 percent) is carried dissolved in the plasma.

The rate of diffusion of oxygen from the alveoli into the capillary is dependent on three factors that can vary with pulmonary pathologies: (1) the surface area of the respiratory units available for gas exchange (A), (2) the thickness of the alveolar capillary membranes (T), and (3) the pressure gradient ($P_1 - P_2$) created between the partial pressure of oxygen within the alveoli (P_1) and that within the pulmonary capillary (P_2). Fick's law describes these relations as follows:

$$^{15}\dot{V}\text{GAS} \propto \frac{A}{T} D(P_1 - P_2)$$

where D is the diffusing constant for a specific gas, in this case, oxygen.

To better understand diffusion during respiration, a further discussion of the variables of Fick's law may be helpful. The lungs' approximately 300 million alveoli correspond to 160 m^2 of alveolar surface area potentially available for gas diffusion.[3] The alveolar capillary membrane that must be permeated to permit the diffusion of oxygen consists of several layers. There is a thin layer of surfactant fluid that lines the inside of the alveoli, an alveolar epithelium, an alveolar epithelial basement membrane, an interstitial space, a pulmonary capillary basement membrane, and a capillary endothelial membrane. Although that seems like an abundance of layers, the approximate thickness of the combined layers is only 0.63 μm.[3]

Determining the partial pressure of oxygen in the ambient environment is the first step in understanding the pressure gradient created by oxygen for diffusion. The total pressure exerted by the atmospheric gases at sea level is 760 mm Hg. Oxygen makes up approximately 21 percent of all of the atmospheric gases; this is called the fraction of inspired oxygen: $F_{IO_2} = 0.21$. The fraction of inspired nitrogen is about 79 percent: $F_{IN_2} = 0.79$. All other gases make up less than 1 percent of atmospheric air. Since all gases combined exert a pressure of 760 mm Hg, the partial pressure exerted by oxygen (P_{O_2}) alone is 21 percent of 760 mm Hg, or 159 mm Hg. As atmospheric air enters the lungs, some oxygen becomes displaced by water vapor (P_{H_2O}) from the humidification process of the upper airway and diluted by carbon dioxide (P_{CO_2}), which is constantly diffusing into the alveoli. The partial pressure of oxygen is thus decreased. In the alveoli, P_{AO_2} (P_1 of Fick's law for oxygen diffusion) is 104 mm Hg[20] (Table 3–1).

The blood within the pulmonary capillary returns from the tissue level with a partial pressure of oxygen (P_{VO_2}) of 40 mm Hg; P_2 of Fick's law is 40 mm Hg (Table

TABLE 3–1 The Approximate Partial Pressures of Atmospheric Air at Sea Level and at Different Points During Ventilation and Respiration

	Dry Atmosphere, mm Hg	Moist Atmosphere, mm Hg	Tracheal, mm Hg	Alveolar, mm Hg	Arterial, mm Hg	Venous, mm Hg	Exhaled, mm Hg
P_{O_2}	159	159	149	104	95	40	120
P_{CO_2}	0.3	0.3	0.3	40	40	45	27
P_{H_2O}	0.0	47	47	47	47	47	47
P_{N_2}	600	597	563	569	569	569	566

*Although single numbers are given for clarity, ranges providing some variability would be more accurate.

3–1). Therefore, the pressure gradient for oxygen diffusion at the alveolar capillary membrane is from 104 mm Hg (arterial side) to 40 mm Hg (venous side).

The blood leaving a fully functioning alveolar capillary unit has a partial pressure of oxygen in the arterial blood (Pao_2) of 104 mm Hg.[3] Diffusion across the pressure gradient has occurred, and most of the blood (98 percent) that enters the left side of the heart has a Pao_2 of 104 mm Hg.[3] The other 2 percent of blood entering the left atrium comes from the bronchial circulation system, which supplies the conducting airways. This blood is venous blood that does not take part in the external respiratory process and therefore has a Po_2 of 40 mm Hg. Mixing the newly oxygenated blood from the pulmonary veins with the venous blood from the bronchial vein causes the partial pressure of oxygen within the left heart to become slightly diluted: The blood within the left side of the heart has a Pao_2 of 95 to 100 mm Hg. (Note that alveolar partial pressures of gas is denoted by "A" and arterial blood partial pressure by "a.")

The oxygenated blood travels out of the left heart into the aorta and through a network of connecting arteries, arterioles, and capillaries until its destination, the tissue, is reached. Internal respiration takes place as the arterial blood reaches the tissue level. Oxygen now diffuses off the gas-carrying sites of hemoglobin, out of the red cells, out of the capillary through the membranes, and into the mitochrondria of the working cells. Again, this process of diffusion is due to differences in pressures. The capillary has a Pao_2 of 95 to 100 mm Hg, since no oxygen has been given off. The interstitial fluid has a partial pressure of oxygen of between 5 and 40 mm Hg.[3] Therefore, the pressure gradient promotes oxygen diffusion from the capillary into the tissues—from an area of high pressure to an area of lower pressure. Blood leaving the cell and going into the venous system has a Pvo_2 of 40 mm Hg.

Carbon dioxide, which is produced at the tissue level as a by-product of metabolism, diffuses out of the cells and back into the capillaries. It is transported through the venous system into the right side of the heart. Once the carbon dioxide makes its way to the pulmonary capillary, it is released through the capillary membrane, through the interstitial space, and into the alveoli, where it is finally exhaled into the atmosphere. The rate of diffusion of carbon dioxide out of the cell, into the capillary, and then out of the capillary into the alveoli depends on all the variables of Fick's law:

$$V_{GAS} \propto \frac{A}{T} D (P_1 - P_2)$$

The surface areas (A) for diffusion of CO_2 are the same as those already described for oxygen. The thicknesses of the membranes T through which diffusion occurs also are the same as those for oxygen. The pressure gradient (T) $(P_1 - P_2)$ created by carbon dioxide are not, however, the same. Blood leaves the tissue and returns to the pulmonary artery and pulmonary capillary with a partial pressure of CO_2 of 46 mm Hg.[3] The alveoli have a partial pressure of CO_2 of 35 to 45 mm Hg. Carbon dioxide diffuses out of the pulmonary capillary and into the alveoli. As blood leaves a functioning alveolar-capillary unit, the partial pressure of CO_2 is 35 to 45 mm Hg. The pressure gradient created by the partial pressure of carbon dioxide is far less than the pressure gradient created by oxygen. The diffusion of CO_2 might not be so complete if the diffusion constant of CO_2 were not so great. In fact, the diffusion constant for CO_2 is 20 times greater than the diffusion constant for O_2. Carbon dioxide diffusion across the lower pressure gradients occurs rapidly and completely.

When the cycle of external and internal respiration has occurred, oxygen has been provided and carbon dioxide has been removed. Of course, this system is dependent on an intact cardiovascular system to pump the blood through the lungs, deliver it to the working cells, and then return it to the lungs—all in a timely fashion.

Perfusion

"Perfusion of the lung" is the term used to describe pulmonary circulation. Blood is ejected from the right ventricle into the pulmonary artery, through which it goes to the lungs. Blood returns to the left heart via the pulmonary veins. The pulmonary circulation is a low-pressure system as compared with the systemic circulation. Normal pulmonary artery pressure is 25/10 mm Hg as compared with the pressure in the aorta, which is 120/80 mm Hg. Gravity affects the low-pressure pulmonary vascular system more than the systemic high-pressure system. The lower areas of the lung, or the gravity-dependent areas, obtain the greatest amount of the blood flow that is due to the effects of hydrostatic pressure (gravity). That is, in the erect standing position, the gravity-dependent areas of the lungs, the bases, receive the greatest amount of blood flow. The apices of the lungs in this position are the most gravity-independent; as such, they receive the least amount of perfusion. In the supine position, the posterior aspect of the lungs is the most gravity-dependent area; it receives the most blood flow whereas the gravity-independent area, the anterior surface, receives the least amount of perfusion. Figure 3–15 shows the effect of body position on areas of gravity dependence and therefore areas of greatest perfusion.

The effects of local stimulation on the pulmonary system are usually opposite that of the systemic circulation. For example, the pulmonary system responds to hypoxemia by vasoconstriction whereas the systemic circulation responds by vasodilation. In the lung, this vasoconstriction acts to reroute (shunt) the pulmonary blood flow from underventilated alveoli (areas of hypoxia) to ventilated alveoli, thereby causing gas exchange to be nearly optimal. In the systemic circulation, hypoxia stimulates vasodilation to reverse the lack of oxygen the tissue is experiencing. Hypercapnea (an increase in carbon dioxide) causes pulmonary vasoconstriction but systemic vasodilation. Other stimuli that may cause opposite reactions are norepinephrine, serotonin, histamine, and acidemia.

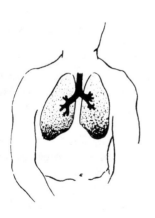 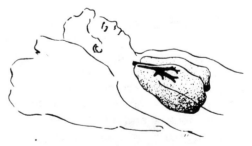

FIGURE 3–15. The effect of body position on pulmonary perfusion. (From Frownfelter, D: Chest Physical Therapy and Pulmonary Rehabilitation: An Interdisciplinary Approach, ed 2. Mosby-Year Book, Inc., Chicago, 1987, p. 51, with permission.)

Ventilation-Perfusion Relationship

At the alveolar capillary level, the ventilation (V) and the perfusion (Q) must be balanced so that optimal gas exchange can occur. Regional differences in pulmonary blood flow that are due to the influence of hydrostatic pressure have been discussed in the section on pulmonary perfusion. Similar differences are found in the ventilatory aspect of the lungs. The regional differences in ventilation are due to an intrapleural pressure gradient that tends to be more negative at the upper part of the lung and less negative at the lower portion of the lung. In the upright standing position, this pressure gradient results in a greater resting expansion in the apical areas of the lung than in the basalar areas. When a breath is inhaled, the apices, being almost full at the onset of inhalation, receive very little of the new volume of air. The bases, however, being almost empty, receive most of the inhaled volume of air. The greatest change in volume, and therefore the most ventilation, occurs at the bases of the lungs, whereas the least change in volume, and therefore the least ventilation, occurs in the apices. When the position is changed, the areas of greatest ventilation also change. For example, in the supine position, the area of greatest volume change will be in the posterior aspect of the lungs and the least volume change will be in the anterior aspect of the lungs.

The relation of pulmonary ventilation (V) to perfusion (Q) is written as the ratio V/Q. In a normal state of health, ventilation and perfusion are balanced. Knowing that ventilation is 4 liters of air per minute (on the average) and perfusion is 5 liters of blood per minute (again, on the average), the ventilation:perfusion relationship in health can be calculated: V/Q = 4/5, or 0.8.

Ventilation-perfusion inequalities occur in diseased states. Three examples of possible relations are shown in Figure 3–16. The first abnormality shows a normally aerated alveolus with no capillary perfusion; it is called a physiologic dead space (V/Q = 4/0 = ∞). The second abnormality shows a fully perfused capillary with no alveolar ventilation; it is referred to as a physiologic shunt (V/Q = 0/5 = 0). The final abnormality is an alveolus with no ventilation and a capillary with no perfusion, which is called a silent unit (V/Q = 0/0 = 0). In disease states the alveolar capillary unit may have slight to severe alveolar capillary abnormalities. The result of these abnormalities can be detected and monitored with the use of arterial blood gas analyses, which will be discussed later in this chapter.

Regulation of Respiration

Neurologic control of ventilation and respiration is multifactorial. Breathing is primarily an involuntary act, and there is no need to cognitively take a breath. The autonomic nervous system has control over breathing, and there is volitional control over ventilation. Chemoreceptors, baroreceptors, and proprioceptors provide the necessary input to assist in the control of breathing.

The respiratory centers are located within the pons and the medulla oblongata.[19] The medulla seems to control the basic rhythm of inspiration and expiration.[20] The pons is divided into two centers that modulate the basic rhythm of the medulla. The apneustic center in the lower pons provides for greater inspiration effort, and the pneumotaxic center of the upper pons seems to inhibit or limit inspiration after it has reached a certain level, which allows exhalation to occur.

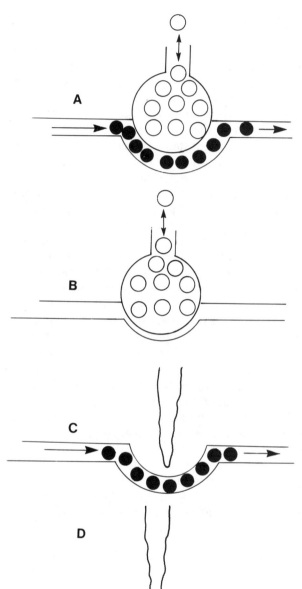

FIGURE 3–16. The ventilation-perfusion relationships that can exist in health and in pulmonary disease. *A*, Healthy alveolar capillary unit. *B*, Normally aerated alveoli with no capillary perfusion–physiologic dead space. *C*, Normally perfused capillary with no alveolar aeration–physiologic shunt. *D*, A nonaerated alveoli next to a nonperfused capillary–silent unit. (Adapted from Price, SA and Wilson, LM: Pathophysiology: Clinical Concepts and Disease Processes, ed 4. Mosby-Year Book, Inc. St. Louis, 1992, with permission.)

The autonomic nervous system is another entity involved in the neural control of ventilation. The sympathetic nervous system, when stimulated, will increase both the depth and frequency of ventilation. It will also increase the size of the bronchial lumen (bronchodilate) and decrease the production of pulmonary secretions. Stimulation of the parasympathetic nervous system will have the opposite effects.

Volitional control by the cerebral cortex, which can override the normal rhythm of breathing, also is present. This volition grants us the ability to phonate, sing a song, or even hold our breath until we "turn blue."

Involuntary stimulus-response types of breathing also are possible. Many types of sensory feedback elicit respiratory responses.[34] For example, imagine that you put your hand on a hot stove. Along with removing your hand, you will find that you take a quick inhalation.

Chemoreceptors respond to changes in the chemical concentration in the cerebral spinal fluid (CSF) and the blood. These are the main receptors for the neurologic control of breathing. The central chemoreceptors line the fourth ventricle of the brain and are sensitive to the changes in CO_2 and H^+ concentrations of the cerebral spinal fluid. The peripheral chemoreceptors are located in the aortic arch and the carotid bodies; they sense changes in the circulating partial pressures of O_2 and CO_2 and the pH. The central chemoreceptors are responsible for the regulation of breathing. Slight variations in the body's $Paco_2$ will begin the firing of the receptors, thereby changing the ventilatory pattern. The oxygen-sensitive aspect of the peripheral chemoreceptors seems to be more of a reserve, or backup system since the partial pressure of oxygen must fall to approximately half of its normal value before the receptors respond and change the ventilatory pattern.

Receptors located within the lung also can exert some control over the ventilatory pattern. The Hering-Breuer inflation receptor is a stretch receptor mechanism that limits inhalation. J receptors, found in "juxtaposition" to the pulmonary capillaries, lie in the alveolar walls close to the pulmonary circulation. The stimulation of these receptors may cause rapid, shallow breathing and bradycardia and may be associated with the sensation of dyspnea. Irritant receptors within the airways can cause bronchoconstriction and hyperpnea.

There are also receptors located outside the lungs that can exert some control over ventilation. Baroreceptors within the aorta and carotid bodies can cause reflex hypoventilation or apnea during an episode of increased arterial pressure or hyperventilation during a period of decreased arterial pressure. Receptors within the respiratory muscles and proprioceptors in the joints of the thoracic cage or exercising limbs may activate a change in the ventilatory pattern.[35,36] The regulation of ventilation is a complex modulation of various stimuli from the receptors. Figure 3–17 integrates these complex interactions into a very simple diagram.

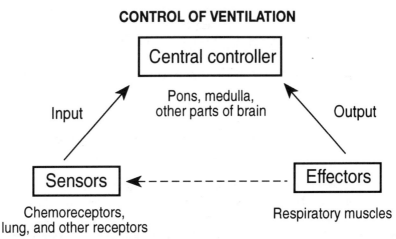

CONTROL OF VENTILATION

FIGURE 3–17. Schematic representation of the regulation of ventilation and respiration. Information from various sensors is fed to the central controller, the output of which goes to the ventilatory muscles. By changing ventilation, the ventilatory muscles reduce perturbations of the sensors (negative feedback). (From West, J: Respiratory Physiology: The Essentials, ed 2. © Williams & Wilkins, Baltimore, p. 115, with permission.)

The three corners of a triangle in Figure 3–17 are labeled the sensors, the central controllers, and the effectors. The sensors are the chemoreceptors, the stretch receptors, the baroreceptors, and the proprioceptors. They send signals to the central controllers: the medulla oblongata, the pons, and the cortex. The central controllers respond by increasing or decreasing the impulses sent to the effectors, which are the muscles of ventilation. The breathing parameters are changed, and the sensors now evaluate the adequacy of the new breathing pattern. The cycle continues sensing and effecting the breathing pattern.

Each breath is initiated, evaluated, and adjusted when necessary to create a breathing pattern that maintains appropriate levels of oxygen and carbon dioxide and provides for hemodynamic stability throughout the body.

ACID-BASE BALANCE

The preceding discussion concerned the role of the partial pressures of oxygen and carbon dioxide in creating pressure gradients that effect diffusion and also stimulate chemoreceptors that regulate ventilation. The partial pressures of gas within the vascular system also have the ability to maintain a stable acid-base balance within the body.

Acid-base balance is of the utmost importance in the maintenance of the body's homeostasis. The acid-base balance of the body hinges on the amount of hydrogen ions (H^+) in the blood. The pH of the body is the negative logarithm of the concentration of the hydrogen ions in the body fluids. A normal range for arterial blood pH is 7.35 to 7.45. Any decrease in blood pH below 7.35 is called acidemia; that is, the blood is more acidic than is normal. Any increase in the blood pH above 7.45 is termed alkalemia; the blood is then more basic than is normal. A small change in the pH in either direction can cause depression or overexcitation of the nervous system; a substantial change in the pH can result in coma or convulsions.

The body has three buffer systems that attempt to maintain and normalize blood pH at all times. The blood buffers provide an immediate defense against an alteration in H^+ concentration. Hemoglobin and other blood proteins can act as buffers, as they have the ability to bind with H^+ and effectively negates its influence on the pH.

The second system that helps regulate the acid-base balance of the body is the respiratory system. By increasing or decreasing alveolar minute ventilation, the respiratory system has the ability to modulate the concentration of carbon dioxide and therefore effect a change in the amount of H^+ in the blood through the following equation:

$$H_2O + CO_2 \rightleftharpoons H_2CO_3 \rightleftharpoons H^+ + HCO_3^-$$

The respiratory system's ability to directly regulate Pa_{CO_2} and thereby indirectly regulate the H^+ concentration, provides an influence on the pH of the body.[37] As previously stated in this chapter, the partial pressure of carbon dioxide in arterial blood (Pa_{CO_2}) is 35 to 45 mm Hg. Hyperventilation is defined as a decrease in the Pa_{CO_2}, which decreases the available H^+. The blood will be less acidic, which will result in a pH greater than 7.45. Hypoventilation is an increase in Pa_{CO_2}, which will cause an increase in available H^+. An acidemia results; it is reflected by a lower pH—one less than 7.35. An inverse relation therefore exists between Pa_{CO_2} and the pH of the blood.

The final body system to be mentioned in the regulation of acid-base balance is the renal system. Serum bicarbonate (HCO_3^-), which is produced and retained by the kidneys, acts as a buffer. The normal level of HCO_3^- in arterial blood is 24 meq per liter. Bicarbonate can combine with H^+ to form H_2CO_3, which effectively eliminates its influence over pH. If the kidneys produce more than the normal amount of bicarbonate, greater than 24 meq per liter, the blood will be more buffered. The result will be an alkalemia. Any decrease in the amount of metabolic buffers results in a decrease in the body pH, and the result is an acidemia. A direct relation exists between the available HCO_3^- and the pH of the blood.

Both the respiratory and the renal systems can cause a primary acidemia or alkalemia. Their responses to changes in pH can also correct alterations in acid-base balance, and therefore either system can be a compensatory mechanism. Within 1 to 15 minutes, the respiratory system can compensate for an alteration in H^+ concentration and return the pH to within the normal range, 7.35 to 7.45.[3] In contrast, several minutes to several days are required for a readjustment of the pH by the serum bicarbonate mechanism.[3]

ARTERIAL BLOOD GAS ANALYSIS

The analysis of the partial pressures of gases within the arterial blood indicates the effectiveness of alveolar ventilation and the role of the ventilation in acid-base balance.[37] Three factors from an arterial blood gas analysis are required to evaluate the acid-base status: (1) the blood pH, (2) the partial pressure of carbon dioxide, and (3) the amount of serum bicarbonate. The pH should be evaluated first. Any change from 7.35 to 7.45, and also the direction of the change, should be noted. By determining the pH, an acidemia, alkalemia, or normal pH can be detected.

The next value to be determined in the assessment process is the $Paco_2$. Again, any change from the normal range, 35 to 45 mm Hg, should be noted. The direction of the change should be compared with the direction of change in the pH. It is important to remember that an inverse relation exists between the $Paco_2$ and the pH. For example, if all other body systems are stable and the $Paco_2$ becomes less than 35 mm Hg, a respiratory alkalosis occurs, whereas an increase in $Paco_2$ produces a respiratory acidosis. An approximate numerical relation also exists between the $Paco_2$ and the pH. For every 10 mm Hg change in the $Paco_2$ value, there should be an approximate change (in the opposite direction) of 0.08 in the pH. For example (using the midrange of 40 mm Hg for $Paco_2$ and the midrange of 7.40 for pH), an increase in the $Paco_2$ to 50 mm Hg would result in a pH decrease to 7.32. Likewise, a decrease in the $Paco_2$ to 30 mm Hg would result in a rise in the pH to 7.48. If the inverse relationship is evident, the alteration in pH is respiratory in origin. If the inverse relationship does not exist, further investigation into the cause of altered acid-base balance is necessary.

The third value to assess when determining acid-base balance is the concentration of the bicarbonate ion (HCO_3^-). Any deviation from 24 meq per liter should be noted, as should be the direction of the change. There is a direct relation between bicarbonate and pH. An increase in bicarbonate concentration results in an increase in pH, and vice versa. When this direct relationship exists, the primary cause of the alteration in pH is of metabolic etiology.

Patients may present with signs and symptoms of an alkalosis and acidosis from either a respiratory or metabolic etiology. Table 3–2 summarizes the alterations in the components of primary, uncompensated alterations in body pH as well as their causes, signs, and symptoms.

There are also compensatory mechanisms to be considered in the acid-base balance.

TABLE 3–2 Abnormalities of Acid-Base Balance

Type	pH	Paco$_2$	HCO$_3^-$	Causes	Signs/Symptoms
Uncompensated respiratory alkalosis	↑	↓	—	Alveolar hyperventilation	Dizziness, tingling, syncopy, numbness, early tetany
Uncompensated respiratory acidosis	↓	↑	—	Alveolar hypoventilation	Early: Anxiety, restlessness, dyspnea, headache. Late: confusion, somnolence, and coma
Uncompensated metabolic alkalosis	↑	—	↑	Bicarbonate ingestion, vomiting, diuretics, steroids, adrenal disease	Vague symptoms: weakness, mental dullness, possibly early tetany
Uncompensated metabolic acidosis	↓	—	↓	Diabetic, lactic uremic acidosis, prolonged diarrhea	Nausea, vomiting, cardiac arrhythmias, lethargy, coma

Source: From Rothstein, JM, Roy, SH, and Wolf, SL: The Rehabilitation Specialist's Handbook, FA Davis, 1991, p 619, with permission.

For example, if the metabolic system causes a change in the pH, the respiratory system has the ability to compensate for that change. The reverse also is true. The respiratory system could be the cause of the pH disturbance, and the metabolic system could compensate. In this way, both the respiratory system and the renal system have the ability to create a compensating acidosis or alkalosis to normalize the original dysfunction.[38] It is helpful to know that the body never *over*compensates for an acid-base disturbance.

The analysis of the arterial blood gas also offers insight into arterial oxygenation. The partial pressure of oxygen within the arterial system of a subject breathing room air ($F_{IO_2} = 0.21$) at sea level has previously been stated to be approximately 95 to 100 mm Hg. "Hypoxemia" is the term used when the amount of oxygen in the blood is below 80 mm Hg.[20] In mild hypoxemia, the Pao$_2$ is less than 80 mm Hg; in moderate hypoxemia, it is less than 70 mm Hg; and in severe hypoxemia, it is less than 60 mm Hg.[20]

There is not a finite relation between the partial pressures of oxygen and CO$_2$ in the blood. Although it is true that if subjects decrease their minute ventilation, Paco$_2$ will rise and Pao$_2$ will fall, the reverse is not true. If minute ventilation is increased, Paco$_2$ will fall but the oxygen tension within the arterial system will stay approximately the

TABLE 3–3 Estimated Fractions of Inspired Oxygen F$_{IO_2}$ with Low-Flow Devices

Nasal Cannula, L/min	Estimated F$_{IO_2}$	Oxygen Mask, L/min	Estimated F$_{IO_2}$	Mask with Reservoir, L/min	Estimated F$_{IO_2}$
1	0.24	5–6	0.40	7	0.70
2	0.28	6–7	0.50	8	0.80
3	0.32	7–8	0.60	9	0.90
4	0.36			10	0.99+

Source: From Rothstein, JM, Roy, SH, and Wolf, SL: The Rehabilitation Specialist's Handbook, FA Davis, 1991, p 623, with permission.

TABLE 3–4 Fraction of
Inspired Oxygen (F_{IO_2})
and the Corresponding Alveolar
Partial Pressure
of Oxygen (P_{AO_2})

F_{IO_2}	Available P_{AO_2}, mm Hg
0.21	104
0.30	167
0.40	239
0.50	311
0.60	384
0.70	456
0.80	528
0.90	601
1.00	673

same. This is in part due to the fixed pool of oxygen in the atmosphere and the efficiency of the system, which is difficult to "improve."

To increase the P_{ao_2} above the normal range, an increase in the fraction of inspired oxygen is needed. Table 3–3 lists estimates of the fraction of inspired oxygen available through different types of oxygen delivery systems.[39]

The amount of oxygen available at the alveoli can be estimated from the F_{IO_2}:

$$P_{AO_2} = F_{IO_2}(P_B - 47) - P_{ACO_2}(F_{IO_2} + 1 - F_{IO_2}R)$$

where P_B is the barometric pressure, which can be assumed to be at sea level, or 760 mm Hg, and R is the respiratory quotient, which can be assumed to be 0.8 in most instances.[1] Table 3–4 illustrates the partial pressure of oxygen available within the alveoli according to the F_{IO_2} present.

CASE STUDIES

It may be helpful to study the following three examples of arterial blood gas analyses to determine their significance in patient diagnoses.

CASE 1

A 45-year-old man with asthma was in his usual state of health until he noticed shortness of breath and wheezing. The arterial blood gas values are shown below.

Arterial Blood Gas Values

	Normal	Case Study #1
F_{IO_2}	0.21	0.21
P_{ao_2} (mm Hg)	95	70
P_{aco_2} (mm Hg)	40	25
pH	7.40	7.50
HCO_3^- (meq/L)	24	24

To determine the acid-base balance, the pH was evaluated first. It was found to be 7.50, which is above the 7.45 upper limit of normal; therefore, there is an alkalemia. The next value assessed was the $Paco_2$, which was 25 mm Hg: a 10 mm Hg decrease from the lower limit of normal. The pH and the $Paco_2$ have changed in opposite directions, so the respiratory system is determined to be the origin of the acid-base problem. (Clinical information also is important in making this conclusion.) For each change of 10 mm Hg in the $Paco_2$ there should be a change of approximately 0.08 in the pH (from midpoint 7.40), which results in a pH value of 7.50. Next, the HCO_3^- concentration was evaluated. It was found to be 24 meq per liter. Compensation by the metabolic system has not yet occurred. Therefore, this gentleman was diagnosed as having an alkalemia caused by a respiratory alkalosis with no compensation by the metabolic system. He is also moderately hypoxemic.

CASE 2

A 25-year-old woman with diabetes was in her usual state of health until 2 days ago, when she noted that her diabetes was no longer in control. She was admitted to the hospital in diabetic ketoacidosis with the arterial blood gas values shown below.

	Arterial Blood Gas Values	
	Normal	Case Study
Fio_2	0.21	0.21
Pao_2 (mm Hg)	95	95
$Paco_2$ (mm Hg)	40	25
pH	7.40	7.32
HCO_3^- (meq/L)	24	18

Again, first her pH was evaluated. It was 7.32, a mild acidemia. Her $Paco_2$ has decreased to 25 mm Hg. There is a decrease in $Paco_2$ and a decrease in pH. The change in pH is not from a respiratory dysfunction. If the respiratory system were the cause of the abnormality, a $Paco_2$ of 25 should result in an alkalemia. The HCO_3^- is 18 meq per liter, less than the normal value of 24 meq per liter. A decrease in HCO_3^- and a decrease in pH mean that there is a metabolic cause for the acid-base disturbance. This ABG shows a metabolic acidosis caused by the diabetic ketoacidosis. For a moment, again consider the $Paco_2$ value. Why would the respiratory system decrease the $Paco_2$? It has effectively created a respiratory alkalosis to help compensate for the metabolic acidosis created by the diabetic ketoacidosis. If the respiratory system had not altered the $Paco_2$, the overall acidemia would be far worse. Summarizing this case study, the patient has a normal Pao_2, a mild acidemia caused by a metabolic acidosis with a partially compensating respiratory alkalosis.

CASE 3

A 65-year-old man with a history of chronic obstructive pulmonary disease presents for a routine physical examination in his usual state of health. His arterial blood gas analysis is shown below.

	Arterial Blood Gas Values	
	Normal	Case Study
F_{IO_2}	0.21	0.21
P_{aO_2} (mm Hg)	95	55
P_{aCO_2} (mm Hg)	40	60
pH	7.40	7.40
HCO_3^- (meq/L)	24	29

Again, first evaluate the pH: it is within the normal range of 7.40. His P_{aCO_2} has increased to 60 mm Hg. The increase in P_{aCO_2} is causing a respiratory acidosis that is not reflected in the pH. The HCO_3^- is 29 meq per liter, greater than the normal value of 24 meq per liter. An increase in HCO_3^- is causing a metabolic alkalosis that again is not reflected in the pH. From the clinical information, it can be assumed that the respiratory system is the primary cause for the acid-base disturbance. It can also be assumed that the metabolic alkalosis is the compensating mechanism that is trying to return the body's pH to normal. Summarizing this case study, the patient has severe hypoxemia, a normal pH, and a respiratory acidosis with a fully compensating metabolic alkalosis.

SUMMARY

This chapter has presented a brief review of respiratory anatomy and physiology. The anatomy of the respiratory system comprises the bony thorax (including the sternum, clavicle, humerus, scapula, ribs, and vertebral column), the lungs, the upper airways (nose, mouth, pharynx, and larynx), the lower airways (trachea, bronchi, and bronchioles), and the respiratory unit (respiratory bronchioles, alveolar ducts, alveolar sacs, and alveoli). The muscles of ventilation include both the muscles of inspiration and those of expiration.

The discussion of physiology includes both ventilation and respiration. Ventilation is the movement of air in and out of the pulmonary system. The ventilation topics discussed include lung volumes, capacities, flow rates, and the mechanics of ventilation. "Respiration" refers to the ability of the pulmonary system to diffuse gas. The respiration topics discussed include diffusion, ventilation-perfusion relations, acid-base balance, and arterial blood gas analysis.

Neurologic control of respiration is provided by a complex group of systems: the cerebral cortex, the pons, the medulla oblongata, the autonomic nervous system, mechanical receptors, and chemical receptors. Their contribution to the regulation of respiration has been presented.

Respiratory diseases can alter the anatomy and physiology of the respiratory system either acutely or chronically, and Chapter 6 will discuss the possible alterations of the respiratory system and the resulting effects.

REFERENCES

1. Harper, R: A Guide to Respiratory Care: Physiology and Clinical Applications. JB Lippincott, Philadelphia, 1981.

2. Loring, S and Mead, J: Action of the diaphragm and rib cage inferred from force-balance analysis. J Appl Physiol 53:756–760, 1982.
3. Guyton, A: Textbook of Medical Physiology, ed 7. WB Saunders, Philadelphia, 1986.
4. Gray, H: Anatomy of the Human Body. In Goss, C (ed). Lea & Febiger, Philadelphia, 1973.
5. Roussos, C: Function and fatigue of the respiratory muscles. Chest (Suppl)88:1245–1335, 1985.
6. Roussos, C and Macklem, P: The respiratory muscles. N Engl J Med 307:786–796, 1982.
7. DeTroyer, A, Kelly, S and Zin, W: Mechanical action of the intercostal muscles on the ribs. Science 220:82–88, 1983.
8. Luce, J and Culver, B: Respiratory muscle function in health and disease. Chest 81:82–89, 1982.
9. Kigin, C: Breathing exercises for the medical patient: The art and science. Phys Ther 70:700–706, 1990.
10. Raper, A, et al: Scalene and sternomatoid muscle function. J Appl Physiol 21:497–502, 1966.
11. Woodburne, R: Essentials of Human Anatomy. Oxford University Press, New York, 1961.
12. Loring, S and Mead, J: Abdominal muscle use during quiet breathing and hyperpnea in uniformed subjects. J Appl Physiol 52:700–704, 1982.
13. DeTroyer, A: Mechanical action of the abdominal muscles. Bull Eur Physiopathol Respir 19:575–581, 1983.
14. Downie, P (ed): Cash's Textbook of Chest, Heart and Vascular Disorders for Physiotherapists. JB Lippincott, Philadelphia, 1982, p 82.
15. Green, J: Fundamental Cardiovascular and Pulmonary Physiology, ed 2. Lea & Febiger, Philadelphia, 1987, p 178.
16. Hobson, L and Dean, E: Review of respiratory anatomy. In Frownfelter, D: Chest Physical Therapy and Pulmonary Rehabilitation: An Interdisciplinary Approach, ed 2. Year Book Medical Publishers, Chicago, 1987.
17. Moore, K: Clinically Oriented Anatomy. Williams & Wilkins, Baltimore, 1980.
18. Youtsey, J: Basic pulmonary function measurements. In C Spearman (ed): Egan's Fundamentals of Respiratory Therapy, ed 4. CV Mosby, St Louis, 1982.
19. West, J: Respiratory Physiology: The Essentials. Williams & Wilkins, Baltimore, 1979.
20. Martin, D and Youtsey, J: Respiratory Anatomy and Physiology. CV Mosby, St Louis, 1988.
21. Zadai, C: Pulmonary physiology of aging: The role of rehabilitation. Topics Geriatric Rehabil 1:49–56, 1985.
22. Berry, R, Pai, U and Fairshter, R: Effect of age on changes in flow rates and airway conductance after a deep breath. J Appl Physiol 68:635–643, 1990.
23. Rahman, M, Ullah, M and Begum, A: Lung function in teenage Bangladeshi boys and girls. Respir Med 84:47–55, 1990.
24. Hepper, N, Black, L and Fowler, W: Relationship of lung volume to height and arm span in normal subjects and in patients with spinal deformities. Am Rev Respir Dis 91:356–362, 1965.
25. Oscherwitz, M, et al: Differences in pulmonary functions in various racial groups. Am J Epidemiol 96:319–327, 1972.
26. Dufetel, P, et al: Characteristics of lung volume and expiratory flow seen in black African adults. Rev Mal Respir 7:215–222, 1990.
27. Morris, J, Koski, A and Johnson, L: Prediction nomograms (BTPS) spirometric values in normal males and females. Am Rev Respir Dis 163:57–67, 1971.
28. Craig, D, et al: Closing volume and its relationship to gas exchange in seated and supine positions. J Appl Physiol 31:717–721, 1971.
29. ATS Statement: Snowbird Workshop on Standardization of Spirometry. Am Rev Respir Dis 119:831–838, 1979.
30. Hodgkin, J and Petty, T: Chronic Obstructive Pulmonary Disease: Current Concepts. WB Saunders, Philadelphia, 1987.
31. Farzan, S: A Concise Handbook of Respiratory Diseases, ed 2. Reston Publishing, Reston, VA, 1985.
32. Kilburn, K and Warchaw, R: Pulmonary function impairment associated with pleural asbestos disease. Chest 98:965–972, 1990.
33. West, J: Pulmonary Pathophysiology: The Essentials. Williams & Wilkins, Baltimore, 1977.
34. McLaughlin, A: Essentials of Physiology for Advanced Respiratory Therapy. CV Mosby, St. Louis, 1977.
35. Cheeseman, M and Revelette, W: Phrenic afferent contribution to reflexes elicited by changes in diaphragm length. J Appl Physiol 69:640–647, 1990.
36. Tallarida, G, Peruzzi, G and Raimondi, G: The role of chemosensitive muscle receptors in cardiorespiratory regulation during exercise. J Auton Nerv Syst (Suppl)30:155–161, 1990.
37. Flenley, D: Blood gas and acid base interpretation. Respir Care 27:311–317, 1982.
38. Milhorn, H: Understanding arterial blood gases. Am Fam Physician 21:112–120, 1980.
39. Rothstein, J, Roy, S and Wolf, S: The Rehabilitation Specialist's Handbook. FA Davis, Philadelphia, 1991.

CHAPTER 4

Physiologic Adaptations to Aerobic Exercise

Rehabilitation management of cardiopulmonary disease is designed to reduce the physical and psychologic impact of a disabling disease, as well as to increase the individual's functional capacity. However, to meet increased demands for energy placed on the body during exercise, several physiologic adjustments must be made. Arm activity and muscular contractions of the isometric type may evoke the Valsalva maneuver, increase muscle pressure on the arteries, and increase blood pressure, and they do not benefit the cardiovascular system.[1-3] For those reasons, activities involving sustained contractions and dynamic overhead arm work are not generally recommended as a major part of cardiopulmonary rehabilitation programs or for older adults.[4-8] Although recent investigation indicates that low-intensity resistive exercise training when combined with aerobic activity has beneficial effects on coronary heart disease (CHD) risk factors,[9] this discussion of physiologic adaptations to exercise (acute and chronic) will be limited to changes that occur during dynamic, rhythmic, and continuous activities of an aerobic nature.[10-15]

ACUTE RESPONSES TO AEROBIC EXERCISE

The acute responses to exercise include the physiologic adjustments that normally occur in response to a single bout of exercise. The major adjustments that must be made include cardiac adaptations, coronary and systemic circulatory adjustments, blood pressure and volume changes, and metabolic adaptations.

Cardiac Adaptations

The rate of contraction of the heart begins to increase before exercise begins (anticipatory rise). As exercise commences and continues, the increase in heart rate is proportional to the intensity of the activity.[6,9,16] If the intensity of the activity is too great, the maximum heart rate will be achieved, exhaustion will ensue, and the exercise will be anaerobic. Aerobically, there is a linear relation between heart rate and oxygen consumption. (See the section on metabolic adaptations.)

The cardiac muscle responds to exercise not only by increasing its rate of contraction but also by increasing its force of contraction. The increased force of contraction results in an increase in the stroke volume, or the amount of blood ejected by the heart per beat. The normal ejection fraction is 0.6 to 0.75, and it increases during exercise.[5,17]

As a result of the increased heart rate and stroke volume that accompany exercise, the cardiac output increases. Cardiac output is equal to the volume of blood pumped by the heart per minute: It is a product of the stroke volume and the heart rate. As presented in Chapter 2, the rate and force of cardiac contraction are regulated by the autonomic system, chemoreceptors, pressoreceptors, and body temperature.[15,18]

Two important aspects of heart rate and cardiac output should be noted. The first is that the maximal heart rate an individual can attain decreases with age; that is, there is an inverse relation. The second is that both heart rate and stroke volume increase when an individual is exercising at 40 to 60 percent of his or her maximum capacity. At higher levels, however, increased cardiac output is accomplished by an increase in heart rate only; stroke volume does not increase.[4,19] Keeping in mind that coronary circulation (circulation to the heart muscle itself) occurs primarily during diastole, it is important to remember that for people with limited ability to increase heart rate (coronary, pulmonary, and/or older patients) exercise must be at comparatively low heart rates.[5,19,20]

Coronary Circulation Adjustments

In response to exercise, the heart muscle must increase its work. It therefore needs more oxygen so its metabolism can produce the energy for it to continue to contract. At rest, the cardiac muscle extracts approximately 70 percent of the oxygen that is delivered to it via the coronary circulation. That leaves little reserve for increasing oxygen delivery to the cardiac muscle by this mechanism. The increased coronary demands of exercise are met by increasing the rate at which blood flows through the coronary arteries and by increased aortic blood pressure, all of which force more blood into the coronary arteries. Any obstruction to coronary blood flow decreases the amount of oxygen delivered to the cardiac tissues and could precipitate an ischemic condition. The literature suggests that high exercising heart rates in cardiopulmonary and older patients make it difficult for the myocardium to continue to receive adequate amounts of oxygen. Therefore, graded exercise testing with ECG monitoring, a scientifically developed exercise prescription based on the exercise test, and careful monitoring during exercise sessions can help to avoid situations in which there may be inadequate blood flow to the myocardium.[6,14,16]

Systemic Circulation Adjustments

During aerobic exercise, the muscles that are actively working need a greater oxygen supply to produce the energy needed for continuing muscular contraction. The increased need for oxygen by the working muscles is met not only by an increase in the cardiac output but also by an increase in blood flow to the active muscles. Because a limited amount of blood must supply all the tissues of the body, the amount of blood flowing to any specific tissue depends on the oxygen need of that tissue. Thus, during exercise, blood is shunted (directed away) from tissues that are less active (such as digestive organs) and to muscles that are actively working and have increased metabolic activity. This shunting is accomplished by a series of chemical (increased CO_2 and lower pH) and reflex adjustments (sympathetic nervous system firing) that cause the dilation of arterioles in the working muscles and a constriction of vessels in inactive regions of the body.[5]

Because blood is shunted to areas of increased activity during exercise, there is also increased blood flow to the lungs. To meet the metabolic demands of the body, both the rate and depth of ventilation and the diffusion of oxygen from the alveoli into the pulmonary capillaries increase with increasing activity.[15]

The increased blood flow to active muscles during exercise thus improves oxygen delivery to the active tissues. In addition, there are increases in the oxygen consumption (metabolism) of the muscle cells, and there is better oxygen extraction by those cells.[14]

To dissipate the heat that is produced during exercise, blood flow to the skin increases. The hypothalamus is responsive to changes in the temperature of the blood. When blood temperature increases, the hypothalamus signals the blood vessels that supply the skin to dilate. More blood can then flow to the surface of the skin so that evaporation of perspiration can occur. The evaporation cools the skin and that, in turn, cools the blood. Exercising in an environment of high humidity impairs the cooling process owing to decreased ability to evaporate sweat. Cardiopulmonary patients should be warned of the dangers of exercising in an environment of high humidity, particularly when high humidity is combined with a high environmental temperature.

Respiratory Adaptations

To supply adequate amounts of oxygen during exercise, there is an increase in all phases of respiration. Therefore, external, internal, and cellular respiration increase in response to increased oxygen demand. Because of an increase in tidal volume and respiratory frequency, the minute volume (VE) may increase from a resting value of approximately 6 liters per minute to above 100 liters per minute during vigorous activity. The primary stimulus for the increase in VE seems to be the concentration of carbon dioxide (CO_2) in the arterial blood ($Paco_2$). A linear relation exists between pulmonary ventilation and increasing levels of activity. Increased ventilation during activity is combined with increased cardiac output, so adequate removal of CO_2, buffering of lactic acid, and maintenance of a constant pH are achieved. In patients with pulmonary disease, breathing rates during exercise increase more rapidly than in normal persons because, in part, there is a smaller than normal increase in tidal volume. At minute ventilations of approximately 40 liters, the breathing rate of the pulmonary-diseased individual may be two times greater than that of a normal person and may approach the maximum voluntary ventilation (MVV). Exercise for the pulmonary patient is usually terminated at a relatively low heart rate because of ventilatory limitations.[21,22]

Blood Pressure Adjustments

In the active muscles during aerobic exercise, the blood vessels dilate. The dilation decreases the resistance to blood flow and tends to cause a decrease in blood pressure. However, the trend toward lower blood pressure during exercise is negated by an increase in cardiac output. The net effect is that the systolic blood pressure increases in normotensive individuals. The increase in systolic blood pressure is normally proportional to the intensity and oxygen demand of the activity. In normotensive individuals, there is little or no increase in diastolic blood pressure with increased aerobic work.[5]

Dramatic declines in systolic blood pressure can be seen when an individual has been exercising intensively and suddenly stops. The resultant pooling of blood in the lower extremities decreases venous return and cardiac output. It may cause fainting associated with poor perfusion to the brain. To avoid that result, especially in cardiopulmonary patients, all aerobic exercise sessions should include a cool-down phase.[5,19]

Exercises involving the arms evoke a greater rise in blood pressure than exercises with the legs. Apparently the difference is at least partially due to the smaller muscles being used for the activity. Although there is dilation of the blood vessels in the arms, there is constriction of the vessels in the inactive, larger leg muscles, and blood pressure increases during arm exercises. For persons with cardiopulmonary disease and older individuals, aerobic activities involving the arms should be cautiously administered. Prolonged intense arm exercises are to be used with care, and patients should be cautioned about performing daily activities involving continued arm work such as shoveling, digging, raking, lifting, and carrying. However, since many leisure and vocational activities require arm activity, arm training may be included as part of a rehabilitation program. Rehabilitation programs should emphasize aerobic activities that utilize the larger leg muscles: walking, jogging, and cycling.[4,5,8,14,16,23]

Blood and Fluid Adaptations

The body cools itself by evaporation of perspiration. Continued aerobic exercise can cause significant loss of body fluid. Consequently, the plasma volume (approximately 90 percent water) may decrease while the protein and cellular components remain relatively unchanged. This state is referred to as hemoconcentration because the solid particles of the blood constitute a relatively higher percentage of whole blood. Hemoconcentration results in "thicker" blood. It can increase the resistance to blood flow and also increase blood pressure. Exercises performed in an environment of high temperature and high humidity can promote further dehydration and fluid loss and are to be avoided.[5]

Metabolic Adaptations

To meet the increased metabolic demands of exercise, the amount of oxygen delivered to the tissues increases as a result of increased cardiac output and increased blood flow to the working muscles.[16] (This assumes that the hemoglobin concentration of the blood is normal and provides adequate oxygen transport.) On delivery to the individual cells, oxygen must be used by those cells to provide energy for continued muscle contraction. Oxygen utilization (oxygen uptake) is determined not only by delivery but also by the number of mitochondria in the cells, the amount of myoglobin, the enzymes of metabolism, the substrates available for metabolism, and probably many other factors. The maximal amount of oxygen (Vo_2max) that can be consumed by an individual is commonly considered to be the best and most accurate indication of cardiorespiratory fitness.[4,6,14,16] Vo_2max is usually expressed as milliliters of oxygen used per kilogram of body weight per minute. Direct measurements of Vo_2max can be made if the arterial-venous oxygen difference is found by sampling inspired and expired air. Because of the expense of the necessary measuring equipment, it is considered acceptable to predict Vo_2max. Predictions are based on heart rate responses to a standard exercise work load as both Vo_2max and heart rate increase in a linear manner in response to increases in exercise intensities.[5,14,24]

It has been suggested that the limiting factor in exercise performance is the ability of the tissues to utilize oxygen.[5,16,24] Compared with the resting state, the arterial-venous oxygen difference during exercise increases by as much as threefold.[4] This ability to use more oxygen during exercise by the active muscles keeps the heart from having to work too hard to supply the necessary circulation for continued muscular contractions. Increased oxygen extraction by the tissues during exercise is enhanced by chemical, temperature, and hormonal changes in the blood.[12]

CHRONIC RESPONSES TO AEROBIC EXERCISE

In recent years, considerable interest has developed in the long-term physiological benefits an individual derives from engaging in a program of dynamic, rhythmic, and continuous activities over a period of time. Although there is considerable controversy on the subject, many researchers feel that cardiopulmonary disease can be prevented and/or reversed with cessation of smoking, regular aerobic exercise (training), and the elimination of or a reduction in the amount of dietary fat, salt, caffeine, and the like.[16,18,25-28] Because of lack of information, there seem to be different opinions about the constituents of a good training program. For clarity, the information presented in this text will be for the purpose of training the cardiopulmonary-impaired individual and will not deal with the training of athletes.

Cardiac Adaptations to Aerobic Training

The individual fibers of cardiac muscle may adapt to aerobic training by becoming larger (hypertrophy) and stronger.[29] Unlike skeletal muscle, cardiac tissue does not seem to respond to training by increasing the number of mitochondria or by increasing the oxidative capacity of the respiratory enzymes.[16]

The hypertrophy of cardiac muscle as a result of aerobic training is accompanied by a larger stroke volume. Thus, at any given work load, the heart does not have to beat as often to supply an adequate volume of blood, and the cardiac output at submaximal work levels may not change compared with pretraining conditions. At maximal work loads, the cardiac output increase is due to the increased stroke volume, whereas the maximal heart rate does not appear to change. Endurance training also causes an increase in recovery heart rates from all levels of work.[14,16]

As yet, there is no clear explanation for the bradycardia that results from aerobic training. Bradycardia is observed at rest and at all levels of work. Bradycardia may be partially due to the increased strength of the myocardial fibers, so that more blood is pumped per beat and the heart does not have to beat as often to supply the same amount of blood. Recent studies indicate an increased vagal tone in response to aerobic training.[4,5,14] This results in a shift away from the sympathetic nervous system's influence (the catecholamines) on the heart in favor of the parasympathetic system, which enhances the influence of the vagus nerve and results in bradycardia. In cardiac patients, the bradycardia that results from training is a major factor in raising the angina threshold—the level of work at which angina occurs.[4,5,14,19,21]

Coronary Circulation Responses

Because aerobic training does not seem to increase the oxygen extraction ability of the myocardium, the increased need of the myocardium for oxygen during exercise must be met by increases in coronary blood flow. Increases in coronary blood flow result from increases in heart rate, stroke volume, and vasodilation. Relatively speaking, however, the bradycardia and increased stroke volume that accompany training result in a longer period of diastole between beats, so there is enhanced perfusion in the coronary arteries as a result of training. These physiologic adaptations to aerobic training are major factors in the improvement of ischemic ECG changes in patients with coronary artery disease (CAD).[14]

There is considerable controversy over whether there is an increase in the diameter of the coronary arteries and/or increased collateral circulation as a result of aerobic training.[16,30] Such increases have been demonstrated to occur in animal experimentation and in some studies with humans, but as yet not consistently in humans.[14,26,31] Current methodologies to determine increased collateral circulation in humans may not be sensitive enough to detect improvements.[13,32,34,35,36]

Pulmonary Responses

The effects of regular aerobic exercise on the pulmonary system are to decrease the rate and increase the depth of ventilation. This training benefit apparently results, in part, from improved efficiency of the respiratory musculature. Increased pulmonary diffusion, not noted at rest or submaximal exercise, is increased during maximal work. It may be a result of increased pulmonary blood flow, which causes greater perfusion of the lung. Decreased lactic acid concentrations and an increased anaerobic threshold with improved functional capacity are other benefits of regular aerobic exercise.[21,22]

Whether aerobic activity improves pulmonary function, as measured by standardized tests, remains controversial. Some studies have reported improvements in lung volume;[37,38] others have shown no improvements in lung function as a result of regular aerobic activity.[39,40] It may be that, at this time, the data are not available, since rehabilitation of the patient with pulmonary disease as part of standard medical treatment for the pulmonary patient is a fairly new concept.

Changes in Systemic Circulation

The capacity for blood flow to skeletal muscles is increased in response to aerobic training by an increase in the number of capillaries that supply the muscle fibers. There is also an increase in the number and size of the mitochondria and the enzyme systems in skeletal muscle that supply energy for contraction.[16] These changes in skeletal muscles account for a greater arterial-venous oxygen difference in response to training. However, during submaximal work, blood flow to the active muscles does not seem to be as important as metabolism in the observed arterial-venous oxygen difference. During maximal work, blood flow and metabolism are considerably increased in response to aerobic training. These physiologic adaptations to training allow for better delivery and utilization of oxygen at the tissue site so that, relatively speaking, the heart does not have to work so hard to deliver an adequate blood supply to the active muscles.[14]

Blood Pressure Changes

Although there is considerable controversy about the long-term effects of aerobic exercise on blood pressure, recent studies have reported a decrease in both systolic and diastolic resting and working blood pressures following periods of consistent training.[41-45] These changes have also been reported in individuals who are hypertensive and medicated.[42,43,46,47] In some cases the blood pressure decreases were so dramatic that the individuals were able to discontinue their medications. The physiologic mechanisms whereby those changes occur are yet to be determined. It may be that aerobic training directly causes improvements in the smooth muscles of the circulatory system, or the reported decreases in blood pressure may be a result of reduction of the risk factors that often accompany training—reduced body fat, cessation of smoking, and the like.[24,43,45,48]

Blood and Fluid Responses

Endurance training causes an increase in the total blood volume of the body. This increase in due largely to an increase in the amount of the plasma portion of whole blood. As a result, aerobic training allows a person to adjust better to environments of high temperatures and high humidities by improving the sweating mechanism.[5,49]

Aerobic training increases the number of red blood cells slightly. Consequently, the amount of hemoglobin increases, although the hematocrit remains relatively unchanged. Whether training causes decreased aggregation of the platelets and thus lessens the chance of forming an intravascular thrombosis remains to be demonstrated, but increasing evidence indicates that exercise enhances fibrinolytic activity.[33,50-53]

Metabolic Adaptations

The increase in Vo_2max that results from aerobic training is due to increases in cardiac output and in the arterial-venous oxygen difference.[14] Measurements of Vo_2max are utilized extensively in the diagnosis of cardiovascular diseases and in the prescription of appropriate exercise programs for persons with cardiovascular disease. Tests for Vo_2max are discussed in Chapter 9.

Training increases the number of mitochondria in the working muscles and enhances the use of oxygen. During submaximal exercise, the lactic acid concentration of the blood does not increase as it does in maximal work because of an adequate oxygen supply and utilization by the mitochondria (steady state). Exercise prescriptions for the cardiac patient should elicit work of a submaximal nature so that metabolic energy comes from aerobic metabolism (Krebs cycle) rather than from anaerobic sources (glycolysis).[14]

Body Composition Changes

It is well established that regular aerobic exercise can be an important factor in helping individuals lose and/or control body fat. Weight loss through exercise is accompanied by a decrease in the percentage of body fat and an increase in lean body mass. For best results, cardiopulmonary patients needing to lose body fat should combine an aerobic exercise program with restricted caloric intake.[18,44,54,55]

Changes in Blood Lipids

The lack of agreement in the literature about the effects of aerobic training on total blood cholesterol, triglycerides, and high-density lipoprotein cholesterol (HDL) most likely is due to lack of control over the experimental variables.[16,28,56-58] Several sources have reported that regular exercise is effective in lowering total blood cholesterol and triglyceride levels and increasing the HDL levels.[42,43,53,57,59-61] These results may be due to dietary modifications that reduce saturated fat intake rather than to exercise effects. Whether dietary modifications can alter cholesterol and other blood lipid levels is itself controversial, although several sources indicate a positive response.[6,57] Current thinking favors a combination of proper nutrition (with reduced fat intake) and proper exercise to reduce blood lipid concentration and to prevent or reverse the atherosclerotic process that leads to heart disease. Although more research is needed in this area, significant positive correlations that link HDL levels with the number of aerobic miles run per week have been reported.[33,42,43,56,62-65]

Training and Stress

There is evidence of a correlation between personality traits and incidence of ischemic heart disease. Individuals with type A personalities have been found to have higher levels of blood catecholamines, higher heart rate, and higher blood pressure responses than those with type B personalities when both types are subjected to the same stress situations. Individuals with type A personalities have been reported to experience twice the ischemic heart disease of type B individuals.[6,66-69] Recent research indicates that individuals with type A personalities who harbor anger and hostility may have significantly more CHD than those who do not.[53,67]

Emotional states such as anxiety and depression also have been found to adversely affect the cardiovascular system.[70,71] It is theorized that these emotional stresses can cause platelet aggregation, evoke an ischemic state, or even precipitate an acute attack. Persons subjected to prolonged adverse emotional states may have a higher chance for developing ischemic heart disease than nonstressed individuals.[7,68,69,72-74]

Although more research is needed in this area, aerobic exercise is valuable to some people in helping to relieve some personality and emotional tensions, perhaps as a result of a decreased catecholamine secretion.[26,54,75-77] Speculations about the "runners' high" include increased levels of endorphins in the blood in response to training. If for no other reason, the fact that aerobic activity undertaken on a regular basis gives individuals a sense of well-being may be sufficient justification for recommending training for persons in stressful situations or those with personalities of the A type.[36,71,75-77]

Training and Ischemic Heart Disease

Ischemia occurs when the myocardial demand for oxygen exceeds the supply and the muscle cells must rely on anaerobic metabolism (glycolysis) for their energy. Ischemia usually is thought to result from atherosclerosis of the coronary arteries, although recent evidence suggests that coronary artery spasm may be responsible for ischemia in some individuals.[78]

Angina occurs when an individual reaches his or her ischemic threshold—a phenomenon dependent on systolic blood pressure and heart rate.[16] Anything that causes an increase in either systolic blood pressure or heart rate can precipitate an attack of angina. Physical activity increases both those parameters and can also cause an anginal attack. Regular aerobic activity, however, has been found to cause physiological changes that lower the heart rate and blood pressure for any given submaximal work load and thus raise the ischemic threshold.[5,19,27,42]

Other beneficial effects of regular exercise include a decreased catecholamine production, increased coronary perfusion, increased functional work capacity, decreased peripheral resistance, possible increased collateral circulation, increased fibrinolysis, and decreased ST-T wave changes. In some cases that have been reported, there is an apparent reversal of the symptoms of ischemic heart disease in individuals who exercise on a regular basis and restrict their dietary fat consumption. More research is needed in this area, because it is a relatively new concept to consider aerobic training seriously as a viable adjunct to traditional medical therapy in the treatment of ischemic heart disease.[6,14,16,23,42,43,51,71,79–81]

SUMMARY

This chapter has presented the major physiologic adaptations made by the body in response to acute and chronic bouts of aerobic exercise. During an acute bout of activity, the heart rate rises in proportion to the intensity of the work load. Cardiac output, dilation of coronary arteries, and blood pressure all increase to allow for increased coronary blood flow. Because coronary circulation occurs during diastole of the cardiac cycle, cardiopulmonary and/or older patients should be exercised at relatively low heart rates to allow for adequate coronary perfusion.

Blood flow during exercise is shunted (directed away) from less active tissues to the more active muscle tissues in which there is also dilation of the blood vessels. Increased rate and depth of ventilation and increased cellular metabolism also occur. The hypothalamus responds to increased heat production by stimulating the sweat glands to increase their output so that evaporation of sweat can promote the cooling process.

Exercise involving the arms and isometric activities should be used with caution in cardiopulmonary patients owing to the dramatic increases in systolic blood pressure that may result. Rehabilitation programs should emphasize aerobic activities that use the larger leg muscles (walking, jogging, and cycling).

In response to chronic bouts of aerobic exercise, cardiac muscle fibers hypertrophy and become stronger. This results in a greater stroke volume and an increase in recovery heart rate. The bradycardia that also results from training seems to be a major factor in raising the angina threshold. It remains to be clearly demonstrated whether increased collateral circulation occurs.

Skeletal muscle capillarization and the number and size of skeletal muscle mitochondria all increase in response to aerobic training. As a result, there is better O_2 delivery and utilization with less lactic acid concentration in the working muscles, and the work load on the heart is reduced. Beneficial effects of aerobic training on both systolic and diastolic blood pressures and better adjustments to high temperatures have been reported.

Aerobic exercise has been found to be very effective in helping individuals control body weight and in increasing the HDL cholesterol levels of the blood. It has also been proved beneficial to persons who are subjected to stress and similar tensions. Chronic aerobic activity has been found to raise the ischemic threshold, decrease catecholamine production, increase coronary perfusion, increase work capacity, decrease peripheral resistance, and decrease ST-T wave ECG changes. It has also been reported that regular aerobic activity can prevent or reverse the symptoms of CHD when combined with dietary and other risk factor modifications and lifestyle changes.

REFERENCES

1. Blomquist, CG: Upper extremity exercise testing and training. In NK Wenger (ed): Exercise and the Heart, ed 2. FA Davis, Philadelphia, 1985.
2. Pendergast, DR: Cardiovascular, respiratory and metabolic responses to upper body exercise. Med Sci Sports Exerc (Suppl)21(5):121–125, 1989.
3. Miles, DS, Cox, MH and Bomze, JP: Cardiovascular responses to upper body exercise in normals and cardiac patients. Med Sci Sports Exerc (Suppl)21(5):126–131, 1989.
4. Astrand, P and Rodahl, K: Textbook of Work Physiology, ed 3. McGraw-Hill, New York, 1986, pp 178–473.
5. deVries, HA: Physiology of Exercise, ed 4. Wm C Brown Group, Dubuque, IA, 1986, pp 113–514.
6. Smith, JJ and Kampine, JP: Circulatory Physiology, ed 3. Williams & Wilkins, Baltimore, 1990, pp 236–276.
7. Strasser, AL: Heart ailments and workplace stress mistakenly called occupational diseases. Occupat Health Safety 54(9):59, 1985.
8. Zamfirescu, NR, et al: Modifications cardiovasculaires determinees par l' effort isometrique (handgrip): Chez Les Malades avec Hypertension Arterielle. Physiol 22(3):197–202, 1985.
9. Goldberg, AP: Aerobic and resistive exercise modify risk factors for coronary heart disease. Med Sci Sports Exerc 21(6):669–674, 1989.
10. Berman, LB and Sutton, JR: Exercise for the pulmonary patient. J Pulmonary Rehabil 6:52–61, 1986.
11. Dehn, MM: Rehabilitation of the cardiac patient: The effects of exercise. Am J Nurs 80:435, 1980.
12. Dehn, MM and Mitchell, JH: Exercise. In The American Heart Association Heartbook. EP Dutton, New York, 1980.
13. Ferguson, RJ, et al: Coronary blood flow during isometric and dynamic exercise in angina pectoris patients. J Cardiac Rehabil 1:21, 1981.
14. Hammond, HK: Exercise for coronary heart disease patients: Is it worth the effort? J Cardiopulmonary Rehabil 5:531–539, 1985.
15. Taylor, JL, et al: The effect of isometric exercise on the graded exercise test in patients with stable angina pectoris. J Cardiac Rehabil 1:450, 1981.
16. Fletcher, GF and Cantwell, JD: Exercise and Coronary Heart Disease, ed 2. Charles C Thomas, Springfield, IL, 1979, pp 11–60.
17. Schlant, RC and Sonnenblick, EH: Normal physiology of the cardiovascular system. In JW Hurst (ed): The Heart, ed 6. McGraw-Hill, New York, 1986.
18. McGandy, RB and Remmell, PS: The dietary management of coronary heart disease. In AN Brest (ed): Coronary Heart Disease. FA Davis, Philadelphia, 1969.
19. Franklin, BA, et al: Exercise prescription for the myocardial infarction patient. J Cardiopulmonary Rehabil 6:62–79, 1986.
20. Getchell, LH: Exercise prescription for the healthy adult. J Cardiopulmonary Rehabil 6:46–51, 1986.
21. Belman, MJ: Exercise in chronic obstructive lung disease. Clin Chest Med 7:585–597, 1986.
22. Wyka, KA: Cardiopulmonary rehabilitation. In LS Craig et al (eds): Egan's Fundamentals of Respiratory Care. CV Mosby, St. Louis, 1990, pp 899–907.
23. Hammond, HK: Regression of atherosclerosis: A review. J Cardiac Rehabil 3:347, 1983.
24. Auchincloss, JH, et al: Cardiac output reserve at exercise. J Cardiopulmonary Rehabil 5:468–473, 1985.
25. Doyle, JT: The prevention of coronary heart disease. In AN Brest (ed): Coronary Heart Disease. FA Davis, Philadelphia, 1969.

26. Ferguson, RJ, et al: Effects of physical training on treadmill exercise capacity, collateral circulation and progression of coronary disease. Am J Cardiol 34:764, 1974.
27. Kattus, AA and McAlpin, RN: Role of exercise in discovery, evaluation and management of ischemic heart disease. In AN Brest (ed): Coronary Heart Disease. FA Davis, Philadelphia, 1969.
28. Miettinen, TA, et al: Multifactorial primary prevention of cardiovascular disease in middle-aged men. JAMA 254:2097–2102, 1985.
29. Hagan, RD, et al: The problems of per-surface area and per-weight standardization indices in the determination of cardiac hypertrophy in endurance-trained athletes. J Cardiopulmonary Rehabil 5:554–560, 1985.
30. Nitzberg, WD, et al: Collateral flow in patients with acute myocardial infarction. Am J Cardiol 56(12):729–736, 1985.
31. Connor, JF, et al: Effects of exercise on coronary collateralization: Angiographic studies of six patients in a supervised exercise program. Med Sci Sports Exerc 8:145, 1976.
32. Andersen, KL, et al: Habitual Physical Activity and Health. World Health Organization, Copenhagen, 1978, p 186.
33. Froelicher, VF: Exercise Testing and Training. Le Jacq, New York, 1983, p 180.
34. Schaper, W and Pasyk, S: Influence of collateral flow on the ischemic tolerance of the heart following acute and subacute coronary occlusion. Circulation (Suppl)53(1):57, 1976.
35. Scheel, KW: The stimulus for coronary collateral growth: Ischemia or mechanical factors? J Cardiac Rehabil 1:149, 1981.
36. Ornish, D, et al: Can lifestyle changes reverse coronary heart disease? Lancet, 336:129–133, 1990.
37. Belman, MJ and Mittman, C: Ventilatory muscle training improves exercise capacity in chronic obstructive pulmonary disease patients. Am Rev Respir Dis 121:273–280, 1980.
38. Rothman, JG: Effects of respiratory exercise on the vital capacity and forced expiratory volume in children with cerebral palsy. Phys Ther 58:421–425, 1978.
39. Keens, TG, et al: Ventilatory muscle endurance training in normal subjects and patients with cystic fibrosis. Am Rev Respir Dis 116:853–860, 1977.
40. Merrick, J and Axen, K: Inspiratory muscle function following abdomen weight exercises in healthy subjects. Phys Ther 61:651–656, 1981.
41. Aaron, DJ: The effects of a 12-week exercise program on the functional capacities, cardiovascular responses and body weights of individuals medicated with beta-blockers. Slippery Rock University, Slippery Rock, PA, 1985. Unpublished thesis.
42. Barnard, JR, et al: Effects of an intensive, short-term exercise and nutrition program on patients with coronary heart disease. J Cardiac Rehabil 1:99, 1981.
43. Hall, JA and Barnard, RJ: The effects of an intensive 26-day program of diet and exercise on patients with peripheral vascular disease. J Cardiac Rehabil 2:569, 1982.
44. Hoglund, JL: The effects of a 12-week cardiovascular exercise program on the resting blood pressure, body weight and resting heart rate levels of hypertensive individuals. Slippery Rock University, Slippery Rock, PA, 1984. Unpublished thesis.
45. McHenry, D: The effects of a twelve-week cardiac rehabilitation program on body composition, heart rate and blood pressure. Slippery Rock University, Slippery Rock, PA, 1981. Unpublished thesis.
46. Gilders, RM, Voner, C and Dudley, GA: Endurance training and blood pressure in normotensive and hypertensive adults. Med Sci Sports Exerc 21(6):629–636, 1989.
47. Leon, AS, et al: Scientific evidence of the value of cardiac rehabilitation services with emphasis on patients following myocardial infarction. Section 1. Exercise conditioning component. J Cardiopulmonary Rehabil 10(3):79–87, 1990.
48. Brannon, FJ and Geyer, MJ: Fitness after fifty-five. Bio-Energetiks Rehabilitation, Prospect, PA, 1980. Unpublished study.
49. Lamb, DR: Physiology of Exercise, ed 2. Macmillan, New York, 1984, p 160.
50. Froelicher, VF and Brown, P: Exercise and coronary heart disease. J Cardiac Rehabil 1:277, 1981.
51. Taylor, HL: Results of physical conditioning in healthy middle-aged subjects. In LS Cohen et al (eds): Physical Conditioning and Cardiovascular Rehabilitation. John Wiley & Sons, New York, 1981.
52. Williams, RS, Scott, E and Andersen, J: Reduced epinephrine induced platelet aggregation following cardiac rehabilitation. J Cardiac Rehabil 1:127, 1981.
53. Miller, NH, et al: The efficacy of risk factor intervention and psychosocial aspects of cardiac rehabilitation. J Cardiopulmonary Rehabil 10(6):198–209, 1990.
54. Bubb, WJ, et al: Predicting oxygen uptake during level 4 walking at speeds of 80–130 m/min. J Cardiopulmonary Rehabil 5:462–465, 1985.
55. Lampman, RM, et al: Exercise as a partial therapy for the extremely obese. Medic Sci Sports Exerc 18:19–24, 1986.
56. Arnold, JD, et al: Lipid profile, physical fitness, and job activity of Canadian postal workers. J Cardiopulmonary Rehabil 5:373–377, 1985.
57. Boyd, GS and Craig, IF: Biochemistry of degenerative vascular disease. In DL Williams and V Marks (eds): Biochemistry in Clinical Practice. Elsevier, New York, 1985.
58. McManus, BM: Defining coronary risks in a reference range for total cholesterol and lipoprotein values: A problem yet to be solved. Am J Cardiol Dec 31, 1985.

59. MacKeen, PC, et al: A 13-year follow-up of a coronary heart disease risk factor screening and exercise program for 40- to 59-year-old men: Exercise habit maintenance and physiologic status. J Cardiopulmonary Rehabil 5:510–523, 1985.

60. Tran, ZV and Brammell, HL: Effects of exercise training on serum lipid and lipoprotein levels in post-MI patients: A meta-analysis. J Cardiopulmonary Rehabil 9(6):250–255, 1989.

61. Palank, EA and Hargreaves, EH: The benefits of walking the golf course. Phys and Sportsmed 18(10):77–80, 1990.

62. Allison, TG, et al: Failure of exercise to increase high density lipoprotein cholesterol. J Cardiac Rehabil 1:257, 1981.

63. Hagan, RD and Gettman, LR: Maximal aerobic power, body fat, and serum lipoproteins in male distance runners. J Cardiac Rehabil 3:331, 1983.

64. Haskell, WL: Influence of habitual physical activity on blood lipids and lipoproteins. In LS Cohen, et al (eds.): Physical Conditioning and Cardiovascular Rehabilitation. John Wiley & Sons, New York, 1981.

65. Rotkis, TC, et al: Relationship between high density lipoprotein cholesterol and weekly running mileage. J Cardiac Rehabil 2:109, 1982.

66. Byrne, DG, et al: Consistency and variation among instruments purporting to measure the type A behavior pattern. Psychosomatic Med 47:242–261, 1985.

67. Dembroski, TM, et al: Components of type A: Hostility and anger in relationship to angiographic findings. Psychosomatic Med 47:219–233, 1985.

68. Velasco, JA, et al: Rehabilitation after myocardial infarction: Prognostic features and psychosocial considerations. J Cardiopulmonary Rehabil 5:427–428, 1985.

69. Williams, RB and Gentry, WD: Psychological problems in the cardiopathic state. In C Long (ed): Prevention and Rehabilitation in Ischemic Heart Disease. Williams & Wilkins, Baltimore, 1980.

70. Adler, HM and Hammett, VBO: The psychosomatics of coronary heart disease. In AN Brest (ed): Coronary Heart Disease. FA Davis, Philadelphia, 1969.

71. Shephard, RJ, et al: Mood state during postcoronary cardiac rehabilitation. J Cardiopulmonary Rehabil 5:480–484, 1985.

72. Blocher, WP: Coronary risk factors. In WP Blocher and D Cardus (eds): Rehabilitation in Ischemic Heart Disease. SP Medical and Scientific, New York, 1983.

73. Leon, GR: Behavior modification in reducing risk factors for ischemic heart disease. In C Long (ed): Prevention and Rehabilitation in Ischemic Heart Disease. Williams & Wilkins, Baltimore, 1980.

74. Willerson, JT, Hillis, LD and Buja, LM: Ischemic Heart Disease. Raven Press, New York, 1982.

75. Dracup, K: A controlled trial of couples group counseling in cardiac rehabilitation. J Cardiopulmonary Rehabil 5:436–442, 1985.

76. Goldwater, BC and Collis, ML: Psychologic effects of cardiovascular conditioning. Psychosomatic Med 47:174–181, 1985.

77. Roth, DL and Holmes, DS: Influence of physical fitness in determining the impact of stressful life events on physical and psychological health. Psychosomatic Med 47:164–173, 1985.

78. Tortora, GJ: Principles of Human Anatomy, ed 5. Harper & Row, New York, 1989, p 362.

79. Dressendoifer, RH, Amsterdam, EA and Mason, DT: Therapeutic effects of exercise training in angina patients. In LS Cohen, et al (eds): Physical Conditioning and Cardiovascular Rehabilitation. John Wiley & Sons, New York, 1981.

80. Levenkron, JC, et al: Chronic chest pain with normal coronary arteries: A behavioral approach to rehabilitation. J Cardiopulmonary Rehabil 5:475–479, 1985.

81. LeMura, LM, et al: Central versus peripheral adaptations for the enhancement of functional capacity in cardiac patients: A meta-analytic review. J Cardiopulmonary Rehabil 10(6):217–223, 1990.

CHAPTER 5

Pathophysiology of Coronary Artery Disease

The American Heart Association estimated that, in 1987, 513,700 individuals died in the United States from coronary heart disease (CHD) and approximately 67 million others (or one of every four Americans) suffer from some form of cardiovascular disease. In 1992, about 1.5 million Americans will have a heart attack and 500,000 of those individuals will die. Although the overall incidence of mortality as a result of coronary artery disease (CAD) declined 28.7 percent from 1977 to 1987, the disease remains the number one cause of sudden death in adults.[1,2]

CAD is an atherosclerotic process that manifests itself in one or more of four clinical syndromes: angina pectoris, myocardial infarction, heart failure, or sudden death. Beginning as early as the second decade of life, atherosclerosis may affect any arterial system in the body, with the most common sites being the aorta, coronary arteries, and cerebral, femoral, and other large to middle-size arteries.[3,4] This disease is characterized by a thickening in the intimal layer of the blood vessel wall owing to the localized accumulation of lipids.

The actual pathogenesis of atherosclerosis remains unknown at this time. Establishing cause and effect has been difficult because the disease begins and progresses insidiously; it exists from months to years prior to the onset of symptoms.[4] Past and current research have closely tied the development of atherosclerotic plaque to a group of coronary risk factors. As discussed in Chapter 13, risk factors are certain characteristics that, through systematic observation and clinical study, have been shown to have a significant relation between their presence and the subsequent development of CAD.[6] The major risk factors are high blood pressure, hyperlipidemia, and cigarette smoking. Risk factors are classified as either modifiable (smoking, blood lipid levels, obesity, inactivity, stress) or nonmodifiable (age, sex, family history of CAD, previous medical history). The presence of more than one risk factor has a synergistic effect on the other risk factors in predicting an individual's risk of CAD.[6]

This chapter reviews the pathophysiology of CAD, beginning with the normal arterial wall structure, and describes the changes that occur with atherosclerosis. The hypothesized pathogenesis of atherosclerosis is briefly reviewed, but most of the chapter is devoted to the clinical manifestations of CAD.

THE ARTERIAL WALL

The normal arterial wall is a smooth muscular wall made up of three distinct layers of tissue: the intima, media, and adventitia. The wall and the individual layers vary in thickness depending on the caliber of the vessel (the larger the inner diameter, the thicker the arterial wall). The layers become progressively less distinct as the vessels reach the level of the arteriole (Fig. 5–1).[8,9]

The intima is a single layer of endothelial cells lining the vascular lumen. It is impermeable to proteins circulating in the blood and is separated from the second layer, the media, by a continuous boundary of elastic fiber known as the internal elastic lamina. The media constitutes the bulk of the arterial wall and is composed almost entirely of smooth muscle cells interspersed with collagen, elastin fibers, and proteoglycans. The media makes the dilation and contraction of the vessel wall possible. The outer layer, the adventitia, is separated from the media by noncontinuous elastin fiber boundary called the external elastic lamina. The adventitia consists primarily of fibrous tissue that gives the arterial wall strength and at the same time provides for some distensibility to prevent rupture in the presence of hypertension.[7]

ATHEROSCLEROTIC LESIONS

Atherosclerosis is a progressive disease with the lesions (or plaque) going through what is hypothesized to be a series of changes that alter both arterial structure and functional capacity.[12,13] The intimal layer of the vessel wall is primarily affected by the atherosclerotic degeneration. The media undergoes some secondary changes as the atheromatous plaque extends into it, weakens the wall, and possibly causes localized dilation or aneurysm formation.[3] These lesions are classified into three morphologic types: fatty streak, fibrous plaque, and complicated plaque or lesion.

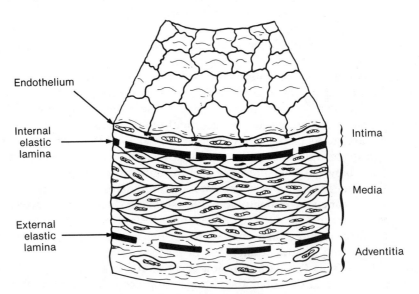

FIGURE 5–1. Structure of normal muscular artery. (Reproduced by permission of the New England Journal of Medicine 294:370, 1976.)

Fatty Streak

The atherosclerotic process begins as a recognizable fatty streak in the intima of the blood vessel. The lesion does not impinge on the lumen of the artery. There are no symptoms at this time. Fatty streaks have been found throughout the arterial tree in individuals from infancy through late adulthood. They most commonly involve the aorta, coronary and cerebral arteries, and the arteries of the lower extremities.[3] Microscopically, these intimal lesions consist of smooth muscle cells with varying proportions of lipid material and fat droplets. They are commonly referred to as "foam cells" because of their tendency to "balloon out."

The lipids are composed mainly of cholesterol, cholesterol ester, phospholipid, and neutral fat. Because of the predominantly fatty content, they are often soft and yellow in appearance.[14] It remains controversial as to whether this lesion progresses to a raised fibrous lesion or is reversible.[8]

Raised Fibrous Plaque

Raised fibrous plaque is the characteristic lesion of atherosclerosis. It is a yellowish-gray elevated lump that thickens and begins to impinge on the lumen of the vessel. As the plaque develops, muscle cells from the intima and media proliferate, and lipids are deposited from the plasma into the lesions. A matrix of collagen, elastin, and connective tissue cells surrounds the plaque and gives it a fibrous cap.[3,9] The central core of the plaque remains mainly a lipid material with various plasma components including white blood cells, albumin, fibrin, fibrinogen, and cellular debris. Although most pathologists believe this plaque is irreversible, some do feel that its progression may be slowed by the appropriate lifestyle modifications.[3,12]

Complicated Plaques

Complicated plaque is a fibrous plaque that has undergone one or more of the following pathologic changes: calcification, necrosis, internal hemorrhage, rupture of the plaque, or thrombus formation over the plaque. The lumen of the vessel is impinged on by these plaques, and the individual may often demonstrate symptoms of decreased or inadequate blood flow in the organ fed by the affected arteries. These structural changes in the intima may progress to affect the medial layer of the wall. Degeneration of a medial muscular layer further affects the arteries' ability to distend and meet the oxygen demand of the cells.[10] The weakened arterial wall may permit localized arterial dilation or ballooning out, that is, an aneurysm, which may rupture and cause hemorrhage. Other complications arise if the plaque has broken through the intima and comes in contact with the flowing blood. The rough surface of the complicated plaque provides a site for platelet aggregation, fibrin deposition, and clot formation. The clot further impinges on the vessel's lumen and may either completely occlude the artery or embolize to occlude a more distal, smaller vessel and cause ischemia. Ischemia is a supply of oxygen to the myocardium that is inadequate to meet metabolic demands. It is due to a functional constriction or actual obstruction of the coronary artery. If ischemia is prolonged, infarction of the adjacent muscle may occur.[15]

All three types of lesions may be present at the same time at various sites in the arterial tree. Unaffected segments may be interspersed with diseased segments.[16] Post-mortem studies indicate that when the coronary arteries are affected, the majority of lesions occur at proximal points in the three major coronary arteries at the points of bifurcation of the arteries.[18] Symptoms in coronary patients usually correlate with lesions that occlude 70 percent of the coronary arterial lumen.[11]

PATHOGENESIS OF ATHEROSCLEROSIS

Although the pathogenesis of atherosclerosis is unknown, there are six accepted hypotheses: response to injury, monoclonal, clonal-senescence, lipid-insudation, thrombogenic, and hemodynamic. Some factors of these hypotheses are interchangeable and have been combined with one another through years of speculation and research. Two hypotheses currently predominate: the response-to-injury and monoclonal hypotheses. They are briefly discussed here, but the reader is referred to other sources for further explanation of these and the remaining four hypotheses.[4,5,12,13,17]

Response-to-Injury Hypothesis

According to the response-to-injury hypothesis, plaque formation begins in response to some type of trauma to the endothelial lining of the vessel wall. The damage may result from any one of a number of mechanical, chemical, hormonal, or immunologic stressors. The turbulence of arterial blood flow in an individual with hypertension, the hydrocarbons from cigarette smoke, and circulating plasma cholesterol have all been hypothesized as causative agents.[14,17] The damaged endothelium then becomes permeable to substances in the blood and provides a site for platelet aggregation. As the platelets aggregate, they release substances that may interact with plasma constituents and cause a proliferation of smooth muscle cells into the intima, forming new connective tissue. Also in response to the injury, the endothelial cells proliferate to repair the damage. Ross and Glosmet[12,13] proposed that, in limited injury, the regeneration of the endothelial layer may limit the smooth muscle proliferation. However, in repeated injury, this relationship may be thrown out of balance, and continual proliferation of smooth muscle and connective tissue cells and additional lipid deposition into the intima may result. The final result is the "growth" of fibrous plaques within the intimal layer of the arterial wall.[4,12]

Monoclonal Hypothesis

The monoclonal hypothesis suggests that each lesion is a result of the proliferation of one smooth muscle cell that has acquired a selective advantage. Benditt[14] suggests that this is a result of some mutagenic agent such as cigarette smoke or a virus. Microscopically, however, neither fibrous plaques nor fatty streaks are of one type of cell origin, which raises serious questions as to the validity of the hypothesis.[4,14]

ATHEROSCLEROSIS AND CORONARY ARTERY DISEASE

Atherosclerosis is a disease that affects people in the middle-to-older age brackets. Although the initial lesion has been isolated in infants, the onset of symptoms is usually in the fourth to fifth decade of life for men and approximately ten years later in women.[15] Although atherosclerotic changes and plaque formation can occur in any artery, this text is specifically concerned with its effect on the coronary arteries and the clinical manifestations of atherosclerosis in CAD.

As CAD progresses, the atherosclerotic lesions develop in the intima of the coronary arteries. As the lesions grow, they thicken and harden the walls of the artery, reduce arterial wall elasticity, and impinge on the lumen of the vessel. These structural changes in the wall result in a decrease in coronary artery blood flow and a decrease in oxygen distribution to the myocardium.

With the coronary circulation compromised and the arteries inelastic, the normal adaptive mechanism (local dilation of the coronary arteries) to increase blood flow through the coronary arteries in response to increasing oxygen requirements is diminished. As the lesions progressively occlude the vessels' lumen and without adequate collateral circulation to provide blood flow to the area, the demands of the heart cannot be met. This causes an ischemic episode (an inadequate supply of oxygenated blood to the muscle) to occur.

Initially, individuals with CAD may be asymptomatic, but as the atherosclerotic lesions progress, the individual becomes symptomatic. Although symptomatology and the progress of the atherosclerotic disease process vary tremendously from one individual to the next, the functional inability of the artery to supply oxygenated blood remains the same. The resulting imbalance in myocardial oxygen demand versus supply is known as ischemia.

Ischemia and Infarction

Ischemia occurs when blood flow to the cell is insufficient to meet cellular needs. Ischemia may be the result of some obstruction to blood flow, an increased metabolic demand that the heart is unable to meet, inadequate hemoglobin content in the blood, or pulmonary disease. The duration and severity of ischemic imbalance determine the pathologic injury to the involved tissue. Transient ischemia is completely reversible. The ischemic tissues do not sustain any permanent damage.[8] When ischemia is prolonged, the tissues undergo a series of changes, including a shift from aerobic to anaerobic metabolism. Prolonged ischemia may ultimately result in irreversible injury or infarction.[9]

Manifestations of ischemia and infarction include pain, elevated serum enzymes (enzymes that are released by the damaged cells into the circulation), and symptoms related to the function of the affected organ or tissues (decreased renal function with renal ischemia; intermittent claudication or muscle cramps with peripheral ischemia). Chronic ischemia may produce a dull pain, whereas acute occlusion causes an intense pain often followed by numbness or absence of sensation. The mechanism of ischemic pain is not fully understood, and it may be a result of one of two phenomena. The peripheral nerve endings may be stretched and stimulated by swelling of the cell caused by the ischemia, or the nerve endings may be stimulated by the localized release of kinins and other chemical mediators that result in the pain sensation.[9]

The transition from ischemia to infarction is not inevitable. Several factors determine whether or not infarction will result. The factors include the rate of onset of the ischemia, the ability of the ischemic tissue to compensate for decreased blood flow, the oxygen requirements of the particular tissue, and the availability of oxygen in the blood.[22] Ischemia that has developed gradually is usually better tolerated because collateral circulation (communicating channels that serve as an alternate pathway to blood flow) may develop and supply the otherwise ischemic areas. Tissues also compensate for decreased oxygen supply by increasing their oxygen extraction from whatever blood flow is available. The heart is unable to compensate in that manner because at rest the heart muscle extracts 65 to 70 percent of the available oxygen, leaving little for reserve in response to decreased blood flow or increased oxygen demand.[9] The overall oxygen requirement of the affected tissue also determines the tissue's vulnerability to infarction. Some tissues, like those in the brain, are very sensitive to decreased oxygen supply; skeletal muscle, on the other hand, has a longer survival time in the presence of decreased oxygen. Finally, the quality of the individual's blood influences the ischemia-to-infarction progression. Anemia, decreased oxygen-carrying capacity, and decreased oxygen diffusion into the blood all reduce potential oxygen availability to the tissue and increase vulnerability to infarction.[22]

Infarction, or cellular death, is identified as a central core of necrotic cells that are electrically and functionally silent. Surrounding this core are cells with gradations of function dependent on the severity of the ischemia to the surrounding area.[20]

Treatment is aimed at reversing the ischemia and preventing further infarction by promoting oxygen supply to the affected area. This is achieved by removing any physical impedance to blood flow and removing any stimulus that may increase metabolic demands to the tissue. Oxygen and pharmacologic agents may be used, as appropriate, to relieve ischemia. If the individual is anemic, transfusion of red blood cells may be necessary to provide sufficient hemoglobin to transport oxygen adequately.

Despite all interventions, cell necrosis may still result. When cells die, they release enzymes that promote cellular destruction and the inflammatory response. Cellular debris is removed via phagocytosis, and the tissues undergo a series of changes ending in the formation of fibrous scar tissue.

Myocardial Ischemia and Infarction

Ischemia occurs when the oxygen demand of a tissue exceeds the oxygen supply. Myocardial ischemia results when an inadequate amount of oxygen is supplied to the heart.

The myocardial oxygen demand (MVO_2) is determined by the heart rate, the myocardial contractility, and the ventricular wall tension.[4,21] The heart rate is the frequency at which the heart pumps. The faster the heart rate, the greater the demand for oxygen. The myocardial contractility is the actual mechanical work of the heart. The work load is determined by the oxygen demands of the tissues. The heavier the work load, the harder the pump has to work and the greater its own demand for oxygen. Ventricular wall tension is directly influenced by preload (the ventricular volume or filling pressure) and afterload (the resistance, primarily the systemic blood pressure, against which the ventricle must pump to expel the blood). As the work load increases, the ventricular wall tension also increases, resulting in an increased myocardial oxygen demand.

The supply of oxygen to the myocardium depends on many factors, including the integrity of the pulmonary system, the hemoglobin content of the blood, the health of the coronary arteries, the heart rate, the blood pressure, and the resistance of the coronary arteries.[4,5,21,25]

An intact pulmonary system ensures that oxygen will diffuse from the lungs into the blood, where it is bound to the hemoglobin and carried to the tissues. If the hemoglobin level is low (anemia), the oxygen-carrying capacity is reduced.

The health of the coronary arteries refers to their ability to dilate in response to demand. In exercise they may need to carry four to five times their normal capacity. Coronary atherosclerosis not only impairs vessels' ability to dilate but also affects redistribution of blood and oxygen within the heart.

Since the myocardium is perfused during diastole, the heart rate is a factor in myocardial oxygen supply and demand. The faster the heart rate, the shorter the period of time for perfusion during diastole (Chapter 2) and the greater the myocardial demand.

Hypotension (low blood pressure) inhibits adequate coronary artery perfusion. Hypertension (high blood pressure) affects the ventricular wall tension by increasing the afterload against which the heart must pump (increasing oxygen demand).

Resistance within the coronary circulation depends on the ventricular wall pressure. During systole, the ventricular wall pressure collapses the coronary arterial walls and occludes the blood flow to the myocardium (Chapter 2). The greatest external wall pressure is on the subendocardial vessels, making the subendocardium particularly vulnerable to ischemia.[5,20,21]

The six factors previously discussed emphasize the interrelatedness of myocardial oxygen demand and supply. The heart's initial response to increased demand (increased heart rate) increases the oxygen supply as well as further increasing the oxygen demand. If the demand continues to exceed the supply, a vicious cycle is established.

When the oxygen demand is increased sixfold to eightfold, the healthy heart responds by increasing the coronary artery flow four to five times its normal level and by increasing its oxygen extraction to make up for the relative deficiency.[5] In a heart with CAD, the diseased vessels are not able to dilate to provide an increased blood flow and therefore the muscle supplied by the stenotic artery becomes ischemic.

CORONARY ARTERY DISEASE: CLINICAL MANIFESTATIONS

CAD is manifested in any of four clinical syndromes: angina, myocardial infarction, sudden cardiac death, and congestive heart failure.[7] To varying degrees, the manifestations are the results of the ischemia-infarction process on the myocardial muscle, which is extremely sensitive to decreased oxygen supply, particularly in the presence of coronary atherosclerosis.

Angina Pectoris

Angina pectoris (literally "strangling of the chest") is a reversible ischemic process caused by a temporary inability of the coronary arteries to supply sufficient oxygenated blood to the heart muscle. There are three basic categories of angina: stable angina, unstable angina, and variant or Prinzmetal's angina. All are results of ischemia to the myocardium and, except for variant angina, occur secondarily to the arterial changes brought on by CAD.[6,28,29] All three are characterized by the sudden onset of anterior chest pain that is relatively diffuse. The pain is usually described as a "squeezing" or pressure sensation. It can also manifest itself as burning in the throat or jaw, discomfort between the shoulder blades, shortness of breath, or many other, equivalent symptoms. The three types of angina differ in their duration intensity, pattern of occurrence, and precipitating factors.

STABLE ANGINA

Stable angina is known as effort angina in that it is most often precipitated by exercise or stress. Individuals who experience stable angina quickly become aware of the specific activities that bring on the pain. Some of the most common precipitating events are exercise (particularly after a large meal), emotional stress, cigarette smoking, and exposure to low temperatures.[23,28] The angina "attack" is characterized by substernal chest pain or pressure that may or may not radiate. The duration of pain is 5 to 10 minutes. Cessation of the activity is often sufficient to relieve the pain; otherwise, rest and sublingual nitrates completely relieve the angina.[7] In stable angina, the episodes of pain are very similar in cause, character, and method of relief.[23,27] Angina brought on by emotional stress may be more difficult to relieve because the stressor itself is more difficult to eliminate.[28]

UNSTABLE ANGINA

Unstable angina also is effort-related, but the episodes of pain occur with increased frequency, intensity, and duration. Angina pectoris at rest that occurs for the first time and is present less than 60 days and effort angina that occurs with an accelerated change in pattern may also be defined as unstable angina. It is also known as crescendo or preinfarction angina. Crescendo angina may indicate progressive CAD and an increased risk of impending myocardial infarction.[21,23] These patients are likely to have a mixture of severe, fixed disease (CAD) and coronary spasm.[7]

The symptoms are less responsive to rest and nitrates. Individuals may require hospitalization for rest and treatment with intravenous nitrates to prevent the myocardial ischemia from progressing to myocardial infarction. Unstable angina is a transient phase because it either progresses to a myocardial infarction or stabilizes because the individual develops collateral circulation[5,18] or receives appropriate medical intervention.[28]

PRINZMETAL/VARIANT ANGINA

Prinzmetal/variant angina, commonly known as rest angina, is caused by coronary artery spasm.[27,28,30] The pain often occurs while the individual is at rest and most frequently in the early morning or on arising. The anginal episodes are cyclic and often occur at the same time each day. Variant angina is unaffected by exertion, but it may be relieved by rest and nitrates. The pain is usually more intense and of longer duration than in stable angina. Variant angina frequently leads to myocardial infarction.[15,21,27,33] Individuals with variant angina often present with both pain and related complaints of syncope and palpitations. Cardiac arrhythmias occur more frequently during episodes of variant angina than during those of effort angina.[21]

Although variant angina may be seen in individuals without CAD, it is often seen in the presence of significant CAD.[7,27] With the advent of coronary arteriography, actual coronary artery spasm has been visualized and documented. During the cardiac catheterization, coronary artery spasm has been provoked by use of ergonovine, an ergot alkaloid that exerts a strong vasoconstricting effect on the coronary vascular system. The spasm of variant angina has been successfully relieved by use of nifedipine, a calcium channel blocker.

DIAGNOSIS AND TREATMENT

The frequency and characteristics of angina attacks vary. The attacks may depend on the degree of coronary insufficiency, the collateral circulation, the response to treatment, and the physical and emotional characteristics of the individual.[18,23] Angina provoked by emotional stress may last longer than episodes brought on by physical activity.

In CAD, the degree of stenosis (structural change) does not always correlate well with the functional impact of the disease because of individual variations in oxygen demand and work load tolerance. Predicting the extent of the coronary artery disease based on the anginal symptoms alone is difficult.

The diagnosis of angina is usually by history alone, because anginal episodes do not usually occur during the physical examination.[7,28] If the individual is examined during an episode of pain, tachycardia and hypertension will be found. During auscultation of the heart, an S_3 or S_4 gallop or a mitral murmur may be heard. These sounds may be secondary to ischemia of the papillary muscle.[21,28] ECG findings during episodes of pain reveal ST-segment elevation in variant angina and ST depression in unstable angina.[21] Exercise tolerance tests and cardiac radionuclide imaging may reveal areas of decreased perfusion. Cardiac catheterization provides a means of definitive diagnosis and treatment. The procedure enables the physician to visualize and evaluate atypical chest pain, coronary anatomy, left ventricular function, and postmyocardial infarction (MI) damage and function. Cardiac catheterization is also the means by which electrophysiologic studies of the cardiac conduction system are done. Direct intracoronary antithrombolytic therapy (streptokinase, urokinase, tPA) and percutaneous transluminal angioplasty (PTCA) are two of the ways catheterization is used as part of the treatment of acute MI. Both therapies are aimed at reperfusion of the ischemic area in an attempt to minimize the damage to the heart muscle.

The treatment of angina (discussed in Chapter 7) is directed toward relieving symptoms and arresting the progress of the disease with medications, surgical procedures, and appropriate lifestyle modifications. Chronic effort angina is treated pharmacologically with beta-blockers, nitrates, and calcium channel blockers, specifically nifedipine. Beta-blockers relieve angina by directly lowering myocardial oxygen demand, but they may aggravate coronary spasm and therefore should be avoided in individuals with rest/variant angina. Nitrates and calcium channel blockers are the drugs of choice in treating variant angina.[7]

Myocardial Infarction

MI, the second manifestation of CAD, is the death or necrosis of some portion of the cardiac muscle secondary to sustained myocardial ischemia. Reduced coronary artery blood flow is most often caused by acute occlusion of coronary arteries at the site where atherosclerotic plaques have significantly compromised the coronary circulation. The acute occlusions may be the result of a coronary artery thrombus or a coronary artery spasm.[5,7] Decreased blood flow associated with hemorrhage or profound shock (hypovolemia) also may result in infarction.

Because the underlying pathologies of angina and MI are similar, the initial clinical presentations may also be similar. The classic presenting symptom of MI is "viselike" retrosternal tightening of the chest. The tightening becomes progressively intense over a period of hours to days until the pain becomes absolutely unbearable. The pain typically radiates to any number of areas, the most common of which are the jaw, upper back, and down the inner aspects of both arms. The pain of the myocardial infarction usually begins at rest and is unrelieved by nitrates, rest, or any other method the individual typically uses to relieve anginal pain.[34]

ASSESSMENT AND DIAGNOSIS

The medical diagnosis of MI is based on the individual's history, current symptoms, serum enzymes, and electrocardiographic (ECG) changes. Positive findings in any two of these three diagnostic parameters are unequivocal evidence of MI.[7,24] However, because of the vulnerability of the myocardium, even suspect MIs are treated as MIs until the diagnosis is ruled out.

HISTORY AND CURRENT SYMPTOMS

Patients with suspect MIs often have histories of angina pectoris. However, a considerable number of patients experience an acute infarct as the first indication of cardiovascular problems.[18,27] Other individuals, about 15 percent of those who have MIs, may experience no discomfort at all ("silent MI").[18,28,29]

The typical patient presents with complaints of severe substernal pressure or pain. He or she may appear to be in acute distress: dyspneic, diaphoretic, with pale, cool, and clammy skin and associated complaints of nausea and vomiting. Extreme weakness and an overwhelming feeling of impending doom may also be expressed.

On examination, an S_3 gallop, indicating decreased compliance of the myocardium, or a mitral murmur, indicating an ischemic papillary muscle, may be auscultated. The blood pressure may be elevated (partially in response to the pain) or may be very low, if the left ventricular function is severely compromised, resulting in a decreased cardiac output. The pulse may be very rapid and feeble. Arrhythmias are very common. They may include premature ventricular contractions, atrial fibrillation or flutter, conduction blocks, ventricular tachycardia, and fibrillation.

There are two particularly vulnerable periods when fibrillation is most likely to occur: within the first 10 minutes following the infarction and during a second period of cardiac irritability beginning 3 to 5 hours after the infarct and lasting for several days. Multiple arrhythmias are often observed.[5]

ELECTROCARDIOGRAPHIC CHANGES

Typical ECG changes are observed in 88 percent of individuals having MIs.[15,29,34] The ECG reflects change in myocardial electrical conduction in the area of the myocardial injury. Ischemia causes the T wave to become enlarged and symmetrically inverted owing to late repolarization. With injury, cells depolarize normally but repolarize more

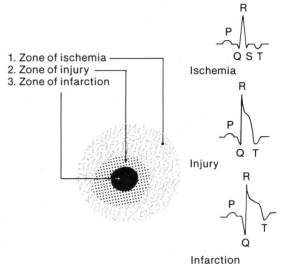

1. Zone of ischemia
2. Zone of injury
3. Zone of infarction

Ischemia

Injury

Infarction

FIGURE 5 – 2. ECG changes of infarction, injury, and ischemia as they correspond to the zones of infarction. (1) Ischemia causes inversion of T wave. (2) Injury causes ST-segment elevation. (3) Infarction causes permanent Q waves. (From Underhill, SL, et al.: Cardiac Nursing. JB Lippincott, Philadelphia, 1983, p. 206, with permission.)

rapidly, resulting in ST-segment elevation. An absence of current flow through the infarcted cells and opposing currents from other parts of the heart cause a permanent Q wave (Fig. 5–2).[35] However, if the infarction is small, an abnormal Q wave may not appear. Approximately 30 percent of abnormal Q waves disappear or revert to border-line significance within 18 months after infarction.[27]

In the MI, the infarcted area is surrounded by a zone of injury, which in turn is surrounded by a zone of ischemia. As the areas of ischemia and injury resolve (usually within 1 to 2 weeks of the MI), the ECG changes associated with them return to normal. The area of infarction is permanent and so therefore is the Q wave most often permanent.[7,35]

SERUM ENZYMES AND ISOENZYMES

Enzymes are groups of proteins found in all cells. The major cardiac enzymes are creatine kinase (CK), lactate dehydrogenase (LDH), and serum glutamic–oxaloacetic transaminase (SGOT). These particular enzymes are found in all cells, but specific forms of them, their isoenzymes, are found only in cardiac cells. With cellular ischemia and death, the enzymes and isoenzymes are released into the serum in a characteristic pattern over the ensuing hours to days following the infarct. Each enzyme has an individual pattern of rise and fall. Serial blood samples can reveal patterns that are diagnostic of acute myocardial infarction (Fig. 5–3).[7,11,26,27] Enzyme elevation patterns may also be indicators of the prognosis following myocardial infarction. Laboratory studies for these specific enzymes (LDH, CK, and SGOT) are sensitive, but they may have a false-positive rate as high as 15 percent.[27] More accurate identification of the enzyme activity indicative of myocardial necrosis can be made from the separation of the total enzyme activity into subunits, isoenzymes. This separation is done by electrophoresis.

CK is found in high concentrations in skeletal muscle, brain, and myocardium, and trauma to any of those tissues will cause an elevation in the total CK. The isoenzymes,

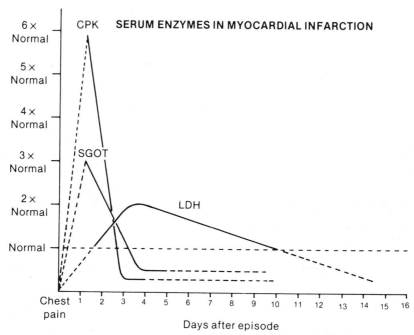

FIGURE 5–3. Serum enzymes in myocardial infarction. (From Vinsant and Spence,[7] p. 185, with permission.)

subunits of CK, are tissue-specific. Therefore, elevations in isoenzymes identify the tissue that has been injured. CK-MM is predominant in skeletal muscle, and CK-BB is predominant in brain tissue. Myocardial tissue is the only human tissue that contains substantial amounts of CK-MB. Elevation in CK-MB is highly specific for myocardial necrosis. The level begins to rise 2 to 4 hours after the infarct, and an increase greater than 5 percent is considered abnormal. Serial CK-MB levels have been correlated with infarct size, arrhythmic complications, and prognosis. CK-MB may also be elevated after cardiac surgery or cardiopulmonary resuscitation and in individuals with muscular dystrophy.[7,27]

LDH can be separated into five separate isoenzymes by electrophoresis. Cardiac tissue is rich in LDH_1 and LDH_2. Normally, LDH_2 activity exceeds LDH_1 activity. Myocardial infarction results in LDH_1 activity exceeding LDH_2 activity, which is referred to as a flipped LDH pattern. Elevated LDH_1 activity is seen within 24 hours and returns to normal in 7 to 10 days. An increase in LDH_1 activity is seen with hemolytic anemias, hemolysis of blood specimens, renal infarction, hyperthyroidism, and cancer of the stomach.

The flipped LDH pattern in combination with at least a 5 percent elevation of CK-MB provides objective evidence of myocardial necrosis.[7,27]

INFARCTION SITES AND MUSCULAR INVOLVEMENT

Myocardial infarcts are identified by their anatomic location and the layers of the myocardium involved. The location is identified by the surface or combination of

TABLE 5-1 Comparison of Right and Left Coronary Distribution

Right Coronary Artery Supplies	Left Coronary Artery Supplies
1. SA node (55%)	1. SA node (45%)
2. AV node	2. Anterosuperior division of left bundle
3. Bundle of His (a portion)	3. Right bundle branch (major portion)
4. Posterior one third of septum	4. Anterior two thirds of septum
5. Posteroinferior division of left bundle (a portion)	5. Posteroinferior division of left bundle (a portion)
6. Inferoposterior surface of left ventricle	6. Anterolateral surface of left ventricle

Source: From Vinsant and Spence,[7] p. 25, with permission.

surfaces of the ventrical that is infarcted: lateral, inferior, posterior, and anterior, septal or anteroseptal, inferoposterior, and so forth. The location of the infarction depends on which coronary artery is occluded and the location of the occlusion within the arterial tree. Occlusions that occur in the large branches of the coronary circulation result in more extensive damage than those occurring in smaller arteries. (Table 5-1 summarizes the areas of the heart that are supplied by the left and right coronary arteries.) It is important to note that 75 to 80 percent of the vessel must be occluded before the myocardial blood flow is diminished.[19] Therefore, significant disease is usually present when symptoms begin to appear. Additional information on myocardial blood supply and MI location can be found in references 7, 11, 26, and 27 at the end of this chapter.

The MI also is identified by the layers of myocardium involved. Transmural infarcts, those that extend from the endocardium to the epicardium, are most commonly diagnosed.[7] Infarcts may be limited to the layers of muscle below the epicardium (subepicardial), in the middle of the heart muscle (intracardial), or the muscle below the endocardium (subendocardial). Because of its poor blood supply and greater ventricular wall pressure, the subendocardial layer is the most vulnerable to ischemia.[5,7,11]

The location, size, and degree of myocardial involvement are determined by the patterns of ECG changes revealed in the various leads of the 12-lead ECG. Knowledge of the location and amount of muscular damage enables health-care providers to anticipate the clinical course, complications, and prognosis following the infarction.[26]

TREATMENT GOALS

The immediate goals of treatment for the individual who has experienced an MI are the following:

1. Rapid management of myocardial ischemia/infarction and related symptoms (pain, dyspnea, nausea/vomiting)
2. Prevention or early detection and treatment of arrhythmias
3. Prevention of complications (See Complications of Myocardial Infarct, page 88.)
4. Rapid reperfusion of the ischemic/infarcted area if possible by use of antithrombolytics and/or PTCA

Clinical Course

UNCOMPLICATED MYOCARDIAL INFARCT

An uncomplicated MI is one in which the infarction is small and no complications arise during recovery.

Initially, the individual is treated in the coronary care unit, where he or she is allowed minimal activity. All efforts are directed toward decreasing myocardial work load and oxygen demand.[5] The patient is treated symptomatically. Oxygen, nitroglycerin, and/or morphine sulfate are given to reduce ischemic pain. Antihypertensives are administered for hypertension (although many people are hypotensive after an MI[18]). Other drugs, such as beta-blockers and calcium channel blockers, are given as necessary (Chapter 7). Beta-blockers reduce myocardial oxygen demand by decreasing the heart rate and contractility. Calcium channel blockers decrease the heart rate and also decrease the work load of the heart by systemic vasodilation (decreased afterload).

Cardiac rhythm is observed for arrhythmias. Of all the people who experience MIs, 90 percent have some type of arrhythmia. Early detection and treatment with appropriate pharmacologic agents have significantly reduced inhospital mortality.[5,27,34] The prophylactic use of lidocaine during the first 24 to 48 hours to prevent ventricular fibrillation is currently being advocated.[7,47]

The individual typically remains in the coronary care unit 2 to 3 days postinfarction and remains in the hospital an additional week. During that time, activity is gradually increased, and the patient is monitored for signs and symptoms of repeat ischemia. The rehabilitation process, which begins in intensive care with low-intensity exercise to prevent complications of bed rest, continues. Education of the individual and his or her family centers on understanding the CAD process, lifestyle modification, and risk factor adjustment.

COMPLICATIONS OF MYOCARDIAL INFARCT

Myocardial infarction has four major complications: arrhythmias, heart failure, thrombolytic complications, and damage to the heart structures.

Arrhythmias

Arrhythmias, caused by abnormalities in impulse generation, conduction, or both, occur in 90 percent of the individuals who have an MI. Although benign arrhythmias are often observed in healthy individuals, there are several (SVT, VT, VF) that are dangerous or life-threatening and require immediate treatment (Chapters 7 and 8). The types of arrhythmias seen as a result of MIs vary with the surface of the heart infarcted and the point on the conduction pathway where the tissue is ischemic or infarcted.

Ischemia of a myocardial cell causes an alteration in the initiation and conduction of impulses throughout that area. Infarcted cells are electrically silent, and they neither initiate nor conduct impulses. Abnormalities in conduction may also result from the elongation of conduction pathways secondary to dilation of the infarcted ventricle.

Heart Failure

Heart failure is a syndrome characterized by the inability of the heart to maintain a cardiac output sufficient to meet the oxygen and nutritional needs of the tissues. Heart failure manifests itself in two ways. First, in an ischemic state the myocardial muscle does not contract normally, and the infarcted myocardium does not contract at all. That results in asynchronous contraction and a low cardiac output. The second way heart failure is manifested is congestive heart failure. This is characterized by hypotension, retention of water and sodium from decreased renal perfusion, and the pooling of blood in either the pulmonary or the systemic venous beds.

Acutely, following an infarct, the cardiac output may be greatly reduced. Sympathetic stimulation increases the heart rate and the contractility within seconds of the infarct in an attempt to maintain cardiac output. (Cardiac output equals stroke volume times heart rate: $CO = SV \times HR$.) The compensatory mechanisms may be adequate to regain a normal cardiac output. If they are not, the kidneys, sensing the decreased renal blood flow, retain water and sodium in an attempt to increase the circulatory volume and venous return to the heart. If the heart is not damaged severely, those changes may be enough to compensate for the diminished pumping ability (even when it is as low as 30 to 50 percent of normal) and bring the cardiac output back to normal.[36] If the heart is severely damaged and neither compensatory mechanisms nor medical intervention can return the cardiac output to normal, the patient deteriorates. When more than 40 percent of the left ventricle is infarcted, cardiogenic shock (low output failure) develops. The condition is associated with an 80 to 90 percent mortality rate. Chronic congestive heart failure, which may develop as a result of an MI, may require continued treatment or may eventually be resolved. As the myocardium heals, the scar contracts and becomes smaller. This allows progressively less systolic bulge at the site of the scar. Systolic bulge is ballooning of the infarcted area of myocardium when left ventricular pressure increases during systole. Over time, the normal areas of the heart hypertrophy to compensate, at least partially, for the scarred musculature, and the heart at rest may have a normal cardiac output.[5,29]

Thrombolytic Complications

Two types of thrombus formation, venous and mural thrombi, may occur after MI. Both are primarily triggered by venous stasis (stoppage of the flow of blood).

Deep vein thrombi usually form in the calf as a result of circulatory stasis imposed by activity restrictions. Mural thrombi form on the areas of relative statis that are present in the ventricular wall after infarction. Both have the potential for embolism.

Emboli from a venous thrombus may result in a pulmonary embolism. Pulmonary embolism, once a major complication and cause of death after MI, now accounts for less than 1 percent of total deaths.[27] Prophylactic antithrombolytic therapy with intravenous heparin, early ambulation for individuals with uncomplicated MIs, and in-bed exercises for patients who are confined to bed have decreased the incidence of deep vein thrombus and recurrent intracoronary thrombosis.

Emboli from a mural wall thrombus may lodge in visceral arteries and result in an infarction of the brain, kidney, spleen, or intestine or lodge in an extremity and cause sudden pain, numbness, and coldness in the affected extremity. Embolectomies may successfully remove the obstruction to the blood flow in extremities.

Heart Structural Damage

Damage to the heart structures as a result of ischemia or infarction is a fourth major complication of MI. Structural damage includes ventricular aneurysm formation, papillary muscle rupture, ventricular free wall rupture, and intraventricular septal rupture. Ventricular aneurysms, the bulging of the wall in the weakened area, occur in transmural infarcts. Papillary muscle dysfunction or rupture occurs with papillary muscle ischemia or infarction. Papillary dysfunction results in mitral valve insufficiency. Ventricular free wall rupture is common in the second week post-MI when the scar is forming. The site is weakened because phagocytosis occurs earlier than collagen scar tissue formation. Rupture of the intraventricular septum, although rare, may also occur as a result of necrosis and the inability of the infarcted area to withstand the repeated pressure generated by the left ventricle during systole.[27,29] The "rupture" is usually a tunnel-like lesion through the septum. Any one of these structural problems may be fatal or result in mild to severe heart failure. Immediate surgical intervention may be required to repair the damage.

Pericarditis, an inflammation of the pericardium, may also occur post-MI. The characteristic symptom is pain over the precordium, which is aggravated by breathing and relieved by sitting up. Pericarditis accompanied by the accumulation of fluid in the pericardial sac is known as pericardial effusion. The accumulation of fluid may be sufficiently slow that the pericardium stretches and accommodates the fluid without interfering with cardiac performance. However, if the onset is abrupt and fluid accumulates rapidly, the heart is compressed and tamponade results. Cardiac tamponade is a life-threatening complication of pericarditis. The increased pressure restricts diastolic filling and results in reduced ventricular volume, elevated ventricular diastolic pressure, and reduced ventricular diastolic compliance. The cardiac output is decreased, as is the arterial blood pressure. Tachycardia is often insufficient to maintain cardiac output even at rest.

The decreased cardiac output is a result not of mechanical pump failure, but of the external restraint to cardiac filling and inadequate ventricular preload. Treatment is by pericardial aspiration. The accumulated fluid is removed to relieve the tamponade. Heart function returns to normal. Further treatment with analgesics, steroids, and antibiotics may be indicated.

Prognosis after Myocardial Infarction

Occasionally after the MI, the heart returns to its full functional capacity. More often, the functional capacity is decreased.[36] The prognosis depends on many factors, the most important of which are the extent of ventricular damage, the remaining cardiac reserve (the ability to respond to increased metabolic demands), and the severity of the CAD.

The medical and surgical management of the individual postinfarct is directed toward maximizing the cardiac function and minimizing any residual effects of the infarct. Cardiac rehabilitation programs, through education, exercise, diet, and risk factor reduction, facilitate lifestyle modifications that may reduce the risk of future infarctions.

SUDDEN CARDIAC DEATH

In addition to the previously discussed clinical syndromes of angina and MI, a third clinical manifestation of CAD is sudden cardiac death (SCD). The common definition of SCD is an unexpected cardiac death occurring in an apparently healthy individual engaging in his or her normal activities of daily living without prior symptoms or with symptoms of less than an hour's duration.[27] The American Heart Association estimated that, in 1987, one of every three individuals who had an MI died. Of those who died, 60 percent died within one hour before they reached the hospital.[1,5,26]

The leading causes of SCD are cardiac arrhythmias, ventricular tachycardia, and ventricular fibrillation, often in the presence of CAD but unrelated to MI.[1,26,27,48] Ventricular tachycardia, often a result of myocardial hypoxia, degenerates to ventricular fibrillation, which is a rapid and chaotic heart rhythm. The ventricle quivers rather than contracts. There is no effective cardiac output. If sustained, death may result within 4 minutes.[5] Prompt initiation of cardiopulmonary resuscitation (CPR) is the only proven means of preventing SCD.

Most victims of SCD are men about 60 years of age. Four characteristics are associated with an increased risk of SCD: ventricular electrical instability, extensive coronary artery narrowing, abnormal left ventricular function, and ECG conduction and repolarization abnormalities.

Four conditions contribute to the heart's tendency to fibrillate. Ischemia of the muscle cells causes the release of potassium into the extracellular fluid, which may increase myocardial irritability. Ischemic muscle remains negatively charged and can elicit abnormal impulses that may cause fibrillation. Sympathetic stimulation resulting from the low cardiac output may increase myocardial irritability. The myocardial infarction itself may, by dilating the ventricle, cause stretching of the conduction pathways or cause routing of impulses along abnormal pathways around the infarcted site. This final factor allows for a cyclic state of myocardial cell excitation. In this situation, impulses reenter muscle during the relative refractory period and set up a cycle of excitation that overrides the normal depolarization-repolarization cycle and allows the heart to fibrillate.[5,11,27]

Recently, the development of the automatic implantable cardioverter defibrillator (AICD), a device that monitors the heart rate through epicardial leads, has drastically lowered the incidence of repeat lethal arrhythmias in patients at high risk for SCD.[48,49] (See Chapter 7.)

CONGESTIVE HEART FAILURE

Congestive heart failure (CHF) is a fourth manifestation of CAD. This syndrome is characterized by the inability of the heart to maintain an adequate cardiac output to meet the demands of the tissue. The heart (the pump) is the direct cause of the imbalance. CHF results in diminished blood flow to the tissues, abnormal retention of sodium and water, and congestion in the pulmonary and systemic circulation. The most common etiology is ischemic heart disease secondary to CAD. CHF may also be associated with hypertension, valvular disease, or congenital heart disease.[5]

The ability of the heart to maintain an adequate cardiac output depends on the heart rate and the stroke volume. The stroke volume is a function of preload, the end-diastolic volume in the left ventricle; afterload, the systemic vascular resistance or the force against which the heart must pump; and contractility, the force of the contraction generated by the myocardium. Alterations in any one of these three factors results in decreased cardiac output. Changes in myocardial contractility are the most frequent cause of heart failure.[5,27]

In the person with CAD, decreases in normal coronary blood flow cause hypoxia and acidosis of the myocardial cells. Contractility is altered by such changes in the cellular environment. Whether the change is gradual or acute, as in MI, there is a resultant change in the cardiac output.

When a reduction in cardiac output occurs, the body immediately brings compensatory mechanisms into play to restore the balance. Compensatory mechanisms are physiologic alterations in the body's functioning that maintain homeostasis or, in this case, cardiac output. These mechanisms include increased sympathetic nervous system stimulation, increased sodium and water retention by the kidneys, increased dilation of the cardiac muscle fibers to accommodate the increased volume, and ventricular hypertrophy. Increased sympathetic activity occurs immediately and causes increased heart rate and contractility. It also increases vascular tone and thereby augments both venous return (preload) and systemic vascular resistance (afterload). The second compensatory mechanism is retention of water and sodium triggered by a drop in kidney perfusion. Initially, the increased circulating volume augments preload, afterload, and contractility. The heart may also dilate or hypertrophy (increase its muscle mass) in response to increased work load.[26,36] These mechanisms may be successful in maintaining a normal cardiac output for some period of time, but they increase myocardial oxygen demand. They may not be able to sustain the cardiac output if the pump function does not improve or if it deteriorates.

TYPES OF HEART FAILURE

There are several types of heart failure. Each is described briefly below.

Acute versus Chronic Failure

Acute heart failure may identify the initial manifestation of heart disease or it may be an acute exacerbation of a chronic cardiac condition. The events that precipitate the symptoms of acute heart failure occur rapidly. The rapid failure of the pump may result in an acute shift of blood from the systemic circulation to the pulmonary circulation before the compensatory mechanisms can be effective. The patient may experience a symptomatic fall in cardiac output and rapid onset of the associated symptoms, including pulmonary congestion and edema.[7]

Chronic heart failure develops gradually and is associated with the chronic retention of fluid and salt by the kidneys and other compensatory mechanisms. With time, the chronic overstimulation of compensatory mechanisms may lead to end organ failure.

Compensated versus Uncompensated Failure

In compensated failure, the heart has been able to maintain adequate cardiac output by means of the compensatory mechanisms described previously. Sympathetic stimulation and renal retention of water and sodium have maintained the cardiac output at normal levels, except for a mild to moderately elevated right atrial pressure ($+4$ to $+6$ mm Hg). Cardiac function at rest appears normal.[5] Symptoms appear when myocardial oxygen demand increases. A rapid heart rate, pallor, and diaphoresis all indicate that the cardiac output cannot meet the increased demand.

Uncompensated failure occurs when a severely damaged heart cannot regain normal cardiac output. Although compensatory mechanisms are at work, normal cardiac output is not attained. Fluid retention worsens because inadequate renal perfusion persists. Gradually the heart is stretched until it is unable to pump even moderate quantities of blood. The heart may fail completely. The patient may die of uncompen sated cardiac failure. Often this progression can be halted or slowed by appropriate pharmacologic therapy. Diuretics and fluid and salt restriction may control circulating volume while cardiac glycosides (e.g., digitalis) are given to improve the contractility. In this way an adequate cardiac output may be maintained. Although digitalis has little effect on the contractility of the normal myocardium, in the failing heart it may double the strength of contraction.[5]

Intractable Heart Failure

Intractable heart failure persists despite application of all therapies. Pulmonary and systemic congestion and a low cardiac output, ejection fraction less than 20 percent, exist even at rest.[27,50] The cause of pump failure is usually ischemic cardiomyopathy from CAD and idiopathic dilated cardiomyopathy. The current treatment of choice, for patients who meet specific medical criteria, is cardiac transplantation with the goals of improving survival, symptoms, and exercise capacity.[50,51]

Left Ventricular Failure versus Right Ventricular Failure

The left and right sides of the heart may fail separately or together. Left-sided failure is more common than right-sided failure, and it frequently leads to right-sided failure.[5,36,39]

Left-sided failure is most frequently seen after MI. When the heart is damaged, it may not pump effectively, and blood can back up in the left ventricle. As the pressure from the increased volume builds, it is communicated in a retrograde fashion to the left atrium and on through the pulmonary capillary beds. Pulmonary capillary pressure builds. The fluid is forced from the capillaries into the interstitial spaces and then into the alveoli. The presence of fluid in the interstitial spaces and the alveoli produces edema, which interferes with the diffusion of gases. Clinically, the patient is dyspneic at rest even when sitting upright. As pulmonary congestion increases, the lungs become stiff and less compliant and dyspnea worsens. A cough is another symptom of CHF. The cough produces frothy pink (blood-tinged) sputum, and rales (abnormal breath sounds from the movement of air through fluid in the alveoli) are audible over the lungs. (Signs and symptoms of left ventricular failure are included in Table 5−2.) If left untreated, acute pulmonary edema ensues, requiring prompt treatment with bronchodilators, vasodilators, and diuretics.

Right ventricular failure may occur unilaterally. This type of failure can result from congenital heart problems or chronic obstructive pulmonary disease (COPD). In the latter, lung compliance decreases significantly, and pulmonary vascular resistance increases significantly. The most common cause of right ventricular failure, however, is left ventricular failure.[5,27,36] Right ventricular failure follows left ventricular failure when the increase of pressure through the pulmonary circulation overloads the right ventricle (Fig. 5−4). The first sign of right ventricular failure is elevated central venous pressure (CVP) and neck vein distention. Liver engorgement, ascites, and peripheral edema of the dependent portion of the body (feet and ankles) also are observed.

All individuals with heart failure complain of fatigue and a decreased tolerance for activity. Treatment of the acute episode is directed toward decreasing circulatory overload, decreasing myocardial work load and oxygen demand, and increasing myocardial

TABLE 5–2 Signs and Symptoms of Cardiac Failure

	Left Ventricular Failure	Right Ventricular Failure
Subjective		
	Dyspnea	Abdominal pain
	Orthopnea	Anorexia/nausea
	Paroxysmal nocturnal dyspnea	Bloating
	Cough	Fatigue
	Fatigue	Ankle swelling (bilateral)
Objective		
	Rales	Distended neck veins
	S_3 gallop	Hepatojugular reflux
	Pleural effusion	Hepatomegaly/splenomegaly
	Peripheral cyanosis	Ascites
	Increased respiratory rate	Elevated CVP, right atrial pressure
	Cheyne-Stokes respirations	S_4 gallop
	Decreased urine output	Peripheral edema
	Pink frothy sputum	Decreased urine output

Source: From Patrick, ML, et al (eds): Medical-Surgical Nursing: Pathophysiological Concepts. JB Lippincott, Philadelphia, 1986, p. 548, with permission.

contractility. These goals may be accomplished with the judicious use of diuretics, water and sodium restrictions, cardiac gycosides (to increase myocardial contractility), and oxygen therapy as necessary.

CHF is usually a recurring phenomenon characterized by repeated exacerbations of symptoms that increase in frequency and severity as the myocardial muscle becomes progressively weaker and distended.[11,27] Chronic management attempts to decrease the frequency and severity of the symptoms.

PHYSIOLOGIC CHANGES IN INDIVIDUALS WITH CORONARY ARTERY DISEASE IN RESPONSE TO PHYSICAL CONDITIONING

The role of exercise in preventing or reversing CAD is undefined. The World Health Organization has concluded that regular vigorous exercise can enhance approaches to treatment and modify risk factors in patients with CAD.[40] There are, however, definite physiologic responses to physical conditioning in the individual with CAD (Chapter 4). The most beneficial physiologic change is an improvement in functional capacity attributable to an increase in myocardial oxygen supply and a decrease in myocardial oxygen demand. This allows the individual to carry higher work loads for longer periods of time without reaching his or her ischemic threshold.[46] The work load can be expressed as the product of the heart rate (HR) and the systolic arterial blood pressure (SBP). This is known as the rate pressure product (RPP) or double product (HR × SBP = RPP; for example, 70 × 100 = 7000 or 70 × 10^2) (Chapter 9). Both the heart rate and arterial blood pressure (BP) are major determinants of the myocardial oxygen consumption during exercise. As they increase, so does the RPP. In the physically conditioned individual with CAD, heart rate and blood pressure are decreased at rest and with

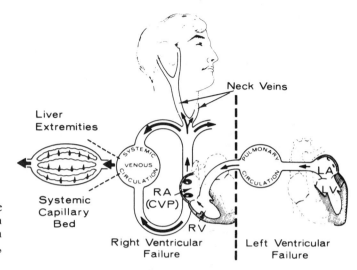

FIGURE 5–4. Retrograde failure of right ventricle from left ventricular failure. (From Vinsant and Spence,[7] p. 385, with permission.)

submaximal exercise. Therefore, the RPP, the myocardial oxygen demand, and the myocardial oxygen consumption are all lower.

Another benefit of training is the increased efficiency with which the peripheral muscles use oxygen.[42] This efficiency has not been documented in the heart as yet,[40,42] but the increased efficiency in the periphery decreases myocardial oxygen demand for any given level of exercise.

Physical conditioning also results in a swifter return to the resting heart rate after exercise. To date, it has not been shown to facilitate the development of collateral coronary circulation,[45,46] but in a recent cumulative analysis by Shephard,[43] the data show that individuals who had undergone physical conditioning not only experienced fewer repeat MIs but also had a smaller percentage of those events with fatal outcome.[43,46] Other studies have indicated that low-intensity, long-duration conditioning may improve myocardial function in a very select group of cardiac patients.[52]

In addition to the physiologic response to exercise, the psychologic satisfaction, the improved sense of well-being, and the decrease in cardiac risk factors that occur as a result of physical conditioning are of great benefit to the individual with CAD.

SUMMARY

In presenting the pathophysiology of coronary artery disease, particular attention was given to atherosclerosis and to the ischemia-infarction process that is the basis for all the related clinical manifestations of CAD.

The clinical manifestations of CAD, including angina, MI, SCD, and cardiac failure, were discussed in relation to the pathophysiology and the progression of CAD, their presenting symptoms, and their major complications.

The major physiologic changes in relation to training and physical conditioning of individuals with CAD were found to be improvement in functional capacity and the increased efficiency with which peripheral muscles use oxygen.

REFERENCES

1. 1990 Heart and Stroke Facts. American Heart Association, Dallas, TX, 1989.
2. Years of life lost from cardiovascular disease. Morbidity Mortality Weekly Report, Mass Med Soc 35:42, 1986.
3. Atherosclerosis; arteriosclerosis. In DG Holvey (ed): Merck Manual, ed 12. Merck, Sharp, and Dohme, Rahway, NJ, 1972.
4. Cowan, MJ: Pathogenesis of atherosclerosis. In SL Underhill, et al (eds): Cardiac Nursing, ed 2. JB Lippincott, Philadelphia, 1989.
5. Guyton, AC: Textbook of Medical Physiology, ed 7. WB Saunders, Philadelphia, 1986.
6. Underhill, SL: Assessment of cardiovascular function. In LS Brunner and DS Suddarth: Textbook of Medical-Surgical Nursing, ed 6. JB Lippincott, Philadelphia, 1987.
7. Vinsant, MO and Spence, MI: Commonsense Approach to Coronary Care: A Program, ed 5. CV Mosby, St Louis, MO, 1988, pp 178–210, 449, 498–500.
8. Chaffee, EE and Greisheimer, EM: Basic Physiology and Anatomy, ed 2. JB Lippincott, Philadelphia, 1969, pp 343–391.
9. Cowan, M: Atherosclerosis. In ML Patrick et al (eds): Medical Surgical Nursing: Pathophysiological Concepts. JB Lippincott, Philadelphia, 1986.
10. Schwartz, CJ: Gross aortic sudanophilia and hemosideria deposition: A study of infants, children and young adults. Arch Path 83:325, 1967.
11. Fowler, NO (ed): Cardiac Diagnosis and Treatment, ed 3. Harper & Row, Hagerstown, MD, 1980.
12. Ross, R and Glosmet, JA: The pathogenesis of atherosclerosis, Part I. N Engl J Med 295:369, 1976.
13. Ross, R and Glosmet, JA: The pathogenesis of atherosclerosis, Part II. N Engl J Med 295:426, 1976.
14. Benditt, E: The origin of atherosclerosis. Sci Am 236:74, 1977.
15. Sokolow, M and McIlroy, MB: Clinical Cardiology. Lange Medical Publications, Los Altos, CA 1986.
16. Wolff, R: Coronary heart disease. Med Clin North Am 57:1, 1973.
17. Glasgov, S: Mechanical stress on vessels and the non-uniform distribution of atherosclerosis. Med Clin North Am 57:1, 1973.
18. Coronary artery disease. In DH Holvey (ed): Merck Manual, ed 12. Merck, Sharp, and Dohme, Rahway, NJ, 1972.
19. Zak, R and Rabinowitz, M: Metabolism of the ischemic heart. Med Clin North Am 57:1, 1973.
20. Solack, SD: Pathophysiology of myocardial ischemia and infarction. In SL Underhill et al (eds): Cardiac Nursing, ed 2. JB Lippincott, Philadelphia, 1989.
21. Tannenbaum, RP, Sohn, CA, Cantwell, R and Rogers, M: Angina pectoris: How to recognize; how to manage it. Nurs 81(11):9, 1981.
22. Rokosky, JS: Ischemia and infarction. In ML Patrick et al (eds): Medical-Surgical Nursing: Pathophysiological Concepts. JB Lippincott, Philadelphia, 1986.
23. Riseman, JEF: Diagnosis of angina pectoris at the present time. Med Clin North Am 58:2, 1974.
24. Altschule, MD: Physiology in acute myocardial infarction. Med Clin North Am 58:2, 1974.
25. Texon, M: Atherosclerosis: Its hemodynamic basis and implications. Med Clin North Am 58:2, 1974.
26. Braunwald, E: Heart Disease, ed 3. WB Saunders, Philadelphia, 1988.
27. Hurst, J, et al (eds): The Heart, Arteries, and Veins, ed 7. McGraw-Hill, New York, 1990.
28. Underhill, SL: Diagnosis and treatment of the patient with coronary artery disease and myocardial ischemia. In SL Underhill et al (eds): Cardiac Nursing, ed 2. JB Lippincott, Philadelphia, 1989.
29. Woods, SL and Underhill, SL: Coronary heart disease: Myocardial ischemia and infarction. In ML Patrick et al (eds): Medical Surgical Nursing: Pathophysiological Concepts. JB Lippincott, Philadelphia, 1986.
30. Heupler, FA and Proudfit, WL: Nifedipine therapy for refractory coronary artery spasm. Am J Cardiol 44, October, 1979.
31. Kannel, WB: Update on the role of cigarette smoking in coronary artery disease. Am Heart J 101:319–328, 1981.
32. Forman, MB, et al: Increased adventitial mast cells in a patient with coronary spasm. N Eng J Med 313:18.
33. Spittle, L: Management of patients with cardiovascular disorders. In LS Brunner and DS Suddarth: Textbook of Medical-Surgical Nursing, ed 6. JB Lippincott, Philadelphia, 1987.
34. Woods, SL: Diagnosis and treatment of the patient with an uncomplicated myocardial infarction. In SL Underhill et al (eds): Cardiac Nursing, ed 2. JB Lippincott, Philadelphia, 1989.
35. Woods, SL: Electrocardiography, vectorcardiography, and polarcardiography. In SL Underhill, et al (eds): Cardiac Nursing, ed 2. JB Lippincott, Philadelphia, 1989.
36. Mechanical complications in coronary heart disease: Heart failure and shock. In MO Vinsant and MI Spence: Commonsense Approach to Coronary Care: A Program, ed 5. CV Mosby, St Louis, 1989.
37. Bopp, DL: Heart failure. In Patrick, ML et al (eds): Medical-Surgical Nursing: Pathophysiological Concepts. JB Lippincott, Philadelphia, 1986.
38. Niles, NA and Wills, RE: Heart failure. In SL Underhill et al (eds): Cardiac Nursing, ed 2. JB Lippincott, Philadelphia, 1989.
39. Sivarajan, ES: Cardiac rehabilitation activity and exercise program. In SL Underhill et al (eds): Cardiac Nursing, ed 2. JB Lippincott, Philadelphia, 1989.

40. Oberman, A: Exercise and the primary prevention of cardiovascular disease. Am J Cardiol 55:100, 1985.
41. Sami, M, et al: Significance of exercise induced ventricular arrhythmias in stable coronary artery disease. Am J Cardiol 54:1182, 1984.
42. Wenger, N and Fletcher, GF: Rehabilitation of the patient with atherosclerotic coronary heart disease. In J Hurst et al (eds): The Heart, Arteries and Veins, ed 7. McGraw-Hill, New York, 1990.
43. Shephard, RJ: The value of exercise in ischemic heart disease: A cumulative analysis. J Cardiac Rehabil 3:294, 1983.
44. Stern, MJ and Cleary, P: National exercise and heart disease project: Psychosocial changes observed during low level exercise programs. Arch Int Med 141:1463, 1981.
45. Wenger, NK: Rehabilitation of the patient with symptomatic coronary atherosclerotic heart disease, Part II. In HD McIntosh (ed): Cardiology Series, Vol 3, No 3. Parke-Davis, Morris Plains, NJ, 1980.
46. Dehn, MM: Rehabilitation of the cardiac patient: The effects of exercise. Am J Nurs 80:435, 1980.
47. Bond, EF: Antiarrhythmic drugs/pharmacologic management of the patient with coronary heart disease. In SL Underhill, et al (eds): Cardiac Nursing, ed 2. JB Lippincott, Philadelphia, 1989, p 629.
48. Lehmen, MH and Steinman, RT: Preventing sudden cardiac death. Postgrad Med 82:7, 1987.
49. Cooper, DK, Valladares, BK and Futterman, LG: Care of the patient with the automatic implantable cardioverter defibrillator: A guide for nurses. Heart Lung 16(6), pt 1:640–648, 1987.
50. Squires, RW: Cardiac rehabilitation issues for heart transplant patients. J Cardiopulmonary Rehabil 10:159–168, 1990.
51. Schroeder, JS and Hunt, S: Cardiac transplantation: Update 1987. JAMA 258:3142–3145, 1987.
52. Ehsani, AA, et al: Improvement of left ventricular function in patients with coronary artery disease. Circulation 74:350–388, 1986.

CHAPTER 6

Chronic Lung Diseases

In this chapter, chronic obstructive pulmonary disease (COPD); its individual components of peripheral airways disease, chronic bronchitis and emphysema; asthma; bronchiectasis; cystic fibrosis; and restrictive pulmonary disease will be discussed. COPD and asthma are the most common chronic lung diseases for which pulmonary rehabilitation is rendered. Bronchiectasis, although it is a chronic pulmonary disease of the obstructive nature, is not a component of COPD, but it may be the presenting diagnosis of a patient enrolled in a pulmonary rehabilitation program. Advances in the care of patients with cystic fibrosis have resulted in increased longevity. Patients with cystic fibrosis are surviving with increased pulmonary dysfunction, making them candidates for pulmonary rehabilitation. Patients with restrictive pulmonary disease have generally been excluded from pulmonary rehabilitation programs because of their exercise intolerance. Recent information provides support for the use of pulmonary rehabilitation with this patient population.[1]

CHRONIC OBSTRUCTIVE PULMONARY DISEASE

Definition

In 1962, the American Thoracic Society defined the clinical conditions of COPD as "damage to the alveolar walls and inflammation of the conducting airways."[2] Numerous revisions of this definition have been published since,[3-5] the most recent of which is taken from the 1987 position statement by the American Thoracic Society. The statement concluded that COPD is a disorder characterized by abnormal tests of expiratory flow that do not change markedly over periods of several months observation.[5] The three pulmonary components that are included in the definition of COPD are chronic bronchitis, peripheral airways disease, and emphysema. Asthma, bronchiectasis, and cystic fibrosis are diagnoses that have been excluded from the term "COPD."[5]

The controversy over definitions and terminologies used to describe chronic pulmonary diseases continues. COPD, chronic obstructive airways disease (COAD), chronic obstructive lung disease (COLD), chronic airflow or airways obstruction (CAO), and chronic airflow limitation (CAL) all refer to the same combination of pulmonary disorders.[6] Since these components can coexist and their clinical signs and symptoms overlap, the term "chronic obstructive pulmonary disease" is useful in the clinical setting.

Etiology

COPD is the most commonly encountered chronic pulmonary disorder, and its prevalence is increasing. It has been estimated that more than 15 million Americans have the disease,[7] and physical disability caused by COPD is second only to disability from heart disease.[8]

Causal agents in the development of COPD include environmental pollutants. Whether from cigarette smoke or industrial sources, pollution is the major contributor to COPD.[9]

Research suggests that peripheral airways disease may actually be a precursor to the development of COPD.[10,11] There is also a relation between chronic bronchitis and the subsequent development of emphysema.[12]

Pathophysiology

The pathophysiology of COPD is a composite of individual components that contribute to the disease process. Chronic inflammation from inhaling environmental pollutants causes bronchial glands and goblet cells to hypertrophy. Excessive secretions that obstruct the airway are then produced. The smooth muscle encircling the bronchiole may become hypertrophied, and the submucosa becomes thickened. These obstructive changes lead to alveolar hypoventilation, weakened bronchiolar walls, and alveolar destruction. The small airways will collapse during expiration, which leads to air trapping and hyperinflation.[13] Ventilation and perfusion imbalances that are due to patchy areas of disease will lead to hypoxemia. As the disease progresses and more areas of the lung become involved, hypoxemia will worsen and hypercapnea will develop. Bronchial hyperreactivity may also be present.

Clinical Presentation

Patients with COPD will present with a variety of symptoms. Chronic cough, expectoration, and exertional dypsnea may all be present in varying degrees. The symptoms relate to their unique combination of chronic bronchitis, emphysema, and peripheral airways disease. For example, if a patient has a large component of chronic bronchitis, the predominant presenting symptoms may be chronic cough rather than shortness of breath. The intensity of symptoms relates to the severity of each component of COPD.

The hallmark of COPD is a significant and progressive decrease in expiratory flow rates as measured by pulmonary function tests, the most important of which is the forced expiratory volume in one second (FEV_1).[5] Pulmonary function studies will also reveal that this airway obstruction does not show a major reversibility in response to pharmacologic agents. Hyperinflation is demonstrated by an increase in residual volume (RV). The diffusing capacity of the lungs for carbon monoxide (DL_{CO}) can be reduced to less than 50 percent of the predicted normative value because of the destruction of the alveoli.[14] (See Chapter 10 for more information relating to DLco).

Arterial blood gas alterations occur in the advanced stages of COPD. Hypoxemia is present in the early stages, and hypercapnia appears as the disease progresses. Because of the chronicity of those changes in advanced disease, the metabolic system compensates for the potential respiratory acidosis by elevating the bicarbonate ion, which allows the arterial blood gas analysis to show a relatively normal pH.

Chest roentgenograms display regional hyperlucency and overinflation as measured by the anterioposterior diameter. Bullous lesions are also a fairly common finding on chest roentgenograms of patients with COPD.

Course and Prognosis

The clinical course of COPD can run for 30 years or more,[6] and the progression of the disease can be monitored by pulmonary function studies.[15] The rate of decrease in FEV_1 is approximately 54 milliters per year,[16] but smoking cessation has been shown to delay that decline in function.[17] Chest roentgenograms do not usually depict the severity of the disease, nor do they indicate the prognosis of COPD.

The components of COPD—peripheral airways disease, chronic bronchitis, and emphysema—will now be discussed individually. Although separating COPD into its basic components allows for a more organized discussion, it must be remembered that, in pulmonary rehabilitation programs, the components appear most often in combinations that are broadly referred to as COPD.

PERIPHERAL AIRWAYS DISEASE

Definition

According to the American Thoracic Society, peripheral airways disease is diagnosed by the abnormalities found in the terminal and respiratory bronchioles. The changes include inflammation, fibrosis, and narrowing of the airways.[5,10]

Etiology

Chronic inflammation seems to be the main etiologic feature in peripheral airways disease. Inflammation may be a result of chronic irritation, as by cigarette smoke. Changes in peripheral airways have been found in smokers less than 40 years of age.[18]

Pathophysiology

The airways that are less than 2 mm in diameter are those that are affected in peripheral airways disease. Inflammatory airflow obstruction of these airways occurs. However, the contribution of these peripheral airways to the total pulmonary airflow is relatively small, and the disease is therefore not readily detectable by using only FEV_1.[19]

Initially in the disease process, squamous cell metaplasia, inflammatory infiltrate, and an increase in connective tissue are observed. As the disease progresses, the amount of connective tissue within the airway walls increases. There is also hypertrophy of the muscle of the airway. Goblet cell metaplasia becomes an important pathological finding in advanced cases.[18]

Clinical Presentation

Symptoms of peripheral airways disease include cough and expectoration. The distribution and severity of the symptoms vary considerably among individuals.

Expiratory flow rates as measured by FEV_1 may be normal. However, by employing more sensitive tests that identify obstruction of small airways, such as single-breath nitrogen washout studies and air and helium closing capacities and by evaluating the middle segment of the forced expiratory flow curve ($FEF_{25-75\%}$), the presence of small airway impairment can be uncovered.[5,18,20,21] Diffusion studies (DL_{CO}) may be slightly below normal values.[20] (See Chapter 10 for more information about these pulmonary function tests.) Physiological or roentgenographic evidence of hyperinflation is not apparent in peripheral airways disease.

Course and Prognosis

It is impossible to predict the course of the peripheral airways disease. Most patients will have symptoms of chronic cough and expectoration for many years without developing any disability or complication.

In some but not all patients, progression of the disease will continue. The pathological changes of the peripheral airways appear to be a precursor to the development of COPD.[5,10,21] Although peripheral airways disease continues to contribute to airflow obstruction in COPD, it is of secondary importance once emphysematous changes have occurred.[22]

Early detection of peripheral airway abnormalities may allow for a timely alteration in the patient's personal environment. Such intervention may halt or even reverse the progression of the peripheral airways disease and prevent COPD.[18]

CHRONIC BRONCHITIS

Definition

Chronic bronchitis is defined by the American Thoracic Society in clinical terms as chronic cough and expectoration when other specific causes of cough can be excluded.[5] "Chronic" means that the cough and expectoration have persisted for at least a 3-month period and this pattern has been repeated for at least 2 consecutive years.[14]

Etiology

The incidence of chronic bronchitis in males is significantly different from that in females. Symptoms of chronic cough and expectoration are found in 25 to 35 percent of all males and 15 percent of all females.[7]

The most important etiologic factor in the development of chronic bronchitis is cigarette smoking. There is a direct relation between the amount and duration of cigarette smoking and the severity of the disease.[7] There is also a significant individual variation in the susceptibility and effect of smoking on the lungs. The etiologic role of other factors, such as agents inhaled from occupational exposure without the effect of smoking, appears to be relatively insignificant.[7,8] Chronic bronchitis is a rare disease among the nonsmoking population.

Pathophysiology

Pathophysiologic changes in chronic bronchitis are related to narrowing of the airways. Chronic exposure to irritants results in chronic inflammation of the bronchial mucosa, which is the major cause of airway narrowing. The airways are further narrowed by hyperplasia of the bronchial mucous glands, hypertrophy of the smooth muscle within the bronchial walls, and an increase in the number of goblet cells. An increased amount of mucus is produced by these glands and cells in response to chronic irritant exposure, which leads to plugging of the smaller airways.[12] Decreases in ciliary function and an alteration in physiochemical characteristics of bronchial secretions impair airway clearance and also affect the airway size.[8] Stagnant bronchial secretions predispose the patient to recurrent respiratory infections. Damaged and inflamed mucosa results in an increased sensitivity of the irritant receptors within the bronchial walls, which in turn causes bronchial hyperreactivity.

During inhalation, airways are pulled open by the surrounding air sacs, which allows air to pass into the alveoli. When exhalation occurs, the airways normally become narrowed. When incomplete obstruction that is due to secretions occurs, exhalation becomes abnormal. Airways take longer to empty, and they often collapse before full exhalation has occurred. That type of incomplete obstruction acts like a ball valve: It allows air into the lungs, but it does not allow air out. The results of the pathology are a decreased expiratory flow rate, hyperinflation of the chest, and an altered ventilation/perfusion ratio that cause abnormalities in the partial pressures of oxygen and carbon dioxide in arterial blood. In advanced stages of chronic bronchitis, destruction of the alveolar capillary membrane may also be present. Increased pulmonary vascular resistance that is due to capillary destruction and reflex vasoconstriction in the presence of hypoxemia and hypercapnia results in right ventricular hypertrophy, or cor pulmonale. Polycythemia, an increase in the amount of circulating red blood cells, is another advanced complication of chronic bronchitis.[12]

Clinical Presentation

The major presenting symptoms in chronic bronchitis are cough and expectoration that appear slowly and insidiously. Dyspnea, another symptom of chronic bronchitis, also begins slowly; it is first evidenced during exertion. Severely involved patients may appear dyspneic even at rest. Chronic bronchitis results in prolonged expiratory wheezing. Crackles also may be present, and they can be altered by coughing. Initially, chest roentgenograms may appear normal, but abnormalities of hyperinflation and increased lung markings may be found with disease progression.

Pulmonary function tests reveal a reduced FEV_1 that does not improve significantly following bronchodilator inhalation. Inspiratory flow rates also are reduced in chronic bronchitis. The narrowing of the airways in chronic bronchitis causes air trapping. An increase in residual volume may be detectable, although the total lung capacity is usually normal or near normal. With advancing disease and increasing airway obstruction, ventilation/perfusion relations are altered and there are resulting changes in the arterial blood gas values of hypercapnia and hypoxemia. Since that is a chronic change, the metabolic system compensates for it by increasing the bicarbonate ion and thereby returning the arterial blood to a relatively normal pH value. The patient with advanced chronic bronchitis is in a chronic compensated respiratory acidosis.

Course and Prognosis

Patients will have symptoms of chronic cough and expectoration for many years before developing signs or symptoms of airway obstruction. The progression of chronic bronchitis is evidenced by an increase in the severity of symptoms that is due to increased airway obstruction, deterioration of pulmonary function, and more frequent respiratory tract infections.[23] Once patients show evidence of pulmonary function abnormalities, the prognosis becomes much less favorable and they may advance to the point of severe respiratory insufficiency and failure. Pulmonary emphysema often develops; it complicates chronic bronchitis and adversely affects the prognosis. Proper medical management and patient compliance in smoking cessation can positively influence the prognosis of chronic bronchitis.[6,18]

EMPHYSEMA

Definition

Emphysema is defined in anatomic or pathologic terms as abnormal enlargement of the acinus, which is accompanied by destructive changes of the alveolar walls without obvious fibrosis.[5] Overdistension of the air spaces without destruction of the alveolar walls, as normally seen in aging, is not included in the definition of emphysema.

Depending on the site of involvement in the distal respiratory unit or acinus, emphysema has been classified into three forms: centriacinar, panacinar, and distal acinar.[5] Centriacinar emphysema often involves the upper lung fields and is almost always associated with chronic bronchitis. Panacinar emphysema is less common, and it affects the entire acinus. It is predominantly found in the lower and anterior aspects of the lungs and is more often associated with the alpha$_1$-antitrypsin deficiency form of emphysema. Finally, distal acinar emphysema affects the distal portion of the acinus, predominately the alveolar ducts and alveolar sacs.

Etiology

The development of pulmonary emphysema has been linked to environmental pollutants. Because of a definite relation between cigarette smoking and chronic bronchitis and an association between chronic bronchitis and emphysema, it has been deduced that smoking is a major etiologic factor in the development of pulmonary emphysema. However, many patients with long-standing chronic bronchitis never go on to develop emphysema. It is also true that emphysema occurs in individuals who have never smoked. Therefore, the etiology of emphysema may not be from pollutants alone, and other as yet unknown factors must be involved in the development of emphysema.

A small number of patients with emphysema are known to have a genetically determined deficiency of alpha$_1$-antitrypsin. This serum enzyme normally inhibits the effect of trypsin, an enzyme that digests the proteins of the lung parenchyma, namely, elastin and collagen. Trypsin is present in the white blood cells and macrophages and may be released during an inflammatory process. Based on this theory, the alveolar destruction that is due to emphysema is caused by the release of trypsin from the inflammatory cells that remains unopposed by alpha$_1$-antitrypsin, its natural inhibitor.[8]

Not all individuals with a deficiency in alpha$_1$-antitrypsin enzyme develop emphysema in the same manner. Again, other factors must be present, factors that cause an inflammatory response and contribute to the development of emphysematous changes. The trypsin/antitrypsin imbalance may be exacerbated by the chronic inflammatory response to respiratory irritants, such as cigarette smoke, and infectious processes. Indeed, smoking appears to be implicated in the development of emphysema in patients with alpha$_1$-antitrypsin deficiency. In nonsmoking patients with alpha$_1$-antitrypsin deficiency, the mean age of onset of dyspnea has been reported to be 51. In smoking patients with alpha$_1$-antitrypsin deficiency, the mean age of onset of dyspnea has been found to be 32.[24] Pulmonary function abnormalities are also more pronounced in smokers as compared with nonsmokers who have the enzyme deficiency.[24,25]

Pathophysiology

Airflow obstruction in emphysema is due to the destruction of pulmonary elastic tissues, which results in a loss of the normal elastic recoil properties of the lungs. During expiration, the airways collapse from a lack of support by the surrounding elastic parenchyma.[8] Premature airway collapse causes hyperinflation or air trapping and reduced expiratory flow rates. Inspiratory flow rates are normal, except when there is associated obstructive bronchitis.[8]

Gas exchange is impaired as a result of the destruction of the alveolar-capillary membrane and ventilation/perfusion mismatches. A reduction in the diffusing capacity of carbon monoxide also occurs in emphysema (Chapter 10).

In advanced stages of emphysema, destruction of the alveolar-capillary membrane is present. Increased pulmonary vascular resistance that is due to capillary destruction and reflex vasoconstriction in the presence of hypoxemia and hypercapnia results in right ventricular hypertrophy, or cor pulmonale. Polycythemia, an increase in the amount of circulating red blood cells, is another advanced complication of emphysema.

Clinical Presentation

The clinical symptom of emphysema is dyspnea. The onset of dyspnea is noted initially during physical exertion, but it can gradually progress so that dyspnea even at rest is present. In patients who do not also have chronic bronchitis, the symptoms of cough and expectoration are absent.

On physical examination, the thorax appears enlarged because of the loss of lung elastic recoil. The anteroposterior diameter of the chest increases; a dorsal kyphosis is noted; the ribs are elevated; and there is flaring of costal margin and a widening of the costochondral angle.[8] Collectively, these anatomic changes give the patient the "barrel chest" appearance. Consistent with hyperinflation of the lungs, breath sounds are usually distant and somewhat difficult to hear. Expiratory wheezing can sometimes be heard, and heart sounds may appear distant. Use of accessory muscles of ventilation, hypertrophy of the accessory muscles, pursed lip breathing, cyanosis, and digital clubbing may be present in the advanced stages of emphysema.

Several radiographic changes occur with emphysema. They include depressed and flattened hemidiaphragms, alteration in pulmonary vascular markings, hyperinflation of the thorax evidenced by an increased anteroposterior diameter of the chest, and an increased retrosternal air space, hyperlucency, elongation of the heart, and right ventricular hypertrophy. Appearance of bullous lesions on x-ray is an unequivocal sign of emphysema.[26]

Pulmonary function tests show an irreversible decrease in FEV_1 and $FEF_{25-75\%}$. There is also an increase in residual volume, which may be several times the normal value.[14] As a result, functional residual capacity also is increased. Despite a reduction in vital capacity that is due to emphysema, total lung capacity is generally increased.[14]

Reduction of diffusing capacity in emphysema usually differentiates the disease from chronic bronchitis and peripheral airways disease.[8] Arterial blood gas analyses may show a reduced arterial Pao_2, and arterial $Paco_2$ may be chronically elevated.

Course and Prognosis

Periods of increased symptoms, usually related to recurrent infections, frequently exacerbate pulmonary emphysema. Expiratory flow rates measured during stable periods are good indicators of the progression of emphysema. There is also a good correlation between the severity of airway obstruction as judged by FEV_1 and mortality from emphysema. With an FEV_1 below 750 milliliters, few patients survive 5 years.[8]

Arterial blood gas changes are related to the severity of the disease, but the severity of dyspnea is not always correlated with the degree of pathologic and physiologic abnormalities that are due to emphysema. Roentgenographic evidence occurs later in the disease and does not relate well with the severity. It is therefore not useful as a prognostic indicator.[26]

ASTHMA

Definition

Asthma is a clinical syndrome characterized by an increase in the reactivity of the tracheobronchial tree to various stimuli.[5] The most remarkable feature of asthma is the episodic attacks of wheezing and dyspnea that improve either spontaneously or with medical therapy and are interspersed with intervals that are symptom-free.

Etiology

Asthma is a common respiratory disease of uncertain etiology that may begin at any age. Depending on race, age, gender, and geographic differences, the prevalence of asthma has been reported to be from 1.5 to 9.5 percent.[27,28] Although the exact mechanism of airway hyperreactivity is unknown, genetic predisposition,[29] environmental contributions,[30] autonomic nervous system imbalance, and mucosal epithelial damage[8] have been implicated in the development of asthma.

Allergy is one of the etiologic or precipitating factors in asthma, especially in children.[31] When there is clear association with allergy, asthma is referred to as extrinsic or allergic. Intrinsic or ideopathic asthma, usually found in older patients, seems to have no relation to allergens, but it does frequently occur with respiratory tract infections. Respiratory infections can be a common precipitating event in allergic asthma.

The airways of asthmatics are hypersensitive to a variety of factors including respiratory irritants, cold air, emotional stresses, and chemical substances. Any or all of these may precipitate or aggravate both the intrinsic and extrinsic forms of asthma.

Common respiratory irritants in the atmosphere include sulfur dioxide, ozone, dust, pollen, and even perfume.[7] Primary and ambient tobacco smoke is a respiratory irritant that may cause asthmatic attacks in smokers and also in nonsmokers.[7,32]

Exercise and cold air are also known to provoke bronchospasm.[33,34] In fact, exercise-induced bronchospasm (EIB) may be the first manifestation of asthma. The conditions that promote EIB are as follows: (1) Exercise has to be vigorous, and the intensity must be approximately 90 percent of the predicted maximum heart rate. (2) Exercise should last at least 8 minutes. (3) The exercise should be performed in a cold, dry environment. (4) Running is the mode of exercise most often associated with exercise-induced bronchospasm. Shortly following that type of activity, bronchospasm will develop in susceptible persons. Pulmonary function tests show that the most impairment occurs 8 to 15 minutes postexercise.[35] Although this description of EIB is "classic," bronchospasm that occurs any time during the exercise session and/or at any time following the exercise session should be considered exercise-induced.[36] The cooling of the airways appears to be the basic mechanism that causes bronchospasm to occur during exercise.[35-39] To prevent bronchospasm, prior to reaching the alveoli, the inspired air should be 37°C in temperature and saturated with water vapor. Because of the increase in minute ventilation during exercise, humidification and warming mechanisms may become inadequate and allow colder air to be delivered to the tracheobronchial tree. This may precipitate a bronchospastic response.

Chemical substances such as histamine and methacholine are known to produce bronchospasm in asthmatics. For diagnostic purposes, a solution containing methacholine can be nebulized and inhaled. A reduction of 20 percent in FEV_1 following the methacholine challenge is a positive diagnostic sign for asthma.[40]

Other chemical substances, such as those found in the workplace, are associated with occupational asthma and lung hypersensitivity. Among the chemical agents are cotton dust, toluene diisocyanate, aspergillus, and moldy hay.[8,41] Occupational asthma and hypersensitivity are characterized by respiratory symptoms of cough, chest tightness, and wheezing that are cyclical in occurrence and coincide with the work schedule. Symptoms may become chronic and somewhat continuous after many years of exposure.[41] In many patients, different etiologic agents in various combinations are responsible for their asthma attacks.

Pathophysiology

The major physiological manifestation of asthma is widespread narrowing of the airways. The airway narrowing is usually due to a combination of bronchospasm, inflammation of the mucosa, and increased secretions. The narrowed airways increase the resistance to airflow and decrease forced expiratory flow rates, thereby causing hyperinflation. These narrowed airways provide an abnormal distribution of ventilation to the alveoli. In asthma, because of narrowed airways and obstruction, there is a ventilation and perfusion inequality that results in the alteration of arterial blood gases and hypoxemia.[8,42]

Clinical Presentation

The clinical symptom of asthma is bronchoconstriction with varying degrees of dyspnea and wheezing. During an acute exacerbation, the chest is usually held in an expanded position, which indicates that hyperinflation of the lungs has occurred. Accessory muscles of ventilation are used for breathing, and expiratory wheezes can be heard over the entire chest. Sometimes, crackles can be heard as well. With severe airway obstruction, breath sounds may become markedly diminished because of poor air movement, wheezing may occur on inspiration as well as expiration, and intercostal, supraclavicular, and substernal retractions may be present on inspiration.[8]

Chest roentgenograms taken during an asthmatic exacerbation usually indicate hyperinflation as evidenced by an increase in the anteroposterior diameter of the chest with hyperlucency of the lung fields. Less commonly, chest x-rays may reveal areas of atelectasis or infiltrates from the bronchial obstruction. Normal chest roentgenograms can be seen between bouts of asthma exacerbations.

The most consistent changes during episodes of bronchospasm are decreased expiratory flow rates that result in the increase in airway resistance. Residual volume and functional residual capacity are increased because of air trapping at the expense of vital capacity and inspiratory reserve volume, which are reduced. During an acute exacerbation, the results of pulmonary function studies appear somewhat similar to the results found in pulmonary emphysema. However, the reversibility of the abnormalities is distinctive of asthma. During remission, the patient with asthma may have normal or near normal FEV_1 values.

During an asthmatic exacerbation, the most common arterial blood gas finding is mild to moderate hypoxemia. Usually some degree of hypocapnea is present because of hyperventilation, which causes an acute respiratory alkalosis. In severe attacks, hypoxemia may be more pronounced. With further clinical deterioration, arterial $Paco_2$ rises, which indicates the patient is exhausted and respiratory failure is imminent.[8,41,42] Even in severe exacerbations, diffusing capacity usually remains normal.[41]

Clinical Course and Prognosis

By the time adulthood is reached, 33 percent of asthmatic children do not have symptoms of asthma.[8] When the onset of symptoms begins later in life, the clinical course is usually more progressive. Pulmonary function tests during periods of remission become less normal; yet, asthma, with no concomitant complicating disease, has a relatively low mortality.[30]

BRONCHIECTASIS

Definition

Bronchiectasis is an anatomic abnormality characterized by dilatation of the bronchial lumen. Associated inflammation and destruction of the bronchial walls also are present. There are three major morphologic types of dilatation of the airway: cylindrical, fusiform, and saccular.

Etiology

The onset of bronchiectasis usually occurs during childhood. Although the exact cause for the condition is not known, a number of mechanisms have been proposed to explain the dilatation of the bronchi.[43] Bacterial infections have been implicated in the development of altered cilia.[44] With impaired cilial function, infected secretions stagnate within the bronchi; they cause further inflammation and the eventual destruction of the bronchial wall. Certainly, not all bacterial pulmonary infections result in bronchiectasis. Tuberculosis, collapse of lung tissue, aspiration of a foreign body, atelectasis, and allergic bronchopulmonary aspergillosis have all been associated with the development of bronchiectasis.[8]

Pathophysiology

Bronchiectasis causes atrophy of the mucosa, and there is a loss of ciliated epithelium in the bronchi. Infiltration of inflammatory cells and squamous cell metaplasia also are present. The dilated bronchial lumen are often filled with purulent material that causes ulcerations and abscess formation on the bronchial walls.[7,8] With progression of the disease, fibrosis occurs and there is a marked increase in the collateral circulation to the involved area of the lung.[45]

Clinical Presentation

The classic sign of bronchiectasis is cough with expectoration. Patients may have relatively small amounts of secretions, termed "dry bronchiectasis," but more commonly, the patient will produce an extraordinary amount of mucopurulent sputum. Hemoptysis commonly occurs, although the amount and frequency of bleeding are variable and unpredictable. Dyspnea may be present in varying degrees.

Signs of bronchiectasis include diminished breath sounds, crackles that can be heard over the involved areas of the lung, cyanosis, and digital clubbing. These signs will vary in intensity and are dependent on the amount of lung involvement.

Chest roentgenograms may show patchy infiltrates, increased lung markings that are due to peribronchial thickening, segmental atelectasis, and occasional cystic changes with air-fluid levels. These changes occur more frequently in the lower lung fields.

Bronchography, which reveals the walls of the bronchi, can easily identify bronchiectatic areas. Although helpful in quantifying the extent of the disease in a patient pending surgical management, bronchography is no longer widely utilized as a diagnostic tool.[43]

Pulmonary function tests will reveal no abnormality in mild and moderate cases of bronchiectasis. Advanced diseased patients may show both obstructive and restrictive changes. Expiratory flow rates, such as FEV_1, are decreased, and residual volume is increased. There is usually no alteration in diffusing capacity, but in severe cases, the ventilatory impairment may cause hypoxemia.

Course and Prognosis

Variations in the severity, extent, and medical management of the disease affect the prognosis of bronchiectasis. In patients with minimal involvement, there will be minimal effects. Some patients in the second and third decade of life show spontaneous improvement.[43] However, the course of the disease is usually exacerbated and results in a slow decline in function. Chronic infection is very common, and pneumonia tends to recur at the same location. Within several years, severely involved patients will usually succumb to respiratory and/or infectious complications.

CYSTIC FIBROSIS

Definition

Cystic fibrosis (CF), or mucoviscidosis, is the most common lethal genetically inherited disease among white children.[46] The disease is characterized by an exocrine gland dysfunction that results in abnormally viscid secretions. The sweat and saliva are not particularly viscid, but they do contain abnormally high amounts of sodium chloride. Although any organ system can be involved, the most common presentation of the disease is involvement of the pulmonary and pancreatic systems.

Etiology

CF is a hereditary disease transmitted as an autosomal recessive (Mendelian) trait. The pattern of inheritance results in a one-in-four chance of two carriers producing a child with the disease (homozygous), a two-in-four chance of producing a child who is a carrier of the disease (heterozygous), and a one-in-four chance of producing a child who is completely free of the trait. The incidence in white children is approximately 1 in 2000 live births. Although less common in the black population, 2.25 percent of all CF patients identified by the CF Foundation in 1979 were black.[47] Cystic fibrosis is rare in the Asian population.[47]

Pathophysiology

The chronic pulmonary involvement of CF results from an abnormally viscous mucus secreted by the tracheobronchial tree and hyperplasia of the mucus-secreting glands. The function of the mucociliary transport is impaired by the altered secretions, and the impairment results in airway obstruction, recurrent infection, bronchiectasis, and hyperinflation. Fibrotic changes also are found in the lung parenchyma.

Incomplete obstruction of the airways reduces ventilation to the alveolar units. A low ventilation/perfusion ratio is present with diffusion abnormalities in both oxygen and carbon dioxide. A "ball valve" situation, caused by incomplete obstruction of an airway, accounts for the hyperinflation seen in these patients. (Refer to the discussion of hyperinflation in the section on chronic bronchitis.) Complete obstruction of the airways will result in absorption atelectasis.

Clinical Presentation

The diagnosis of CF may be suspected in patients who present with a positive family history of the disease, with pneumonia or recurrent respiratory infections that are due to *Staphylococcus aureus* or *Pseudomonas aeruginosa* or with a diagnosis of malnutrition and/or failure to thrive.

The "sweat" test is diagnostic for CF. A sodium chloride concentration of 60 meq per liter in the perspiration of children is positive for the diagnosis of CF.

Acute pulmonary infections may be the first radiographic sign of the disease. Diffuse hyperinflation, increased lung marking, and atelectasis are common in advanced disease.

Pulmonary function studies show obstructive impairments, decreased FEV_1, a decreased forced vital capacity (FVC), and an increased residual volume and functional residual capacity (FRC).

Arterial blood gas values also show alterations that are due to the abnormal ventilation/perfusion relation within the lungs. Hypoxemia and hypercapnia with a chronically compensated respiratory acidosis are present.

As the disease progresses, destruction of the alveolar capillary network, hypoxemia, and hypercapnia cause pulmonary hypertension and cor pulmonale.

Course and Prognosis

Life expectancy of patients with CF has continued to increase because of advances in diagnosis and treatment. Although some patients still die in infancy and early childhood, the majority survive into adulthood.[48]

Gastrointestinal dysfunctions as a result of CF can be improved by proper diet, vitamin supplements, and the replacement of pancreatic enzymes. Treatment of the pulmonary dysfunction caused by CF centers around removal of the abnormal secretions and prompt treatment of pulmonary infections. In 90 percent of cases, pulmonary involvement is the primary cause of death.[46]

RESTRICTIVE LUNG DISEASE

Definition

Restrictive lung disease is actually a group of diseases with differing etiologies. The common link among these disorders is a difficulty in expanding the lungs and a reduction in lung volume. The restrictions can come from diseases of the alveolar parenchyma and/or the pleura that result in fibrosis of the alveoli, interstitial lung parenchyma, and pleura. The restrictions can also be caused by changes in the chest wall or in the neuromuscular apparatus.[49] For the purpose of this text, the diseases most likely to be encountered in a pulmonary rehabilitation setting will be presented, that is, restrictive diseases of the lung parenchyma and pleura. Diseases of the chest wall, such as ankylosing spondylitis and scoliosis, and neuromuscular diseases, such as Guillain-Barré, will not be discussed.

Etiology

Restrictive lung disease has a variety of causes. Numerous agents, such as x-radiation therapy, inorganic dust, inhalation of noxious gases, oxygen toxicity, asbestos exposure, and tuberculosis can damage the pulmonary parenchyma and pleura. Petty categorizes the etiology of parenchymal restriction in four ways:[50] (1) the pneumoconioses (the dust diseases leading to pulmonary fibrosis), (2) the immunologically mediated cryptogenic fibrosing alveolitis, (3) the collagen diseases, and (4) pulmonary fibrosis of unknown etiology. Pleural thickening and fibrosis can restrict the movement between the lung and the thoracic wall and thereby cause another type of restrictive disease. Radiation therapy and asbestos exposure are two of the more common causes of pleural thickening.

Pathophysiology

The particular changes occurring within the lungs depend on the etiologic factors of restrictive disease. Parenchymal changes will result in alveolar fibrosis, whereas pleural disease will cause pleural thickening and fibrosis.

Parenchymal changes often begin with chronic inflammation and a thickening of the alveoli and interstitium. As the disease progresses, distal air spaces are destroyed and replaced by fibrotic tissue, which results in an increase in the elastic recoil property of the lungs. Consequently, lung volumes are reduced. A reduced pulmonary vascular bed eventually leads to hypoxemia and cor pulmonale.

In pleural diseases, thickened plaques of collagen fibers cause fibrosis that may be found in various locations. In asbestos exposure, for example, the plaques are found on the parietal pleura. The mechanism responsible for plaque development is not completely clear. There may also be parenchymal alterations that accompany pleural diseases. These changes may be due to injury or inflammatory reactions that lead to fibrosis.

Clinical Presentation

Dyspnea is the classic symptom of restrictive lung diseases. A nonproductive cough is often encountered, and weakness and easy fatigue are common.

Signs of restrictive lung disease include rapid, shallow breathing, limited chest expansion, fine-end expiratory crackles (especially over the lower lung fields), digital clubbing, and cyanosis.

In the early stages of parenchymal restrictive disease, the chest x-ray reveals fine interstitial markings that look like ground glass. Long-standing fibrosis has radiographic evidence of diffuse infiltrates and has been likened to a honeycomb. Reduction in lung volumes can be seen serially on the chest x-ray. Roentgenographic evidence of pleural thickening also can be seen, especially on oblique films.

Pulmonary function tests reveal a reduction in vital capacity, functional residual capacity, and total lung capacity. Residual volume may be normal or near normal, and expiratory flow rates remain normal in pulmonary fibrosis. Lung compliance is significantly reduced, and diffusing capacity is diminished. Arterial blood studies show varying degrees of hypoxemia and hypocapnia. Hypoxemia is usually exacerbated by exercise. Exercise may significantly lower Pao_2 even in patients with normal resting Pao_2. Hyperventilation, which results in a lower than normal $Paco_2$, often occurs.

Course and Prognosis

Restrictive pulmonary disease may have a slow onset, but it is chronic and progressive in nature. Survival depends on the type of restrictive disease, the etiologic factor, and the treatment. Chest roentgenograms are insensitive indicators of the extent of the disease.[45] Hypercapnea is an ominous sign of the terminal stage of pulmonary fibrosis.

SUMMARY

In summary, the etiology, pathophysiology, clinical presentation, and prognosis for several diseases of the lungs were presented in this chapter.

COPD is a combination of pulmonary disorders. All types of obstructive lung diseases are associated with hyperinflation of the chest that is due to air trapping, increases in pulmonary volumes and capacities, abnormal ventilation/perfusion ratios, abnormal roentgenograms, and abnormal arterial blood gas values.

Restrictive pulmonary disease results in reduced lung volumes and capacities from a variety of causes: parenchymal disease, pleural disease, and chest wall deformities. Changes can be seen in the pulmonary volumes and capacities, roentgenograms, and arterial blood gas values.

An understanding of the underlying lung disease and its severity allows for the development of realistic patient goals and appropriate treatment programs.

REFERENCES

1. Foster, S and Thomas, H: Pulmonary rehabilitation in lung disease other than chronic obstructive pulmonary disease. Am Rev Respir Dis 141:601–604, 1990.
2. American Thoracic Society: Definitions and classification of chronic bronchitis, asthma, and pulmonary emphysema. Am Rev Respir Dis 85:762–768, 1962.
3. Petty, T (ed): Management of Chronic Obstructive Lung Diseases. Conclusion of the Eighth Aspen Emphysema Conference. US Public Health Service Publication No 1457, May 1966.
4. National Heart, Lung and Blood Institute, Division of Lung Diseases Workshop Report. The definition of emphysema. Am Rev Respir Dis 132:182–185, 1985.
5. American Thoracic Society. Standards for the diagnosis and care of patients with chronic obstructive pulmonary disease (COPD) and asthma, 1987. Am Rev Respir Dis 136:1987.
6. Hodgkin, J and Petty, T: Chronic Obstructive Pulmonary Disease. Current Concepts. WB Saunders, Philadelphia, 1987.
7. Sharma, O and Balchum, O: Key Facts in Pulmonary Disease. Churchill Livingstone, New York, 1983.
8. Farzan, S: A Concise Handbook of Respiratory Diseases. ed 2. Reston Publishing, Reston, VA, 1985.
9. Prince, S and Wilson, L: Pathophysiology: Clinical Concepts of Disease Processes, ed 3. McGraw-Hill, New York, 1986.
10. Thurlbeck, ZW: Chronic airflow obstruction in lung disease. In Major Problems in Pathology, Vol V. WB Saunders, Philadelphia, 1978.
11. Niewoehner, D, Kleinerman, J and Rice, D: Pathologic changes in the peripheral airways of young cigarette smokers. N Engl J Med 291:755–758, 1974.
12. Sheldon, J: Boyd's Introduction to the Study of Disease, ed 10. Lea & Febiger, Philadelphia, 1988.
13. Chronic Obstructive Pulmonary Disease: A Manual for Physicians, ed 3. National Tuberculosis and Respiratory Disease Association, 1972.
14. Morris, J (chairman): Chronic Obstructive Pulmonary Disease. American Lung Association Publication, 1981.

15. Burrows, B: Prognostic factors in chronic obstructive pulmonary disease. Prac Cardiol 6:61–69, 1980.
16. Travers G, Cline, M and Burrows, B: Predictors of mortality in chronic obstructive pulmonary disease. Am Rev Respir Dis 119:895–902, 1979.
17. Nemeny, B, et al: Changes in lung function after smoking cessation: An assessment from a cross sectional survey. Am Rev Respir Dis 125:122–124, 1982.
18. Cosio, M, et al: The relationship between structural changes in small airways and pulmonary function tests. N Engl J Med 298:1277–1281, 1977.
19. Macklen, P and Mead J: Resistance of peripheral airways measured by a retrograde catheter. J Appl Physiol 22:395–401, 1967.
20. McFadden, E, et al: Small airway disease: An assessment of the tests of peripheral airway function. Am J Med 57:171–182, 1974.
21. Wright J, et al: The detection of small airways disease. Am Rev Respir Dis 129:989–994, 1984.
22. Nagai, A, West, W and Thurbeck, W: The National Institute of Health: Intermittent positve pressure breathing trial, Pathology Study II. Am Rev Respir Dis 132:946–953, 1985.
23. The fate of the chronic bronchitic: A report of the 10 year follow-up in the Canadian Department of Veterans' Affairs coordinated study of chronic bronchitis. Am Rev Respir Dis 108:1043–1065, 1973.
24. Hutchinson, D, et al: Longitudinal studies in alpha$_1$-antitrypsin deficiency: A survey by the British Thoracic Society. In Taylor, J and Mittman, C: Pulmonary Emphysema and Proteolysis: 1986. Academic Press, London, 1987.
25. Janis, E, Phillips, N and Carrell, R: Smoking alpha$_1$-antitrypsin deficiency and emphysema. In Taylor, J and Mittman, C: Pulmonary Emphysema and Proteolysis: 1986. Academic Press, London, 1987.
26. Pugatch, R: The radiology of emphysema. Clin Chest Med 3:433–442, 1983.
27. Burr, M, et al: Changes in asthma prevalence: Two surveys 15 years apart. Arch Dis Child 64(10):1452–1456, 1989.
28. Gergen, P, Mullally, D and Evans, R: National survey of prevalence of asthma among children in US, 1976–1980. Pediatrics 81:1–7, 1988.
29. Sibbald, B, et al: Genetic factors in childhood asthma. Thorax 35:671–674, 1980.
30. Burney, P: Prevalence and mortality from asthma. In P Vermeeire, M Demedts, and J Vernault (eds): Progress in Asthma and COPD. Elsevier, Amsterdam, The Netherlands, 1989.
31. Stevensen, D, et al: Provoking factors in bronchial asthma. Arch Intern Med 135:777–783, 1975.
32. Fielding, J: Smoking: Health effects and control, Part I. N Engl J Med 313(8):491–498, 1985.
33. Anderson, S, et al: Exercise induced asthma: A review. Br J Dis Chest 69:1–39, 1975.
34. Tal, A, et al: Response to cold air hyperventilation in normal and asthmatic children. J Pediatr 104:516–521, 1984.
35. Gilbert, I, Fouke, J and McFadden, E: Heat and water flux in the intrathoracic airways and exercise induced asthma. J Appl Physiol 63:1681–1691, 1987.
36. Berman, B and Ross, R: Exercise induced bronchospasm: Is it a unique clinical entity? Ann Allerg 65(2):81–83, 1990.
37. Anderson, S: Current concepts of exercise induced asthma. Allergy, 38:289–302, 1983.
38. Strauss, R, et al: Influence of heat and humidity on the airway obstruction induced by exercise in asthma. J Clin Invest 61:433–440, 1978.
39. Noviski, N, et al: Exercise intensity determines and climatic conditions modify the severity of exercise induced asthma. Am Rev Respir Dis 136:592–594, 1987.
40. Matheson, D and Stevensen, D: Bronchopulmonary diseases: Immunologic perspectives. Post Grad Med 54:105–111, 1973.
41. Burki, N: Pulmonary Diseases. Medical Examination Publishing, Garden City, NY, 1982.
42. Berte, J: Critical Care: The Lungs, ed 2. Appleton-Century-Crofts, Norwalk, CT, 1986.
43. Daves, P, et al: Familial Bronchiectasis. J Pediatr 102:177–185, 1983.
44. Corbeel, L, et al: Ultrastructural abnormalities of bronchial cilia in children with recurrent airway infections and bronchiectasis. Arch Dis Child 56:929–933, 1981.
45. Williams, M: Essentials of Pulmonary Medicine. WB Saunders, Philadelphia, 1982.
46. Wood, R, Boat, T and Doershuk, C: State of the art: Cystic fibrosis. Am Rev Respir Dis 113:833, 1976.
47. Tecklin, J: Pediatric Physical Therapy. JB Lippincott, Philadelphia, 1989.
48. Murphy, S: Cystic fibrosis in adults: Diagnosis and management. Clin Chest Med 8:695, 1987.
49. West, J: Pulmonary Pathophysiology: The Essentials. Williams & Wilkins, Baltimore, 1977.
50. Petty, T: Chronic Lung Disease: A Practical Office Approach to Early Diagnosis and Management. Breon Laboratories Inc, New York, 1975.

CHAPTER 7

The Medical and Surgical Management of Cardiopulmonary Disease

CORONARY ARTERY DISEASE

The medical and surgical management of coronary artery disease (CAD) is as diverse as the symptoms displayed by individuals with the disease. Each year, as surgical techniques are more finely perfected and new pharmacologic agents are developed and tested, the outlook becomes brighter for individuals with CAD. In all cases, treatment is aimed at relieving symptoms and slowing the progression of the disease. Many individuals have had their symptoms managed by a variety of therapies, and the therapies coupled with appropriate lifestyle modifications have allowed them to obtain and maintain an optimal level of well-being.

In this chapter, the pharmacologic agents commonly used in the medical management of acute and chronic CAD and medications administered in pulmonary disease are reviewed. Surgical interventions, including myocardial revascularization and percutaneous transluminal angioplasty, are discussed. The identification of cardiac rehabilitation as an important adjunct to therapy is addressed.

Medical Management

The main thrust of the medical management of CAD concerns the various pharmacologic agents specifically used in the long-term treatment of CAD and its symptoms: nitrates, beta-blocking agents, antiarrhythmics, cardiac glycosides, calcium channel blockers, and antihypertensives. Treatment is directed toward preventing myocardial ischemia and infarction while maximizing and improving the existing cardiac function.

114

NITRATES

Nitrates are classified in two groups: those that act rapidly to eliminate acute anginal attacks and those that are of prolonged duration to prevent anginal attacks. Table 7–1 outlines various preparations of nitrates.

Actions and Uses

Nitrates are vasodilators used in the first-line management of all types of angina. By acting directly on the smooth muscles of the vessel walls, nitrates cause general vasodilation throughout the body. This peripheral vasodilation results in venous pooling, decreased blood return to the heart, decreased left ventricular dimensions, and decreased diastolic filling pressure. The decreased preload, together with decreased afterload (a result of decreased arterial wall tone), significantly reduces the myocardial oxygen demand and may relieve angina or delay its onset. Nitrates may also dilate normal coronary arteries and cause redistribution of blood flow to ischemic areas.[2]

Contraindications and Side Effects

The side effects of nitrates include tachycardia, hypotension, flushing, and headache, all related to generalized vasodilation.

Effects on Exercise in Individuals with Coronary Artery Disease

Anginal pain, often experienced at low levels of exercise by individuals with CAD, results from inadequate cardiac reserve. The heart cannot meet the increased oxygen demand of exercise. Nitrates, given prior to exercise or administered chronically, reduce cardiac work load and improve exercise performance. This is evidenced by an increased tolerance for activity before the onset of anginal pain and/or ischemic electrocardiographic (ECG) changes.

Nitrate Therapy Management

Careful consideration should be given to the following:

1. Administer sublingual nitrate, if prescribed, at the onset of chest pain.
2. Monitor blood pressure. Observe for symptoms of hypotension (light-headedness, dizziness, decreased urine output). Have the individual lie down.
3. If pain is unrelieved by three doses of nitroglycerin (one tablet every 5 minutes), institute the appropriate procedure for obtaining emergency medical care.

BETA-BLOCKING AGENTS

Actions and Uses

Beta-blocking agents (Table 7–2) reduce myocardial oxygen demand by decreasing the heart rate and depressing contractility. They increase diastolic fill and perfusion time

TABLE 7–1 Nitrates: Acute and Chronic Management[1,2,5,25]

Generic Name (Trade Name)	Mode of Administration and Dosage	a. Onset b. Peak Action	Duration of Action	Implications for the Individual with CAD
Acute Management				
Nitroglycerin (Nitrostat)	Sublingual: $\frac{1}{100}-\frac{1}{400}$g prn (for acute anginal pain) IV dosage titrated to relieve pain	a. 2 min b. 5 min a. Immediate	10–15 min 10 min	Nitroglycerin should be taken with onset of chest pain and repeated every 5 min × 3 doses. Additional medical attention should be obtained if pain is not relieved after 15 min.
Isosorbide dinitrate (Isordil)	Sublingual/ chewable: 2.5–5.0 mg	a. 3–5 min b. 15–30 min	1–2 hr	Individual should be seated to prevent light-headedness. Keep nitroglycerin in dark-glass bottle
Chronic Management				
Isosorbide dinitrate (Isordil, Sorbitrate)	po: 5–30 mg QID	a. 20 min b. 30–45 min	½–2 hr	Tolerance may develop.
Nitroglycerin (sustained-release) (Nitro-Bid, Nitrospan)	po: 2.5–6.5 mg tablet q8–12 hr	a. 30 min b. 3–4 hr	8–12 hr	
Nitroglycerin (Topical) (Nitro-Bid, Nitrol)	Topical: ½–4 in ribbon of ointment	a. 30 min	3–4 hr	Ointment may be placed on any body part. Ointment should be covered with a plastic-coated paper for better absorption.
Nitroglycerin transdermal patches (Nitro-Dur, Transderm)	Topical patch: QD 26–154 mg	a. 30 min	24 hr	Ease of administration may increase compliance. Placing patches on the upper thigh may decrease headache. Some individuals experience without compromising effectiveness.

TABLE 7–2 Beta-Blocking Agents[1,3–6]

Generic Name (Trade Name)	Dosage	Therapeutic Uses	Implications
Propranolol hydrochloride (Inderal)	10–12 mg BID to QID. Extremely variable dosages and varied uses.	Hypertension, angina, some arrhythmias (PAT). Postinfarct to prevent reinfarction. Migraine headaches.	Limit smoking because it may result in elevated blood pressure.[3] Caution patient that sudden cessation of drugs may cause an exacerbation of angina.
Metoprolol (Lopressor)	100–450 mg/day single dose or TID. Cardioselective at lower doses.[1]	Hypertension, angina, some arrhythmias	Cardioselective beta-blockers should be administered to individuals with lung disease.
Nadolol (Corgard)	40–320 mg/day single dose or TID	Hypertension, angina, some arrhythmias	
Timolol (Blocadren)	10 mg BID Ophthalmic— 0.25% solution	Postinfarction to prevent reinfarction. To decrease intraocular pressure. Hypertension, angina.	
Atenolol (Tenormin)	50–100 mg/day single dose Cardioselective at low doses.	Hypertension, angina	
Pindolol (Visken)	10–60 mg TID or QID	Hypertension, some arrhythmias	This beta-blocker possesses some intrinsic sympathetic activity (ISA), which is most apparent at rest, producing less resting bradycardia.[1]
Labetolol (Trandate/ Normadyne)		Hypertensive crisis	Alpha-blockade causes vasodilation.
Sotalol	80–320 mg BID	Arrhythmias (SVT/ VT) hypertension	Both beta-blockade and antiarrhythmic properties.[33] Class III antiarrhythmic.
Esmolol (Brevibloc)	IV only	Postoperative atrial fibrillation and flutter	Cardioselect. Only for intravenous use; extremely brief half-life (<10 min)
Acebutolol (Sectral)	200–600 mg BID	Cardioselect	ISA

(thereby increasing blood supply to the myocardium) as a result of decreasing the heart rate. Competing with epinephrine for available beta-receptor sites in the heart and other tissues, beta-blockers inhibit the normal response to adrenergic stimuli. Blocking the beta receptors of the sympathetic nervous system decreases the heart rate, atrioventricular (AV) conduction, contractility, and automaticity in the heart and bronchoconstriction in the lungs. There are $beta_1$ and $beta_2$ receptor sites. $Beta_1$ sites are primarily in the heart, and $beta_2$ sites are in the lungs and throughout the body. Beta-blockers that work specifically on $beta_1$ sites are referred to as cardioselective.

Beta-blockers are used in combination with nitrates for the treatment of chest pain in effort angina. They relieve chest pain by decreasing oxygen demand and restoring the balance of oxygen demand and supply.

Beta-blockers are contraindicated in Prinzmetal angina/variant angina because they allow alpha-adrenergic activity (vasoconstriction) to predominate. They are used in the treatment of mild hypertension and cardiac arrhythmias because they decrease sinoatrial (SA) node automaticity and slow conduction through the AV node. They also affect etiologic factors (i.e., catecholamine release) responsible for arrhythmias. Following an acute myocardial infarction (MI), beta-blockers can be used to salvage ischemic myocardium by decreasing myocardial oxygen demand.

Many of the beta-blockers currently available are listed in Table 7–2. Pindolol (Visken) possesses some intrinsic sympathetic activity (ISA). Beta-blockers with ISA may be advantageous in that little, if any, slowing of the heart rate, depression of contractility, or slowing of AV conduction occur at rest when sympathetic activity is low. The effects of beta-blockers with ISA are similar to the effects of other beta-blockers during exercise.[1] The slightly higher than anticipated resting heart rate in individuals taking pindolol reflects this intrinsic sympathetic activity.[1]

Contraindications and Side Effects

Beta-blockers must be used cautiously in patients with chronic lung disease because blockade of $beta_2$ receptor sites in the lung may cause bronchospasm. Cardioselect beta-blockers may be preferred for individuals with insulin-dependent diabetes because $beta_2$ receptors control glucose release from glycogen stores, so nonselect beta-blockade may prolong insulin-induced hypoglycemia. Patients with mild congestive heart failure (CHF) may benefit from the decreased heart rate caused by beta-blockers, but beta-blockers are contraindicated in individuals with more severe CHF. In the latter individuals, beta-blockers further decrease contractility and the cardiac output and, therefore, further increase the failure. Beta-blockers are also contraindicated in variant angina.

Side effects of beta-blockers include bronchospasm, hypotension, drug fever, gastrointestinal disturbances, transient thrombocytopenia, fatigue and sleep disorders, and sexual disorders. Abrupt cessation of beta-blockers may bring on a recurrence of anginal pain, arrhythmias, or sudden death. Individuals should be cautioned about the importance of titrating the drug when it is to be discontinued.

Effects on Exercise in Individuals with Coronary Artery Disease

Therapy with beta-blockers results in increased exercise tolerance and increased aerobic capacity.[9] The individual taking beta-blockers experiences a decrease in both resting and submaximal heart rate and blood pressure. Therefore, there is a decrease in the rate pressure product (the cardiac work load) and myocardial oxygen demand. Higher levels of activity are attained before the individual's ischemic threshold is reached and anginal pain or ECG changes occur.

Beta-Adrenergic Blockade Therapy Management

Careful consideration should be given to the following:

1. Individuals should be cautioned never to abruptly stop taking beta-blockers.
2. Increases in heart rate normally seen with exercise are lower in individuals on beta-blockers.
3. Changes in beta-blockade therapy necessitate a repeat graded exercise test and reassessment of the exercise prescription.
4. Observe for any change in respiratory effort, dyspnea.

CALCIUM CHANNEL BLOCKERS

Calcium channel blockers (Table 7-3) inhibit the flow of calcium ions across the membranes of myocardial and vascular smooth muscle cells. Calcium plays an important role in myocardial contractility, vasomotor tone, and cardiac electrical activity (Chapter 2).

TABLE 7-3 Calcium Channel Blockers[1,3,5,8]

Generic Name (Trade Name)	Dosage	Therapeutic Uses	Effects on Cardiovascular System
Diltiazem (Cardizem)	30 mg TID to QID (to maximum of 240 mg/24 hr)[5]	Angina and hypertension, some arrhythmias	Dilates coronary arteries. Antiarrhythmic action. Some decrease in contractility.
Nifedipine (Procardia)	Initially 10 mg TID. Maintenance 10-30 mg TID or QID	Angina, hypertension	Potent peripheral vasodilator. Dilates coronary arteries.
Verapamil (Calan, Isopton)	Initially 80 mg q 6-8 hr; 320-480 mg in divided doses	Angina, tachyarrhythmias	Slows AV conduction (negative chronotropic* effect; negative inotropic* effect). Some peripheral and coronary dilation. May cause rise in serum digoxin level.

*The effects of autonomic stimulation on the heart may be classified as (1) chronotropic — affecting heart rate and (2) inotropic — affecting contractility. "Positive" and "negative" are used to describe the responses of the heart to a drug. (For example, a drug that increases contractility has a positive inotropic effect.)[7]

There are four categories of calcium channel blockers: (1) cardioactive agents, (2) dihydropyridine vasoactive agents, (3) piperazine vasoactive agents, and (4) mixed sodium and calcium channel blockers. Currently, only three calcium channel blockers are approved for use in the treatment of hypertension, angina, and heart arrhythmias: verapamil (Isopton, Calan/Category I), nifidipine (Procardia/Category II), and diltiazem (Cardizem/Category I). All other agents, including all those in categories III and IV, were still under investigation in 1989.[39]

Verapamil, the prototype drug for this category, decreases myocardial oxygen demand in three ways. It decreases afterload by peripheral vasodilation and it decreases heart rate (negative chronotropic effect) and contractility (negative inotropic effect). Verapamil is used in the treatment of arrhythmias, specifically, supraventricular tachycardias. Diltiazem acts through these same mechanisms, but the effects are not as strong as those of verapamil.

Nifedipine is a strong peripheral vasodilator, and it decreases myocardial oxygen demand by that mechanism. However, it has no direct effect on heart rate or contractility, and it has no antiarrhythmic properties. It may cause a reflex increase in heart rate in response to vasodilation. Nifedipine is the calcium channel blocker most safely used in individuals with CHF and is a preferred therapy in the treatment of variant angina.

Calcium channel blockers are also used in the treatment of hypertension. They can be used in combination with nitrates to treat effort angina and the angina of coronary artery spasm. They may also be used in combination with beta-blockers in the treatment of effort angina because they permit the use of lower doses of the beta-blockers and avoid the undesirable effects of beta-blockade.[1] Calcium channel blockers neither constrict the bronchial tree nor aggravate coronary and peripheral vascular spasm, characteristics that make them more desirable than some beta-blockers. Calcium channel blockade therapy results in decreased myocardial contractility, vasomotor tone, peripheral vascular resistance, and heart rate, the latter because of slower impulse conduction. The result is a decrease in myocardial oxygen demand.

Contraindications and Side Effects

Calcium channel blockers are contraindicated in moderate to severe CHF, significant hypotension, aortic stenosis, and sick sinus syndrome.

Side effects occur in approximately 17 percent of individuals on calcium channel blockade therapy.[3] They include hypotension, reflex tachycardia, peripheral edema, and headache. Central nervous system side effects include tremors, mood changes, and fatigue. Gastrointestinal distress and skin reactions also have been reported. Nifedipine can cause significant noncardiac pedal edema.

Effects on Exercise in Individuals with Coronary Artery Disease

The decreased myocardial oxygen demand and improved myocardial blood supply may improve an individual's tolerance for activity.

Calcium Channel Blockade Therapy Management

Careful consideration should be given to the following:

1. Observe the individual for symptoms of postural hypotension (light-headedness upon arising, tachycardia, and pallor).

2. Monitor blood pressure (poorly tolerated hypotension has occurred during initial titration or at the time of subsequent upward dosage adjustment and may be more likely to occur in individuals on concomitant beta-blockers).

CARDIAC GLYCOSIDES

The most common cardiac glycosides include digitalis, digitoxin, digoxin (Lanoxin), and Quabain.

Actions and Uses

The exact mechanism of action of cardiac glycosides is unknown. They are believed to increase the influx of calcium into the myocardial cell. They also alter the electrochemical properties of the cell by their effect on the active transport of sodium and potassium.

Cardiac glycosides have both a positive intropic effect (increasing the contractility) and a negative chronotropic effect (decreasing the heart rate). The associated decreased heart rate may result from the vagal stimulation initiated by carotid baroreceptors when increased systolic pressure is sensed.[5] Although these effects are seen in the healthy heart, they are more significant in the failing heart.[3] Increased contractility increases the cardiac output and decreases preload, cardiac work load, and myocardial oxygen demand. That, in turn, reduces CHF.

Cardiac glycosides act directly on the heart rate by increasing the refractory period of the AV node and Purkinje fibers. They also increase the excitability of the Purkinje fibers, but they have only a variable effect on the excitability of the ventricles and have no effect on the excitability of the atrium. Cardiac glycosides have little effect on the pacemaker automaticity of the SA node, but they increase the automaticity of the Purkinje fibers.

Cardiac glycosides are the drugs of choice in the treatment and control of CHF. The increased contractility improves oxygen delivery to all tissues. Increased renal perfusion results in a diuretic effect, which decreases circulating blood volume. Circulatory volume is further decreased by diuretic therapy administered in conjunction with the cardiac glycosides in the treatment of heart failure. Although they relieve the symptoms of CHF, cardiac glycosides do not relieve the cause.

Cardiac glycosides are also used to treat and control certain arrhythmias, including atrial fibrillation, atrial flutter, and atrial tachycardia. Digoxin (Lanoxin) is the most commonly prescribed cardiac glycoside.

Contraindications and Side Effects

In general, the aforementioned drugs have a relatively narrow margin of safety between therapeutic range and toxic range. Levels near or in the toxic range may be very poorly tolerated. Toxicity is assessed on the basis of blood levels. Characteristic ECG changes associated with toxicity include bradycardia, prolongation of the PR interval (first-degree heart block), and a shortening of the QT interval. Other arrhythmias may be observed as the conduction blockade at the AV node increases. Premature ventricular contractions, ventricular tachycardia, and supraventricular tachycardia may all be caused by the alteration in conduction in digitalis toxicity. Because it can precipitate almost any arrhythmia, digoxin must always be viewed as suspect when an individual taking digoxin suddenly develops an arrhythmia.[42] Other side effects include nausea, vomiting, anorexia, drowsiness, fatigue, and confusion. Visual disturbances, such as seeing yellow or green dots and experiencing double vision, are common.[3] Toxicity is facilitated by electrolyte imbalances, particularly hypokalemia.

Cardiac glycoside therapy is contraindicated in individuals with idiopathic hypertrophic subaortic stenosis (IHSS), diffuse cardiomyopathies, and constrictive pericarditis. Cardiac glycosides are contraindicated in preexisting AV block. They are also contraindicated in individuals with increased cardiac automaticity, in which increased AV conduction time may precipitate tachyarrhythmias. In acute MI, cardiac glycoside therapy may be contraindicated because the increased contractility increases myocardial oxygen demand and may extend an infarction.

Effects on Exercise in Individuals with Coronary Artery Disease

The individual with CHF receiving cardiac glycoside therapy will demonstrate increased exercise tolerance because of the increased efficiency of the ventricular function and oxygen utilization. The ST-T wave changes associated with cardiac glycoside therapy may mimic the ECG changes of ischemia. Evaluation of the individual's rhythm strip or 12-lead ECG at rest and exercise will permit definitive diagnosis.

Cardiac Glycosides Therapy Management

Careful consideration should be given to the following:

1. Familiarity with the effect of cardiac glycosides on the ECG is essential. The sagging ST segment may be mistaken for the ST-depression seen in ischemia.
2. Arrhythmias associated with cardiac glycosides may be precipitated by exercise, especially if the patient is hypokalemic.
3. Individuals should learn to check their peripheral pulses daily and report bradycardia or sustained tachycardia.
4. Nausea and vomiting are classic signs of digoxin toxicity. (Hypokalemia from persistent vomiting may precipitate toxicity.)
5. Maintenance doses of digoxin, the most commonly prescribed cardiac glycoside, are 0.125 to 0.25 mg QD. Elderly individuals usually require smaller doses.
6. Caution should be taken during exercise because of the potential visual disturbances associated with cardiac glycosides.

ANTIARRHYTHMICS

Antiarrhythmic drugs alter the conductivity and automaticity of the myocardium to correct abnormalities in electrical activity. Generally, they suppress ectopic stimuli (impulses arising outside the sinoatrial node, the normal pacemaker of the heart), slow the rate of impulse generation and conduction, and decrease myocardial irritability.

There are four recognized classes of antiarrhythmics (Table 7–4). They are classified according to their mechanism of action.[1,38,39]

TABLE 7–4 Common Antiarrhythmics

Generic Name (Trade Name)	Dosage	Class	ECG Changes	Implications/Side Effects
Quinidine sulfate (Quinidex)	200–400 mg q 4–6 hr	IA	Prolonged QT interval.	Severe nausea and diarrhea may make it intolerable.
Quinidine gluconate (Quinaglute)	324 mg q 6 hr	IA	Widened QRS complex.	Observe ECG for prolonged QT interval of greater than 25%
Procainamide hydrochloride (Pronestyl)	250–500 mg q 3–4 hr	IA	Prolonged QT interval. Does increase AV conduction.	Use cautiously in digoxin toxicity, CHF.
Sustained release (Procan SR)	500–1000 mg q 6 hr	IA		IV injection can cause severe hypotension. Systemic lupus erythematous syndrome may develop.
Disopyramide (Norpace)	400–800 mg/day in divided doses	IA	Significant widening of QRS. May cause second- or third-degree heart block.	Use cautiously with urinary retention or glaucoma. Specific for ventricular arrhythmias. May cause cardiac decompensation.
Lidocaine (Xylocaine)	50–100 mg IV rapidly. Repeat if necessary, followed by continuous intravenous drip titrated to control PVCs	IB	Negligible ECG effects. Decrease or elimination of ventricular ectopy.	May cause disorientation, seizures. IM injection may be used to control PVCs (for 1 hr) until emergency center is reached.[3] May cause hypotension.
Mexiletine (Mexitil)	300–900 mg QD in 3–4 doses	IB	Usually no change	Well absorbed in GI tract. Best efficacy when given with class IA agent. Minimize GI symptoms by giving with food. Lower doses used when given in combination with another drug (Class IA or beta-blocker) are better tolerated.[40]

Continued

123

TABLE 7–4 Common Antiarrhythmics *Continued*

Generic Name (Trade Name)	Dosage	Class	ECG Changes	Implications/ Side Effects
Encainide (Enkaid)	25 mg TID up to 200 mg TID (Dosage increased gradually to prevent overshooting of desired effects or proarrhythmic effects[39]	IC	Widened QRS (dose-dependent)	Has few or no clinically significant hemodynamic effects with chronic therapy. Neurotoxicity prominent.[39]
Flecainide (Tambocor)	100–200 mg BID (dosage increased gradually because of proarrhythmic effect)	IC	PR, QRS, and QT intervals are prolonged (dose-dependent). Greater than 25% increase indicates toxicity.[39]	Few hemodynamic effects. Effective in suppressing arrhythmias refractory to other drugs. Has proarrhythmic effect, so benefit of therapy must outweigh this risk. Proarrhythmic effect; benefit of therapy must outweigh risk. May worsen arrhythmias 10–15%
Propranolol (Inderal)	10–30 mg TID or QID	II	Increases PR interval. Slight decrease in the QT interval.	High doses may be necessary to control SVT. Observe for hypotension. Increases in heart rate with exercise will be less than in individual not on beta-blockade.
Bretylium (Bretylol)	5–10 mg/kg IV over 30 min (Acute care setting only)	III	May potentiate digitalis toxicity. Observe for prolonged PR interval. Resolution of ventricular arrhythmias.	May be used in stress-related or sympathetic-nervous-system-triggered arrhythmias. Used in the acute care setting to treat refractory VT and VF. Hypotension is common. Nausea/vomiting may occur with rapid infusion; relieved by decreasing rate of infusion.

124

Drug	Dosage	Class	ECG Effects	Comments
Amiodarone (Cordarone)	200–400 mg/day (greater than 400 mg/day associated with an increase in morbidity)	III	Slightly prolonged PR interval. Marked prolongation of QT. Prominent U waves in precordial leads. Sinus rate decreased 15–20% Severe bradycardia with toxicity	Not well tolerated chronically because of multiple side effects.[39] Toxicity has limited its utilization. Increases serum digoxin levels. Interferes unpredictably with coumadin. Little hemodynamic effect. Toxicity occurs over wide range of plasma concentrations, even clinically useful levels. Most patients experience side effects. Most common is pulmonary infiltrates (10%–20%). All side effects resolve slowly with discontinuation of drug (over 6–12 mos.)[38,39] Recurrence of life-threatening arrhythmias remains high (approx. 40%).[38]
Verapamil (Calan, Isopton)	IV 0.1 to 0.15 mg/kg to treat SVT initially; maintenance oral dose 40–160 mg q 8 hr	IV	Decreased heart rate. Control of SVT. Increased PR interval.	Observe for hypotension (infrequent). Contraindicated in CHF, cardiogenic shock, hypotension. Observe for reflux increase in heart rate with decreased cardiac output. Superior to digoxin in controlling atrial fibrillation.[3]

Class I agents: Suppress sodium (Na^+) channels and reduce conduction velocity.

IA: Quinidinelike drugs: Depress cell membrane responsiveness by depressing the voltage-dependent sodium current; delay repolarization and lengthen action potential.

IB: Inhibit the current in the fast sodium ion channels; accelerate depolarization and shorten action potential duration.

IC: Inhibit the fast inward sodium current and inhibit conduction to the His-Purkinje system; QRS prolongation.

Class II agents: Beta-blocking agents; block sympathetic receptors.

Class III agents: Act selectively on repolarization and reentry circuits and are most effective in abolishing ventricular fibrillation; prolong action potential.

Class IV agents: Depress calcium (Ca^{2+}) channels; calcium channel blockers.

Antiarrhythmics are used to restore normal heart rhythm. This benefits the individual hemodynamically by allowing the heart to work efficiently and therefore, the individual experiences an improved activity tolerance. Asymptomatic arrhythmias or those that do not leave the individual at substantial risk for a life-threatening arrhythmia may be left untreated. It must be remembered that all antiarrhythmics are cardiac depressants and must be administered with caution when either electrical or mechanical depression of the myocardium is present.[1] In addition, all antiarrhythmics may potentiate or generate the very arrhythmias they are designed to suppress, which is known as their proarrhythmic effect.

Currently, an explosion of antiarrhythmic agents are being developed and tested, many for the treatment of ventricular arrhythmias. The agents discussed in this chapter are only those currently approved for use in clinical situations.

Class I

All class I antiarrhythmics suppress sodium (Na^+) channels, but they differ in regard to depolarization and repolarization. They are therefore divided into classes IA, IB, and IC.

CLASS IA

Class IA drugs are effective in the treatment of both atrial and ventricular arrhythmias, including atrial fibrillation, premature ventricular contractions, and ventricular tachycardia. Because they have little or no effect on the SA node, they are not effective against disturbances in SA node function. They cause a prolongation of the relative refractory period and a dose-related slowing of the AV junctional and interventricular conduction. Initial therapy may accelerate AV conduction, and therefore digitalis is always administered prior to these drugs in treatment of supraventricular arrhythmias.[1]

Two marked ECG changes seen with class IA antiarrhythmics are a 25 to 50 percent elongation of the QRS complex and QT interval. Therapy with these antiarrhythmics should be discontinued if ECG changes are observed because the increase in the vulnerable period of the ventricle can lead to the development of polymorphous ventricular tachycardia (VT), or torsade de pointes. Characterized by bursts of VT and an undulating QRS axis that cannot be converted by conventional antiarrhythmics, torsade de pointes is usually associated with bradycardia, prolongation of the QT interval, and hypokalemia. Progression to ventricular fibrillation is common and life-threatening.[47] Class IA antiarrhythmics are administered with caution to patients with CHF. Table 7–4 includes some of the common class IA antiarrhythmics.

Quinidine is one of the best-known class IA antiarrhythmics. The drug is used only to treat atrial arrhythmias, although it is also effective for ventricular arrhythmias. It is contraindicated in patients who are hypersensitive to it or who have conduction defects of the AV node, digitalis toxicity, or potassium imbalance. The most common side effects are severe nausea, diarrhea, and arrhythmias, including torsade de pointes. Quinidine is now used less often in the treatment of certain arrhythmias because of the development of other equally effective drugs that do not cause as significant side effects.

Procainamide is another class IA antiarrhythmic commonly used in the treatment of both atrial and ventricular arrhythmias. It is, however, more specific to ventricular arrhythmias. It controls cardiac arrhythmias by decreasing myocardial automaticity, decreasing conduction velocity, and increasing the relative refractory period of the myocardial cells. It does not cause a change in myocardial oxygen demand during dynamic exercise, but it may mask ST depression. Gastrointestinal disturbances and fatigue are common side effects. Chronic therapy may result in systemic lupus erythematosus (SLE) syndrome.

Class IA Antiarrhythmic Therapy Management

Careful consideration should be given to the following:

1. Observe the ECG for prolongation of the QRS or QT interval.
2. Observe ECG for the development of new or recurrent arrhythmias.
3. Quinidine may reduce the risk of exercise-induced arrhythmias, but it may result in exertional ST-segment depression.
4. With procainamide, arthriticlike joint pains may be the first sign of SLE syndrome.
5. Observe for CHF, because class IA antiarrhythmics are myocardial depressants.

CLASS IB

Class IB agents accelerate repolarization as well as shorten action potential duration. The QT segment is therefore not prolonged. The agents are specific to ventricular arrhythmias. Lidocaine, mexiletine, tocainide, and phenytoin sodium are the currently available class IB agents (Table 7–4).

Lidocaine is the antiarrhythmic most commonly used in the treatment of acute premature ventricular contractions and ventricular arrhythmias. It is also used prophylactically to prevent ventricular arrhythmias in the first few days after an MI. Lidocaine is administered only intravenously; it acts specifically on the Purkinje fibers. The sinus rate and atrial arrhythmias do not appear to be affected by lidocaine.[38]

Tocainide and mexiletine, given orally, act similarly to lidocaine and are used in the chronic management of ventricular arrhythmias. Although class IB agents rarely cause adverse cardiac effects, they may cause numerous neurological and gastrointestinal (GI) side effects, including nausea, vomiting, tremors, confusion, and seizures.

Dilantin (phenytoin sodium) depresses impulse formation and accelerates AV conduction. The drug is used primarily to treat arrhythmias associated with digitalis toxicity.

Class IB drugs are often used in conjunction with class IA drugs for maximum control of arrhythmias with minimal dosage.

Class IB Antiarrhythmic Therapy Management

Careful consideration should be given to the following:

1. Give mexiletine and tocainide with food to minimize GI upset.
2. Monitor blood pressure (BP) with lidocaine, because the drug may cause severe hypotension.
3. Do not give lidocaine for idioventricular rhythm, because it may cause asystole.
4. In the cardiac rehabilitation setting, parameters for administration and the dosage of lidocaine should be identified for each individual depending his or her individual rhythm and pattern of ectopy. (The rule of thumb is lidocaine 1 mg/kg of body weight intravenous push for greater than three PVCs in a row or six PVCs per minute.)
5. Observe for mental status changes.

CLASS IC

Only two agents are currently approved for class IC use: flecainide (Tambocor) and encainide (Enkaid). They are the most potent class I antiarrhythmics. Class IC agents inhibit His-Purkinje conduction and cause a widening of the QRS complex, but they have little effect on repolarization. They are usually not the initial therapy for arrhythmias because they are highly proarrhythmic. Side effects include visual disturbances and negative inotropic effects on the myocardium.

Class IC Antiarrhythmic Therapy Management

Careful consideration should be given to the following:

1. Monitor for proarrhythmic effects (increased ventricular ectopy).
2. Administer with caution to individuals with CHF.

Class II

Antiarrhythmics in class II are beta-blockers. They block sympathetic stimulation at the SA node, increase the effective refractory period of the AV node, and reduce automaticity in the Purkinje fibers. Propranolol (Inderal) is currently the only beta-blocker approved by the Food and Drug Administration (FDA) for use as an antiarrhythmic.[3]

Propranolol effectively slows ventricular response in individuals with supraventricular tachycardias (SVT). The drug is effective in the treatment of SVT precipitated by CAD or exercise.

Contraindications include heart block, CHF, and bradyarrhythmias that are due to the negative inotropic effect of propranolol. Propranolol is given with caution to diabetic patients because their sympathetic responses to hypoglycemia may be masked.

Side effects include an exacerbation of CHF secondary to the negative inotropic effects and all other side effects previously identified for beta-blockers.

CLASS II ANTIARRHYTHMIC THERAPY MANAGEMENT

Careful consideration should be given to the following:

1. An abrupt cessation of propranolol may exacerbate anginal pain in individuals with CAD.

2. Observe ECG for bradyarrhythmias and heart block associated with beta-blockade therapy.
3. There is a decrease in resting and submaximal heart rate and blood pressure with beta-blockers.
4. Decreased contractility and preload result in decreased myocardial oxygen demand and an increased tolerance for activity.

Class III

Only two class III drugs are currently available: bretylium tosylate and amiodarone. Bretylium, an intravenous sympathetic blocking agent, is used in the emergency treatment of ventricular arrhythmias refractory to treatment with other antiarrhythmics. Bretylium may potentiate digitalis toxicity (cardiac glycoside) because it causes a transient increase in norepinephrine release. Therefore, it should be administered with caution to individuals receiving digitalis. Side effects include severe hypotension and the related symptoms of light-headedness, dizziness, and vertigo.

Amiodarone (Cordarone) is a powerful antiarrhythmic that is effective in the treatment of both supraventricular and ventricular arrhythmias, but its potential for toxicity of multiple organ systems has thus far limited its use. It has a very slow onset of action (4 to 10 days) and therefore is not appropriate for the acute management of ventricular arrhythmias. Amiodarone prolongs the refractory period throughout the entire conduction system, thereby reducing heart rate and decreasing myocardial oxygen demands. The ECG changes with amiodarone include a slowed sinus rate, prolonged PR and QT intervals, T wave abnormalities, and presence of a U wave. There is no change in the QRS. The ECG changes are usually seen before the therapeutic effects are evident.[38] Amiodarone is associated with many severe but reversible side effects, the most dangerous of which is pulmonary infiltrates, which occur in 10 to 20 percent of individuals.[3,10,33] Side effects are slow to resolve, often more than 6 months, when the drug is discontinued because of the extended half-life of amiodarone.

CLASS III ANTIARRHYTHMIC THERAPY MANAGEMENT

Careful attention should be given to the following:

1. Observe for pulmonary symptoms. Encourage the individual to inform the physician of new onset of fever, cough, or shortness of breath.
2. Be alert for visual difficulties that are a result of corneal microdeposits.
3. Encourage use of sunscreen because amiodarone causes skin photosensitivity[40] and a gray-blue discoloration of the skin.

Class IV

Class IV antiarrhythmics are the calcium channel blockers, of which only verapamil and diltiazem have significant electrophysiologic effects. Verapamil, accepted for use as an antiarrhythmic, blocks the flow of extracellular calcium into cardiovascular cells in the SA and AV nodes. This drug action prolongs SA and AV node refractory periods and conduction time. It effectively decreases ventricular response in supraventricular tachycardias. Verapamil also decreases myocardial contractility and is, therefore, contraindicated in CHF, severe hypotension, and cardiogenic shock. Side effects include hypotension, a reflex increase in heart rate, constipation, vertigo, and tremors. Diltiazem is not yet recommended for the treatment of arrhythmias.

CLASS IV ANTIARRHYTHMIC THERAPY MANAGEMENT

Careful attention should be given to the following:

1. Observe for signs of hypotension: light-headedness, dizziness, fatigue.
2. Monitor blood pressure.
3. Observe for symptoms of CHF (dyspnea, cough, decreased activity tolerance, peripheral edema).

HYPOLIPIDEMIC AGENTS

It is well documented that elevated cholesterol (> 200 mg per dl) is a risk factor for the development of coronary heart disease. Dietary reduction of cholesterol is the major means of decreasing serum cholesterol. For individuals who are unable to lower their cholesterol level despite diet, exercise, and weight reduction, drug therapy is available.

Six major cholesterol-lowering drugs are recommended by the National Cholesterol Education Program coordinated by the National Heart, Lung, and Blood Institute. All are effective in lowering LDC-C (low-density lipoprotein-cholesterol). Table 7–5 re-

TABLE 7–5 Cholesterol-Lowering Drugs

Drug	Lowers LDL-C[53]	Actions	Additional Information
Cholestyramine (Questran) Colestipol (Colestid)	15–30%	Binds bile acids in GI tract, prompting liver to produce more bile acids from cholesterol.	May increase triglyceride levels. Digoxin absorption may be altered. Can alter absorption of other drugs; patient should take 1 hr before other drugs. May interfere with coumadin action.
Nicotinic acid (Nicobid, Nicolar)	15–30%	Lowers LDL-C and triglycerides by slowing hepatic production of very low density lipoprotein cholesterol (VLDL-C)	Water-soluble B vitamin. Least expensive. Can cause severe flushing and itching. May be hepatotoxic. Should not be taken by individuals with cardiac arrhythmias, diabetes, gout.

Continued

TABLE 7–5 Cholesterol-Lowering Drugs *Continued*

Drug	Lowers LDL-C[53]	Actions	Additional Information
Lovastatin (Mevacor)	25–45%	Blocks HMG-CoA reductase—an enzyme necessary for cholesterol production in the liver. Increases rate of LDL-C removal from plasma.	HMG-CoA reductase inhibitor may cause drop in triglycerides
Gemfibrozil (Lopid)	5–15%	Reduces VLDL-C, raises HDL-C, and modestly lowers LDL-C.	May cause 38–51% decrease in hypertri-glyceridemia; minimal lowering of LDL-C. Used when individual cannot tolerate other cholesterol-lowering drugs. Relatively safe; few side effects.
Probucol (Lorelco)	10–15%	Inhibits cholesterol transport from intestine and may decrease cholesterol synthesis. Speeds the breakdown of LDL-C and inhibits tissue deposition of LDL-C.	Contraindicated in individuals with arrhythmias. Usually well tolerated. May also reduce HDL-C as much as 25%.[53]
Clofibrate (Atromid-S)	Minimal decrease in LDL-C. 22–40% decrease in triglycerides.	Inhibits platelet aggregation in addition to hypolipidemic action.	Most widely used drug.

views some of the specifics of those drugs, all of which cause GI side effects including nausea, bloating, and constipation. Patients who have severe hypercholesterolemia may be treated with more than one of the drugs at a time. Combinations of drugs have lowered LDL-C as much as 70 percent in some patients.[53]

ANTIHYPERTENSIVES

A wide variety of medications are used for the treatment of hypertension in the individual with CAD. Many of those drugs, including calcium channel blockers and beta-blockers, have been discussed previously.

The goal of antihypertensive therapy is to obtain and maintain a diastolic pressure of less than 90 mm Hg without producing intolerable side effects.[3] The antihypertensive medications lower the blood pressure, decrease myocardial work load, and control some of the complications of hypertension. There are four types of antihypertensives, and they are categorized by mechanism of action: (1) centrally or peripherally acting sympathetic nervous symptom inhibitors, (2) peripheral vasodilators, (3) inhibitors of the renin-angiotensin mechanism of the kidney, and (4) diuretics. The reader should consult the references for further information on specific antihypertensive agents.[1,3,5,6,12,23,34,36,40]

ADDITIONAL MEDICATIONS

Many other medications, either over-the-counter or prescription drugs, may impact cardiac function and exercise tolerance; they include caffeine, nicotine, alcohol, and psychotropic drugs (phenothiazines and tricyclic antidepressants). The tricyclic antidepressants have a potent vagotonic effect and in toxicity may cause complete heart block. Lithium and phenothiazines alter ventricular repolarization.[41] Because of the actions and interactions of many of these drugs, it is important that cardiac rehabilitation personnel monitor medication changes and make appropriate modifications in exercise prescriptions in relation to the changes.

THROMBOLYTIC THERAPY FOR MYOCARDIAL INFARCTION

Three agents are currently approved for thrombolysis in acute MI: streptokinase, urokinase, and recombinant tissue plasminogen activator. All three in some way activate the body's fibrinolytic or clot lysis system. Autopsy studies have shown that 85 to 95 percent of patients dying from transmural MI have a fresh thrombotic occlusion of a large epicardial coronary artery.[45]

Streptokinase

Streptokinase is a systemic thrombolytic enzyme effective in dissolving thrombi and restoring patency to an occluded coronary artery during the early hours of an acute MI. The drug can be administered indirectly by the intravenous route or directly by cardiac catheterization. Streptokinase therapy promotes the lysis of fibrin and circulating fibrinogen.[40] In coronary artery occlusion, the goal of streptokinase therapy is to restore coronary perfusion and minimize the size of the MI. Most guidelines suggest that to be effective it should be initiated within 3 to 6 hours after the onset of chest pain.[42,44] A delay in therapy significantly decreases the potential to salvage myocardium. Streptokinase effectively lyses new clots for approximately 14 hours. The effect of this therapy is evaluated within 30 to 60 minutes after the start of therapy. Criteria for effectiveness include abrupt abatement of chest pain, resolution of ST-segment elevation and T wave changes, and abrupt and rapid increase in the release of creatine kinase (CK) into the blood.[44]

Randomized studies of intravenous and intracoronary streptokinase therapy have shown a reperfusion rate (reestablishing perfusion of the obstructed vessel) of 80 to 90 percent,[46] and others report results of 40 to 60 percent for intravenous streptokinase alone.[40] The clinical impact of this therapy depends specifically on how soon after the occlusion reperfusion is achieved. Therapy initiated within 4 to 6 hours after the onset of chest pain has been shown to decrease both inhospital and first-year mortality.[42]

There are several contraindications to streptokinase therapy: individuals with a predisposition to intracranial hemorrhage, infective endocarditis or known left ventricular thrombus, tuberculosis or bronchopleural fistula, recent surgery, severe liver impairment, and previous streptokinase infusion in greater than 5 days and less than 6 months. Streptokinase stimulates an immunological response and an increased titer of neutralizing antistreptokinase for up to 6 months; therefore, additional therapy with streptokinase may be ineffective.

The major side effects of streptokinase therapy include hemorrhage, arrhythmias, recurrent thrombosis, severe hypotension, and allergic reaction. Arrhythmias are a result of a reperfusion phenomenon from the alteration in electrical conduction in ischemic cells.

Urokinase

Urokinase is another systemic thrombolytic agent. It is a naturally occurring human enzyme derived from kidney cells. It acts similarly to streptokinase, but it is nonantigenic and is better tolerated than streptokinase. Intravenous urokinase and streptokinase produce reperfusion of totally occluded infarct vessels in 40 to 55 percent of individuals.[45]

Recombinant Tissue Plasminogen Activator

Recombinant tissue plasminogen activator (tPA) (Activase) is a clot-specific thrombolytic agent. Administered intravenously, the drug activates plasminogen, a fibrinolytic enzyme, only after binding to the plasminogen bound to fibrin contained in the existing thrombus. Recombinant tissue plasminogen activator is a naturally occurring substance found in endothelial, blood, and other human cells and therefore is nonantigenic. Intravenously, tPA is more effective than streptokinase and urokinase: It achieves reperfusion in 70 to 80 percent of cases, but because of the cost of isolating it, it is 10 to 15 times more expensive than streptokinase.[1,43,45] Bleeding is the major complication with this agent as with all thrombolytic agents.

In many instances, physicians are now following thrombolysis treatment with percutaneous transluminal angioplasty and systemic heparin therapy to prevent repeat thrombus and occlusion.

PHARMACOLOGIC MANAGEMENT OF PULMONARY DISEASE

Pharmacologic management of chronic pulmonary disease includes a variety of drugs specifically used to optimize the ventilatory capacity of the respiratory system. The goal is to maximize a patient's functional abilities while minimizing the drug's possible side effects. The three major categories of these drugs are bronchodilators, anti-inflammatory agents, and cromolyn sodium.

Bronchodilators

There are neural and chemical influences on the contractile property of the bronchial smooth muscle. Neural control is mediated by the autonomic nervous system (ANS). Both sympathetic (adrenergic) and parasympathetic (cholinergic) receptors have been identified in the bronchial smooth muscle. These two branches of the ANS have antagonistic effects over the size of the airway lumen.

Stimulation of the sympathetic portion of the ANS causes relaxation of the bronchial smooth muscle, which results in bronchodilation. The postganglionic beta$_2$ adrenergic receptors of the sympathetic nervous system release the chemical norepinephrine, which results in an increased amount of cyclic adenosine 3'5'monophosphate (cAMP). An increase in cAMP is associated with bronchial smooth muscle relaxation[54] (Fig. 7–1).

Stimulation of the parasympathetic system results in bronchoconstriction. The postganglionic cholinergic receptors of the parasympathetic nervous system release the chemical acetylecholine, which increases the level of cyclic 3'5' guanosine monophosphate (cGMP). An increase in cGMP is associated with contraction of the bronchial smooth muscle[55] (Fig. 7–2).

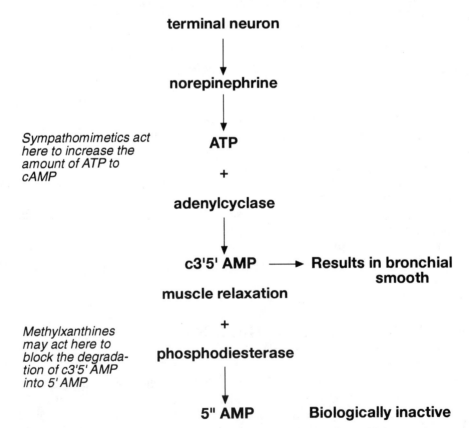

SYMPATHETIC NERVOUS SYSTEM

FIGURE 7–1. The effect of the sympathetic nervous system on bronchial smooth muscle and the potential site of action of sympathomimetics and methylxanthines.

PARASYMPATHETIC NERVOUS SYSTEM

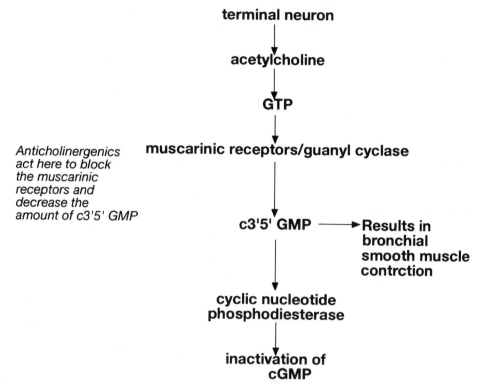

terminal neuron

acetylcholine

GTP

muscarinic receptors/guanyl cyclase

*Anticholinergenics
act here to block
the muscarinic
receptors and
decrease the
amount of c3'5' GMP*

c3'5' GMP ⟶ **Results in bronchial smooth muscle contrction**

cyclic nucleotide phosphodiesterase

inactivation of cGMP

FIGURE 7–2. The effect of the parasympathetic nervous system on bronchial smooth muscle and the potential site of anticholinergic action.

The parasympathetic nervous system innervates the bronchial smooth muscle, and the sympathetic system indirectly affects the bronchial smooth muscle. The airways normally demonstrate intrinsic tone, suggesting that parasympathetic control is more dominant.[56]

Bronchospasm occurs when there is a greater than normal contraction of the bronchial smooth muscle. Pharmacologic therapy of chronic obstructive pulmonary disease is directed toward relieving the bronchospasm.[57] Pharmacologic enhancement of bronchodilation can be accomplished by stimulating the sympathetic nervous system to promote the relaxation of the bronchial smooth muscle or by blocking the influence of the parasympathetic nervous system, which also will promote relaxation of the bronchial smooth muscle. The drugs that assist the sympathetic nervous system are of two types: sympathomimetics and methylxanthines. The drugs that block the parasympathetic nervous system are called anticholinergics.

SYMPATHOMIMETICS

Actions and Uses

Sympathomimetic drugs are the most widely used first-line agents in the management of obstructive pulmonary disorders[57] (Table 7–6). Sympathomimetics mimic the

TABLE 7–6 Sympathomimetic Bronchodilators

Generic Name (Trade Name)	Primary Receptor	Route of Administration	Adult Dosage
Isoproterenol (Isuprel)	Beta$_1$, beta$_2$	Inhaled (MDI)	80–160 μg, repeat in 5 min, 4–6 times per day
Epinephrine (Ephedrine, Bronkaid)	Alpha, beta$_1$, beta$_2$	Inhaled (MDI)	160–250 μg, repeat in 1 min, every 4 hr
Isoetharine (Bronkosol)	Beta$_2$	Inhaled (MDI)	340–680 μg, repeat in 1–3 min, every 4 hr
Metaproteranol (Alupent)	Beta$_2$	Inhaled (MDI) / Oral	1.3–1.95 mg, repeat 2–3 times, every 3–4 hr, 20 mg TID
Terbutaline (Brethine)	Beta$_2$	Inhaled (MDI) / Oral	400 μg, repeat in 1–10 min, 4–6 times per day 2.5–5 mg TID
Albuterol (Proventil, Ventilin)	Beta$_2$	Inhaled (MDI) / Oral	180 μg, repeat in 1–10 min, 4–6 times per day, 2–4 mg TID

action of the sympathetic nervous system and stimulate the beta$_2$ receptors of the bronchial smooth muscle. This increases the activity of the enzyme adenyl cyclase, which causes adenosine 5'-triphosphate (ATP) to be converted to cAMP. Sympathomimetics, also called beta-adrenergic agonists, produce relaxation of the bronchial smooth muscle by increasing the amount of cAMP.

Contraindications and Side Effects

The side effects of sympathomimetics depend on the drugs' selectivity of beta$_2$ receptors and the route of administration. As indicated earlier in the section on cardiac beta-blocking agents, there are beta$_1$ and beta$_2$ receptor sites in the heart and lungs. Stimulation of beta$_1$ receptors affects cardiac parameters, whereas stimulation of beta$_2$ receptors is responsible for alterations in the pulmonary system. The more beta$_2$ selective a drug is, the fewer cardiac side effects are observed. The ingestion of sympathomimetics, especially the nonselective sympathomimetics, produces the systemic side effects of tachycardia, palpitations, angina, GI distress, nervousness, muscle tremor, headache, dizziness, anxiety, sweating, and insomnia. Inhaled beta-adrenergic agonists may cause bronchial irritation with prolonged use but minimize the systemic side effects. The metered dose inhaler (MDI), with its ability to deliver sympathomimetics topically with minimal side effects, has gained acceptance as the best route for administration of sympathomimetic drugs.[57]

The cardiovascular side effects are the most dangerous of the reactions. Caution should be exercised in older patients, particularly those with hypertension, diabetes, and CAD.[58] Patients with hypoxemia from their pulmonary disease or those with an irritable myocardium from associated heart disease are at higher risk for the side effects of tachycardia, arrhythmias, angina, and myocardial necrosis.[54]

Effects of Sympathomimetics on Exercise in Individuals with Pulmonary Disease

There is often an elevated resting heart rate in patients who are taking systemic sympathomimetics. By using the Karvonen formula for calculation of target heart rate

(THR), this heart rate elevation is taken into consideration. When a heart rate increase is observed, it is important to use the rate of perceived shortness of breath scale as an indicator of exercise intensity. (See Chapter 11, Exercise Prescription.)

By using an MDI of a sympathomimetic prior to exercise, the symptoms of exercise-induced bronchospasm can be minimized.

Sympathomimetic Therapy Management

Careful consideration should be given to the following:

1. Administration of sympathomimetics is based on relief of symptoms while minimizing side effects. Careful examination of symptomatic relief and untoward effects is important in determining the amount of drug required.
2. When inhalation is the route of administration, the mouth should be rinsed with water after each dose to minimize both oral irritation and ingestion of the drug.

METHYLXANTHINES

Actions and Uses

Methylxanthines also produce bronchodilation, and there are a number of theories to explain their action (Table 7–7). The most widely held postulate is that methylxanthines block the enzyme phosphodiesterase, which converts cAMP into cGMP.[55] There is a resultant accumulation of cAMP that promotes relaxation of the bronchial smooth muscle. Current research suggests that drugs of the xanthine group block the binding of adenosine to the smooth muscle and thus block smooth muscle contraction.[59] Other theories are that the xanthines inhibit intracellular calcium release, which does not allow constriction of the smooth muscle, and/or that xanthines may be responsible for prostaglandin inhibition.[59] Regardless of the action of drugs of the xanthine group, bronchodilation, increased ciliary action, and stabilization of the mast cells are accomplished with their use.

Methylxanthines have been observed to increase the contractility of skeletal muscles, including the diaphragm, in patients.[56] There has also been found to be an increase in the amount of work performed by the skeletal muscle while it is under the influence of methylxanthines, that is, a resistance to muscle fatigue.[56]

TABLE 7–7 Methylxanthine Bronchodilators

Generic Name (Trade Name)	Route of Administration	Maintenance Dosage
Aminophylline		
(Aminodur)	Oral-time release	PO preparations: 16 mg/kg or 400 mg
Aminophylline suppository	Rectal	(whichever is less) per day
Theophyllin		
(Theodur)	Oral-time release	Time released: 12 mg/kg or 400 mg
(Aerolate)	Oral	(whichever is less) per day
(Slo-phyllin)	Oral	
(Elixophyllin)	Oral	
(Fleet Theo-phylline)	Rectal	Rectal preparations: 16 mg/kg or 400 mg (whichever is less) per day
Oxtriphyllin (Choladril)	Oral	
Dyphyllin	Oral-time release	Adjust dosage according to serum levels

Contraindications and Side Effects

Methylxanthines are not inhaled; they are given systemically, by ingestion, injection, or rectal absorption. The systemic effects of methylxanthines (theophyllin preparations) produce bronchodilation but also affect other organ systems, namely, the central nervous, cardiovascular, renal, musculoskeletal, and gastrointestinal systems.

The therapeutic effects of the theophyllin are directly related to the serum concentration of the drug. Improvement in pulmonary function begins at a blood level as low as 5 μg per milliliter. Even at those low levels of serum theophyllin, headache, restlessness, anxiety, insomnia, and hyperactivity may all be reported.[56]

Improvement in pulmonary function increases proportionately to the serum concentration. The therapeutic range for theophyllin is 10 to 20 μg per milliliter, but toxicity may appear at the upper level of the therapeutic range, that is, 15 to 20 μg per milliliter. Gastrointestinal signs appear as the upper level of therapeutic range is reached; among them are anorexia, nausea, vomiting, and abdominal discomfort.[56]

Serious central nervous system (CNS) effects (e.g., grand mal seizures) and serious cardiovascular effects (e.g., palpitations, tachycardia, and arrythmias) may occur when the serum level exceeds 20 μg per milliliter.[56,59]

Effects on Exercise in Individuals with Pulmonary Disease

There is often an elevated resting heart rate in patients who are taking methylxanthines. By using the Karvonen formula for calculation of the THR, the heart rate elevation is taken into account. When a heart rate increase is observed, it is important to use the rate of perceived shortness of breath scale as an indicator of exercise intensity. (See Chapter 11, Exercise Prescription.)

Methylxanthine Therapy Management

Careful consideration should be given to the following:

1. The mean plasma half-life of theophyllin in adults ranges from 3 to 9½ hours. (Pediatric plasma half-life ranges from 1 to 9½ hours). Therefore, the variability of serum plasma levels requires that serum drug levels be individually titrated and closely monitored to assure that the drug is at a therapeutic level. Attention to signs and symptoms of theophyllin toxicity by health professionals involved in the patient's care may prevent any untoward effects.
2. Methylxanthines are metabolized in the liver; therefore, alcohol consumption and liver disease increase the half-life of the drug.
3. Cigarette smoking has been shown to decrease the metabolism of the drug. It is important to carefully monitor any patient who changes smoking habits during the course of pulmonary rehabilitation for signs and symptoms of theophyllin toxicity.

ANTICHOLINERGICS

Actions and Uses

The parasympathetic nervous system contains cholinergic receptors. The subcategory of cholinergic receptors specific to airway smooth muscle is termed "muscarinic." Anticholinergic pharmacologic agents block the muscarinic cholinergic receptors and thereby decrease the parasympathetic tone within the airway smooth muscle.[59] The result is bronchodilation. There is also a decrease in the secretion of the mucous glands with the use of anticholinergic agents (Table 7–8).

TABLE 7-8 Anticholinergic Bronchodilators

Generic Name (Trade Name)	Route of Administration	Dosage
Atropine sulfate	IM/IV	For preoperative and postoperative control of secretions 0.4 mg.
Ipratropium bromide (Atrovent)	Inhaled	40 μg QID

Contraindications and Side Effects

The severity of side effects from anticholinergic drugs depends on the route of administration and the preparation of the drug. Atropine sulfate, even though used by respiratory patients as an inhalant, has significant systemic absorption. The side effects include dry mouth, throat irritation, constipation, urinary retention, tachycardia, blurred vision, photophobia, and confusion. Ipratropium (Atrovent) is an inhaled agent with little systemic absorption and is therefore relatively free from side effects.[58]

Effects on Exercise in Individuals with Pulmonary Disease

Inhaled ipratropium, which inhibits bronchoconstriction and mucus production, may assist the patient in prolonging the exercise session.

Anticholinergic Therapy Management

Since inhalation is the route of administration, after use, the mouth should be rinsed with water to minimize irritation of the mouth and throat and any possible ingestion of the drug.

Anti-inflammatory Agents

The integrity of the airways is also affected by the inflammatory cells within the lungs.[60] Histamine, slow-reacting substance of anaphylaxis (SRS-A) from the mast cell, neutrophils, lymphocytes, eosinophils, macrophages, plasma cells, and monocytes can all take part in the inflammatory response within the airways. An increase in reactivity of the inflammatory response within the airways is commonly seen in asthma and other obstructive pulmonary diseases. The inflammatory response results in vascular engorgement and in swelling and hypersecretion of the mucous glands.[54] All these contribute to a decrease in the size of the airway lumen. By reducing the amount of inflammation within the airways, relief of symptoms and improved ventilation can be obtained.

CORTICOSTEROIDS

Actions and Uses

Corticosteroids are the most potent anti-inflammatory drugs available.[61] They have many possible actions such as stabilizing the leukocyte lysosomal membranes, inhibiting the accumulation of macrophages, preventing the release of acid hydrolases, reducing leukocyte adhesion to capillary endothelium, reducing capillary wall permeability, and depressing tissue reactivity to antigen-antibody interactions.[58] By reducing this inflammatory response within the airways, bronchoconstriction is discouraged. There are also reduced capillary engorgement, a decrease in mucosal edema, and a decrease in secre-

TABLE 7–9 Anti-Inflammatory Agents

Generic Name (Trade Name)	Route of Administration	Adult Dosage
Beclomethasone (Beclovent, Vanceril)	Inhalation	2 sprays TID-QID
Betamethasone	Oral	0.6–7.2 mg/day
Dexamethasone (Decadron)	Inhalation	3 sprays TID-QID (300 μg)
Flunisolide (AeroBid)	Inhalation	250 μg/2 sprays BID
Methylprednisolone	Oral	2–60 mg/day
Prednisone	Oral	5–60 mg/day
Triamcinolone (Azmacort)	Inhalation	100 μg 2 sprays TID
	Oral	4–48 mg/day

tion production. These collectively increase the inner diameter of the airways and decrease airway obstruction (Table 7–9).

Contraindications and Side Effects

The side effects of corticosteroids are dependent on (1) dosage and duration of therapy and (2) the route of administration. Short-term use of systemic steroids, even in high doses, is unlikely to produce harmful effects.[58] However, prolonged systemic use of the drug can result in hypertension, nausea, GI irritation, headache, hypercholesterolemia, moon face, skin breakdown, bruising, muscle atrophy, osteoporosis, delayed wound healing, and an increased susceptibility to, and masking of, infection. Aerosolized corticosteroid preparations (metered dose inhalers) have become a mainstay in the treatment of airway reactivity, since they effectively treat the cause topically while avoiding the serious adverse systemic side effects.[62]

Effects on Exercise in Individuals with Pulmonary Disease

The side effects of corticosteroids may affect the type of exercise chosen for patients who are receiving systemic corticosteroids. Long-term steroid use can alter the musculoskeletal system, and pathologic fractures secondary to osteoporosis are possible. Activities that produce excessive stress to skeletal structures should be avoided.

Corticosteroid Therapy Management

Careful consideration should be given to the following:

1. Patients should be advised that steroid dosages must always be tapered, not stopped abruptly. Rebound effects and tachyphylaxis are possible when proper tapering is not performed.
2. When the route of administration of corticosteroids is by inhalation, the mouth should be rinsed with water after each dose to minimize fungal growth and irritation.

Cromolyn Sodium

Cromolyn sodium is neither an anti-inflammatory agent nor a bronchodilator. It seems to be, so far, in a category all by itself.

ACTIONS AND USES

Histamine and SRS-A are chemical mediators of bronchoconstriction found within the mast cell. When an antigen is exposed to the body, these mediators are released from the mast cell and cause bronchoconstriction.

Cromolyn sodium acts to stabilize the mast cell membrane and prevent the release of histamine and SRS-A when an antigen is exposed to the body.[55] Because of its action, the drug is used prophylactically rather than reactively in the treatment of bronchospasm. That is, once bronchoconstriction has occurred, stabilizing the membrane is of no therapeutic value.

Cromolyn sodium seems to be most effective in the treatment of children or young adults with allergic asthma and exercise-induced bronchospasm.[55]

CONTRAINDICATIONS AND SIDE EFFECTS

Cromolyn sodium, in powder form, is used in a device called a Spinhaler for inhalation. This powder can actually produce bronchospasm, irritation of the bronchi, cough, and nausea. More recently, cromolyn sodium is available in a metered dose inhaler (Intal). Contraindications are drug hypersensitivity and lactase deficiency.[58]

EFFECTS ON EXERCISE IN INDIVIDUALS WITH PULMONARY DISEASE

Patients can use an inhalant of cromolyn sodium prior to the initiation of exercise in an effort to avert exercise-induced bronchospasm.

CROMOLYN SODIUM THERAPY MANAGEMENT

Careful consideration should be given to the following:

1. Since cromolyn sodium is used to prevent bronchoconstriction, patients should be advised to continue its prophylactic use, especially when feeling well.
2. Improvement may take from 1 to 4 weeks from initiation of the drug, so patience is in order.
3. Cromolyn sodium should not be instituted during an acute period of bronchospasm, because it may increase the bronchospasm.[55]

Other Additional Medications

Many other drugs are used in the management of lung disease. Some of the additional pharmacologic agents that may be used in the management of a patient with pulmonary disease are described below.

Infection is a contributory cause of bronchospasm and respiration dysfunction.[63] Antibiotics are used in the prevention as well as the treatment of pulmonary infections. Antibiotics can be classified into different types: penicillins, tetracyclines, cephalosporins, aminoglycosides, sulfonamides, and erythromycins. The penicillin group includes such antibiotics as penicillin G, ampicillin, ticarcillin, amoxicillin, and carbenicillin. Although the penicillin group of antibiotics rarely has side effects, hypersensitivity reactions from skin rashes to anaphylactic reactions have been reported. Tetracyclines include such drugs as tetracycline, doxycycline, and methacycline. The most common side effects of the tetracyclines are GI disturbances: nausea, vomiting, and diarrhea. The cephalosporin drugs, such as ceftazidine, ceftriaxone, cefaclor (Ceclor), cephalexin (Keflex), and cefamandole, have few frequent side effects. They include pain from injection site, transient elevation of liver enzymes, and superinfections with prolonged use. Aminoglycosides include the antibiotics Amikacin, gentamicin, tobramycin, streptomycin, and neomycin. Some of the side effects found with the use of aminoglycosides are nephrotoxicity, ototoxicity, and damage to cranial nerve VIII resulting in partial or complete hearing loss. Finally, erythromycin is in a category practically by itself even though there are other drugs in the family (Estolate, ethylsuccinate, Gluceptate) that are rarely prescribed. The side effects of erythromycin most usually seen are GI: cramping, nausea, vomiting, and diarrhea. Additional antibiotics used to treat infections that do not fit into the aforementioned categories include clindamycin, polymixin B, and chloramphenicol. These antimicrobial drugs decrease the morbidity and mortality of patients with pulmonary dysfunction. Laboratory sensitivity studies on the infecting organism(s) are necessary to ensure that the appropriate antibiotic will be selected and will be effective.

Anti-infection agents that are not antibiotics are also prescribed to treat various infections. Antifungals are used to treat fungal infections such as *Aspergillus* and *Candida*. The most commonly used antifungal agent is amphotericin B. Antituberculins are used in the treatment of tuberculosis. The most commonly used drugs in this category are streptomycin, ethambutol, isoniazid (INH), and rifampin. Two or more of these drugs are usually prescribed concurrently for long durations (6 months to 2 years) in order to combat the disease. Alcohol consumption causes a drug interaction that may increase the risk of hepatotoxicity. An antiprotozoal agent is used in the treatment of pneumocystis carinii pneumonia (PCP), aerosolized pentamidine isoethionate. Some of the side effects of aerosolized pentamidine are fatigue, a metallic taste, and possible shortness of breath, presumably due to bronchospasm. It is not uncommon to prescribe a sympathomimetic metered dose inhaler (i.e., Ventilin MDI) along with aerosolized pentamidine to relieve any shortness of breath that the pentamidine may cause.

Antitussive drugs, decongestants, antihistamines, mucolytics, and expectorants are available as over-the-counter preparations. They may have interactions with prescription drugs, and some of them have unwanted effects for patients in pulmonary rehabilitation programs. It is important that patients (and pulmonary rehabilitation personnel) be aware and be cautioned about the possible interactions and side effects.

THERAPEUTIC PROCEDURES AND SURGICAL INTERVENTION IN CORONARY ARTERY DISEASE

Surgical intervention and therapeutic procedures in CAD do not alter the atherosclerotic disease process. They improve the quality of life by relieving the symptoms of CAD (angina) and restoring myocardial perfusion. Both types of intervention contribute to improving the individual's tolerance for activity. Coronary disease is treated surgically with myocardial revascularization by coronary artery bypass grafting and by heart transplant. Special therapeutic techniques used both acutely and electively to alter structural changes contributing to coronary stenosis are percutaneous transluminal coronary angioplasty (PTCA), laser angioplasty, and athrectomy.

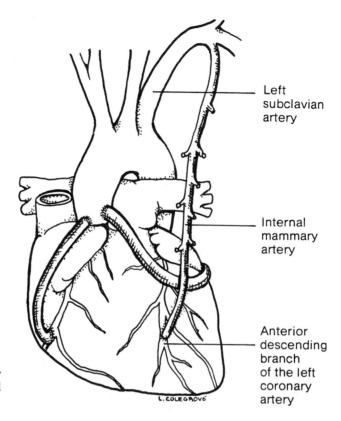

Left
subclavian
artery

Internal
mammary
artery

Anterior
descending
branch
of the left
coronary
artery

L. COLEGROVE

FIGURE 7–3. Coronary artery bypass graft using the SVG and IMA.

Coronary Artery Bypass Grafting

Coronary artery bypass grafting (CABG) is surgical revascularization of the myocardium (Fig. 7–3). Revascularization is accomplished by one or both of the following methods: (1) anastomosing grafts, usually the individual's own saphenous vein (SVG), to the aortic root and to the coronary artery distal to the stenosis and/or (2) direct revascularization by anastomosing the distal end of the internal mammary artery (IMA) to the coronary artery distal to the lesion. The use of the IMA graft is becoming more popular because studies indicate that the IMA conduit has an 85 to 95 percent patency rate 7 to 10 years postbypass as opposed to the SVG rate of 60 percent.[19,22,45,47]

Postoperatively, the SVG conduits show progressive intimal proliferation and atherosclerotic plaque development. Atherosclerosis is rarely observed in IMA conduits.[15,22] Loop and others[22] found that individuals with IMA grafts over the first 10 years postsurgery had not only a higher graft patency rate but also a lesser incidence of late MI, reoperation, and death than those who had only SVG conduits. The IMA is, however, limited by its length and anatomical position. It may be used to revascularize only the anterior portion of the heart and must be grafted to the left anterior descending coronary artery. In addition, the IMA is more difficult to dissect from the chest wall and may extend the length of surgery up to 1 hour.[19,45] In dissecting the IMA, most often the pleural space must be entered to ensure appropriate dissection, although no increase in the incidence of postoperative pulmonary complications has been documented.[22]

Use of the IMA is contraindicated in patients with severe vascular disease of the upper extremities and in individuals who are unstable in surgery and to whom the extra time necessary for an IMA dissection and anastomosis would be detrimental.[19,20,22] Overall, the improved long-term results, which are primarily due to minimal graft atherosclerosis in the IMA conduit, may lead to more widespread use of the IMA graft.[24,52]

There are many indications for CABG surgery, and the criteria for patient selection vary among institutions. The use of CABG surgery is changing as PTCA has become increasingly more popular as an alternative. PTCA allows patients with single or multiple high-grade lesions to undergo a less traumatic procedure to relieve coronary artery occlusion. The criteria for patient selection for CABG generally include:

1. Stable angina with a high grade left main trunk (LMT) lesion
2. Stable angina with triple vessel CAD
3. Unstable angina with triple vessel CAD or severe two-vessel disease
4. Recent MI with continued angina
5. Ischemic heart failure with shock[15]

The location and degree of stenosis caused by the lesion, the amount of myocardium served by the affected artery, and whether the individual has had a previous MI are considered when evaluating the need for surgical intervention. Usually a lesion of greater than 70 percent occlusion of the coronary artery is cause for consideration of surgical intervention. When the occlusion is in the LMT, surgery is considered earlier in the course of CAD. Surgery unquestionably enhances survival when a 50 percent or greater occlusion of the LMT is present.[13,17] In most individuals the LMT and its branches deliver 80 percent of the blood supply to the left ventricle and therefore, with a high-grade lesion, the risk of death from coronary artery occlusion is greater than the risk of surgery.[14,17]

Individuals are evaluated for surgery on the basis of their presenting symptoms, the coexistence of other chronic disease, and a battery of medical tests. The tests include blood studies, pulmonary function studies, electrocardiograms, and, most important, coronary arteriography and a left ventriculogram. Arteriography, performed under fluoroscopy, allows direct visualization of the extent and location of lesions and the status of the coronary circulation distal to the obstruction. Visualization allows the surgeon to determine if bypassing the lesion will permit effective revascularization or if the disease process is so diffuse that grafting would have little value. The ventriculogram allows for visualization of the left ventricular muscle function, identification of hypokinetic, poorly moving or akinetic, immobile segments, and measurement of pressures in the heart chambers, all of which provide vital information regarding the heart's effectiveness as a pump.

In CABG surgery, with the patient under anesthesia, a median sternotomy is performed. This allows direct visualization of the heart. The circulation is supported by means of an extracorporeal oxygenation pump (cardiopulmonary bypass pump) that allows the blood to bypass the heart, become oxygenated, and then flow to the systemic circulation. The heart is paralyzed by administration of a cold, hyperkalemic solution (cardioplegia) instilled into the coronary arteries.[18] The motionless heart allows the surgery to be performed more easily. From one to seven grafts are placed, using the SVG or the IMA as conduits. Four is the average number of grafts.[24] Following the procedure, the heart is rewarmed, and the blood is again circulated through it. The heart beat either begins spontaneously or is initiated by means of internal defibrillation with a 5 to 20 watt-seconds stimulus.

Improvements in surgical techniques, coronary bypass pumps, cardioplegia, and myocardial preservation have decreased perioperative morbidity and mortality. The same improvements have safely allowed extended operative time to do more complete revascularizations.[24]

Operative mortality is 1 to 3 percent nationally,[24,45,47] with perioperative infarction and neurological incidents (secondary to some type of embolic episode) the greatest complications of CABG surgery.

Following uncomplicated CABG surgery, individuals progress rapidly. They are usually out of bed within 24 to 48 hours, ambulating the next day, and discharged from the hospital on the seventh to tenth day. Activities, particularly lifting, are restricted for 6 weeks to 3 months. Return to work is usually dictated by the patient's occupation, rate of recuperation, and duration of unemployment prior to surgery. Statistics indicate that the longer the individual is unemployed prior to surgery, the less likely he or she is to return to work.[13] Postoperative recurrence of angina has also delayed the return to work for some individuals.[13]

The improved myocardial blood supply that is due to the revascularization is intended to provide for improved left ventricular function, decreased incidence of MI, and thus an increase in life expectancy.[25] The most direct explanation for the "relief" of anginal pain is successful coronary revascularization and elimination of myocardial ischemia. There is excellent correlation between anginal relief and graft patency, but other mechanisms, including the infarction of angina-producing myocardium, the transection of afferent cardiac nerves during the procedure, and placebo effect of surgery itself, are offered as explanations for the 70 to 80 percent success rate for relief of angina with CABG.[14,15,24,25] Improved exercise tolerance has also been associated with complete revascularization.

Ten-year survival (excluding deaths within the postoperative hospital stay) has been found to be 86 percent with IMA grafts and 76 percent with SVG grafts. Graft patency observed in postoperative arteriography is the crucial determinant of longevity and freedom from other cardiac events.[14]

Again it should be emphasized that revascularization is not a cure for the atherosclerotic process. As evidenced by postsurgical coronary arteriography, atherosclerosis of the native vessels and of the grafts continues.[24,25] Lifestyle modifications to reduce CAD risk factors are an important adjunct to surgery for the CAD patient.

Percutaneous Transluminal Coronary Angioplasty

PTCA is an invasive but nonsurgical technique used to dilate coronary arteries (Fig. 7–4). Initially it had somewhat limited application, but with revised smaller balloon designs, steerable guide wires, and more advanced skill on the part of the practitioners, the technique can now be used to treat both multiple lesions and lesions virtually anywhere in the coronary circulation.[44]

Under fluoroscopy, a small balloon-tipped catheter is inserted via the femoral artery and advanced in a retrograde fashion to the coronary arteries. The catheter is advanced across the stenotic area, and the balloon is intermittently inflated. The original belief was that the soft noncalcified plaque was compressed into the intima of the coronary artery, but more recent studies reveal two hypotheses that explain immediate and long-term effects. Intimal disruption or a controlled intimal tear is the primary mechanism of dilation of the vessel, and stretching of the vascular media and adventitia results in a localized ballooning or aneurysm formation.[44,45]

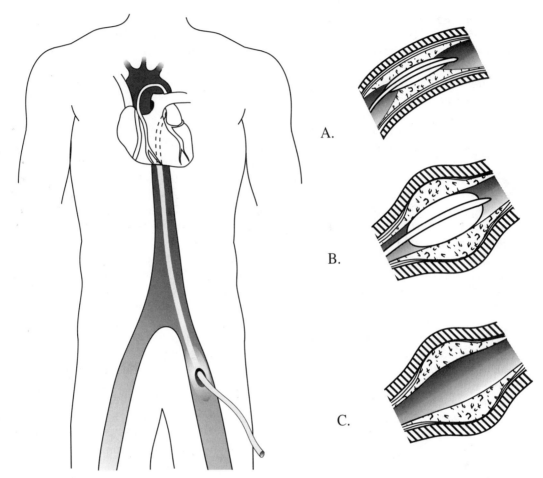

FIGURE 7–4. Mechanism of percutaneous transluminal coronary angioplasty (PTCA). The balloon catheter is inserted in the femoral artery and advanced to the coronary artery. *A*, The balloon is positioned at the site of the atherosclerotic lesion. *B*, The inflated balloon. *C*, The enlarged vessel lumen after PTCA. (From Underhill, SL, et al: Cardiac Nursing, ed 2. JB Lippincott, Philadelphia, 1989, p. 532, with permission.)

Nearly 50 percent of people who need coronary revascularization are candidates for PTCA.[44] Individuals with complex coronary anatomy, multivessel disease, post–coronary artery bypass grafting, and bifurcation lesions have all been successfully treated with PTCA. Individuals with total occlusions who have adequate resting collateral circulation but who cannot tolerate physical activity without developing anginal symptoms also can benefit from PTCA. Angioplasty is also being used in the acute treatment of unstable angina refractory to medical therapy and in conjunction with thrombolysis therapy in an acute MI to recanalize the occluded vessels and prevent rethrombosis and occlusion.

Complications of PTCA include acute occlusion of the coronary artery by spasm, clot, or collapse, coronary artery dissection or rupture, MI, bleeding at the arterial puncture site, internal hemorrhage from systemic anticoagulation, and compromise of the circulation distal to the catheter insertion site. Immediate open heart surgery is necessary should the coronary artery rupture.

Postprocedure, the individual is observed in a specialized care unit for 24 to 48 hours for any sign of arterial reocclusion or other complications. Upon discharge, patients generally have minimal activity restrictions, and most individuals return to work within a week. Initial research has shown that because of the minimal disability suffered with PTCA there is a correspondingly lower incidence of psychological problems in PTCA individuals as compared to individuals who undergo CABG.[31]

Success rates for PTCA in all elective situations and in unstable angina approach 90 percent,[44-47] but restenosis occurs at a rate of 30 percent in the first 4 to 6 months. These reocclusions do respond to repeat balloon angioplasty.[45,49]

Long-term effects of PTCA are not yet known. There are questions regarding the extent of the vascular damage and the interaction between the catheter and the vessel. Laser angioplasty and coronary athrectomy are now being used selectively, and it is believed that because they result in a smoother lumen they may have a significantly lower incidence of restenosis.[44,52] It is known, however, that PTCA has resulted in improved myocardial blood flow, and individuals have reported immediate relief of their anginal pain while experiencing minimal surgical discomfort.[30] It should also be emphasized that PTCA does not change or arrest the atherosclerotic process and that appropriate risk reduction techniques must be encouraged.

Heart Transplantation

Heart transplantation is now the treatment of choice in end-stage myocardial disease in which the left ventricular ejection fraction is less than 20 percent, medical therapies are ineffective, and there is no expectation of recovery. The underlying disease process is either idiopathic cardiomyopathy or ischemic cardiomyopathy from CAD.

Patient selection is done carefully because the surgery and postoperative management are complex and the risk is high. Individuals are usually less than 50 to 60 years old, free of other chronic diseases, infection, and donor-specific antibodies, emotionally stable, and have a strong psychosocial support system.[17,34]

Transplantation is performed through a median sternotomy. The heart is removed from the donor by transecting the great vessels and the atria dorsal to the atrial appendages. The recipient's heart is removed while he or she is maintained on cardiopulmonary bypass. The donor heart is anastomosed in the appropriate anatomical position.

The two major complications postoperatively are infection and rejection. Immunosuppressive therapy is used to minimize rejection; protective isolation is used to minimize the risk of infection. The survival rate at the end of 1 year is greater than 80 percent and at the end of 5 years greater than 50 percent.[45] Ongoing improvements in immunosuppressive therapy and the advent of transvenous endomyocardial biopsy have allowed for early and more aggressive treatment of acute rejection. Chronic rejection is a more challenging complication. It is manifested as accelerated atherosclerosis of the coronary arteries of the transplanted heart, unassociated with the normal risk factors of CAD.[47] Although the mechanism of chronic rejection is unknown, there is a marked intimal hyperplasia with or without lipid deposits. The clinical manifestations are the same as with CAD except that with a denervated heart there is no chest pain.[50] Of all the operated individuals, 60 to 80 percent develop CAD by 5 years after transplant. The lesions are diffuse and begin distally, so bypass surgery or angioplasty is rarely appropriate. Retransplant is the only definitive treatment.[50]

Rehabilitation is an important adjunct to medical therapy posttransplant, and in some centers it is a mandatory component of the pretransplant contract. Although the heart itself is healthy, the individual benefits from a prudent cardiac lifestyle.

Rehabilitation is similar to that of any patient with CAD except for the heart's response to exercise. The response of the denervated heart is very different from that of the normal heart. The resting heart rate is higher (usually about 100 bpm, the intrinsic rate of the SA node without vagal stimulation) and with exercise there is initially no increase in heart rate. Cardiac output increases as a result of preload augmentation from increased venous return from muscular activity. Heart rate increases and cardiac output increases further after several minutes of exercise because of a rise in circulating catecholamines. With the cessation of exercise the heart rate gradually returns to baseline as the plasma catecholamine levels decrease. Because of this response to exercise, the exercise prescription is usually based on Borg's scale of perceived exertion and other indices of oxygen consumption.[50] Despite the delayed response, the transplanted heart is ultimately effective in supporting the physiologic demands of exercise and stress.[50,51] The reader is referred to references following the chapter for further detail on rehabilitation of the heart transplant individual.

Two of the major limitations to heart transplantation are the availability and the difficulty of procuring organs. Currently, research is ongoing in the use of the artificial heart as a mechanism to bridge the waiting period between the time when the individual's own heart fails and when a donor heart is available. Many surgeons presently feel that only temporary use of the artificial heart is appropriate because the quality of life with it does not make its long-term use acceptable. The cost in dollars, resources, and complications also weighs heavily against its use.[35]

Heart-Lung Transplantation

Recently, in individuals with severe pulmonary hypertension or those with combined cardiopulmonary disease, heart-lung transplantations are being performed at a few major centers. In addition, some transplantations are being done for advanced cystic fibrosis.

The criteria for patient selection are essentially the same as for heart transplantation. The patients suffer from the same set of problems as heart transplantation patients because of similar long-term immunosuppressive therapy. In addition, three problems are specific to the lung transplantation patients: (1) problems with the healing of the tracheal anastomosis site, (2) reversible pulmonary gas exchange deficit similar to that of pulmonary edema, and (3) bronchiolitis obliterans, possibly the pulmonary equivalent of late chronic rejection of the heart. As with heart transplantation, a major limitation of heart-lung transplantations is the availability of organs.

CARDIAC REHABILITATION AND CORONARY ARTERY DISEASE

The World Health Organization defines rehabilitation as the "sum of activity required to ensure patients the best possible physical, mental, and social conditions so that they may, by their own efforts, regain as normal a life as possible, a place in the community, and lead an active and productive life."[39] Cardiac rehabilitation is an important adjunctive therapy in both the medical and surgical management of CAD and a mandatory adjunct posttransplantation. Medical and surgical interventions are designed to relieve the symptoms an individual experiences as a result of atherosclerosis. They do not alter the cause or the progression of the atherosclerotic process unless CAD patients concurrently recognize their individual risk factors and modify their lifestyles to reduce their risk. With intensive education and appropriate professional support, individuals are able to make and maintain specific changes in their lifestyles in the general areas of diet, exercise, stress management, and compliance with medical therapy in order to reduce their own cardiac risk factors.

SUMMARY

Medical and surgical management of the individual with CAD disease was presented. Emphasis was placed on the following classes of drugs: nitrates, beta-blockers, calcium channel blockers, cardiac glycosides, antiarrhythmics, hypolipidemics, and antihypertensives. Various combinations of these are used to control the symptoms of CAD, including angina, arrhythmias, CHF, and hypertension. Actions of the medications as well as common side effects and effects on exercise were reviewed. The use of thrombolytic agents in acute coronary artery occlusion was included.

The discussion of pharmacologic agents commonly used to treat patients with pulmonary disease emphasized the medications that increase the ventilatory capacity of the respiratory system while minimizing side effects. Three major categories of medications were discussed: (1) bronchodilators, including sympathomimetics, methylxanthines, and anticholinergics, (2) anti-inflammatory agents (corticosteroids), and (3) cromolyn sodium. Actions, side effects, and effects of these drugs on exercise were presented.

CABG and PTCA as effective means of attaining symptom relief were explained, and it was emphasized that the two techniques are not cures for the progression of atherosclerosis. Organ transplantation was discussed as a recognized treatment of end-stage cardiac and cardiopulmonary disease.

Cardiac rehabilitation and risk factor reduction were briefly identified as important adjuncts to both medical and surgical management of cardiopulmonary disease.

REFERENCES

1. Vinsant, MO and Spence MI: Pharmacological intervention in coronary artery disease. In MO Vinsant and MI Spence (eds): Commonsense Approach to Coronary Care, ed 5. CV Mosby, St Louis, 1989.
2. Tannenbaum, RP, et al: Angina pectoris: How to recognize; how to manage it. Nursing 81(11):9, 1981.
3. Mathewson, MK and Umhauer, MA: Drugs affecting the cardiovascular system. In Mathewson, MK: Pharmacotherapeutics: A Nursing Process Approach. FA Davis, Philadelphia, 1986.
4. Spencer, RT: Drugs affecting the nervous system: Autonomic drugs. In Spencer, RT: Clinical Pharmacology and Nursing Management, ed 2. JB Lippincott, Philadelphia, 1986.
5. Spencer, RT: Cardiovascular drugs: Drugs affecting the heart. In Spencer, RT: Clinical Pharmacology and Nursing Management, ed 2. JB Lippincott, Philadelphia, 1986.
6. Shepherd, JT: Circulatory response to beta adrenergic blockade at rest and during exercise. Am J Cardiol 55:810, 1985.
7. Silke, B, et al: The effects on left ventricular performance of verapamil and metoprolol singly and together in exercise induced angina pectoris. Am Heart J 109:1286, 1985.
8. Bigger, JT: A Primer of Calcium Ion Antagonists. Knoll Pharmaceutical Co., Whippany, NJ, 1980.
9. Froelicher, V, et al: Can patients with coronary artery disease receiving beta blockers obtain a training effect? Am J Cardiol 55:155D, 1985.
10. DeAngelis, R: Amiodarone. Crit Care Nurs 6:12, 1986.
11. Fletcher, GF: Exercise training during chronic beta blockade in cardiovascular disease. Am J Cardiol 55:1100, 1985.

12. Bruce, RA, et al: Excessive reduction in peripheral resistance during exercise and risk of orthostatic symptoms with sustained-release nitroglycerin and diltiazem treatment of angina. Am Heart J 109:1020, 1985.
13. Wenger, NK: Rehabilitation of the patient with atherosclerotic heart disease. In McIntosh, HD (ed): Cardiology Series, Vol 3, No 3. Parke-Davis, Morris Plains, NJ, 1980.
14. Winer, HE, Glassman, E and Spencer, FC: Mechanism of relief of angina after coronary bypass surgery. Am J Cardiol 44:202, 1979.
15. Wulff, KS and Hong, PA: Surgical intervention in coronary artery disease. In Underhill, SL et al (eds): Cardiac Nursing, ed 2. JB Lippincott, Philadelphia, 1989.
16. Kneisl, CR and Ames, SW: Adult Health Nursing. Addison-Wesley, Reading, MA 1986.
17. Wulff, KS: Management of the cardiovascular surgery patient. In Brunner, LS and Suddarth, DS: Textbook of Medical-Surgical Nursing, ed 6. JB Lippincott, Philadelphia, 1987.
18. Woods, SL and Underhill, SL: Coronary heart disease: Myocardial ischemia and infarction. In Patrick, ML et al (eds): Medical, Surgical Nursing: Pathophysiological Concepts. JB Lippincott, Philadelphia, 1986.
19. Lewis, MR and Dehmer, GJ: Coronary bypass using the internal mammary artery. Am J Cardiol 56:480, 1985.
20. Barbour, DJ and Roberts, WC: Additional evidence for relative resistance to atherosclerosis of the internal mammary artery compared to the saphenous vein when used to increase myocardial blood supply. Am J Cardiol 56:488, 1985.
21. Kern, MJ, Eilen, SO and O'Rourke, R: Coronary vasomotion in angina at rest and effect of sublingual nitroglycerin on coronary blood flow. Am J Cardiol 56:488, 1985.
22. Loop, FD, et al: Influence of the internal mammary artery graft on 10-year survival and other cardiac events. N Engl J Med 314:1, 1986.
23. Fowler, NO: Cardiac Diagnosis and Treatment, ed 3. Harper & Row, Hagerstown, MD, 1980.
24. Johnson, WD, Kayser, KL and Pedraza, PM: Angina pectoris and coronary artery bypass surgery: Patterns of prevalence in occurrence in 3105 consecutive patients followed up to eleven years. Am Heart J 108:1190, 1984.
25. Kominski, K and Preston, T: Rehabilitation of the patient with coronary artery disease: Medical versus surgical. In Underhill, SL, et al (ed): Cardiac Nursing. JB Lippincott, Philadelphia, 1982.
26. Loop, FD: Atherosclerosis of the left main coronary artery: 5 year results of surgical treatment. Am J Cardiol 44:195–201, 1979.
27. McGoon, DC: Cardiac surgery. In Brest, AN (ed): Cardiovascular Clinic. FA Davis, Philadelphia, 1982.
28. Behrendt, DM and Austen, WG: Patient Care in Cardiac Surgery, ed 3. Little, Brown & Co, Boston, 1980.
29. Warren, SC and Warren, SG: Coronary angioplasty: Current concepts. Am Fam Physician 32:145, 1985.
30. Hall, DP and Gruentzig, AR: Techniques of PTA of the coronary, renal, mesenteric and peripheral arteries. In Hurst, JW (ed): The Heart, Arteries and Veins, ed 7. McGraw-Hill, New York, 1990.
31. Raff, D, et al. Life adaptation after PTCA and CABG. Am J Cardiol 56:395, 1985.
32. David, P, et al: Percutaneous transluminal angioplasty with variant angina. Circulation 66:695, 1982.
33. Vinsant, MO and Spence, MI: Diagnosis of coronary artery disease. In Vinsant, MO, and Spence, MI (eds): Commonsense Approach to Coronary Care. CV Mosby, St Louis, 1989.
34. Sokolow, M and McIlroy, MB: Clinical Cardiology. Lange Medical Publishers, Los Altos, CA, 1986.
35. A critical look at the artificial heart. In Hospital Ethics, American Hospital Association, Chicago, Jan/Feb, 1986.
36. Oberman, A: Exercise and the primary prevention of cardiovascular disease. Cardiol 55:100, 1985.
37. Wenger, NK and Fletcher, GF: Rehabilitation of the patient with atherosclerotic coronary heart disease. In Hurst, JW (ed): The Heart, Arteries and Veins, ed 5. McGraw-Hill, New York, 1986.
38. Bond, EF: Antiarrhythmic drugs. In Underhill, SL, et al (eds): Cardiac Nursing, ed 2. JB Lippincott, Philadelphia, 1989, pp 629–642.
39. Charrow, B (ed): Essentials of critical care pharmacology. Abridged from The Pharmacologic Approach to the Critically Ill Patient, ed 2. Williams & Wilkens, Baltimore, 1989.
40. Manolis, AS, et al: Mexiletine: Pharmacology and therapeutic use. Clin Cardiol 13:349–359, 1990.
41. Dunn, MI and Lipman, BS: Lipman-Massie Clinical Electrocardiology, ed 8. Year Book Medical Publishers, Chicago, 1989, pp 232–247.
42. Thompson, J, et al: Mosby's Manual of Clinical Nursing, ed 2. CV Mosby, St. Louis, 1989.
43. Civetta, J, Taylor, RW and Kirby, RR: Critical Care. JB Lippincott, Philadelphia, 1988.
44. Sipperly, ME: Expand the role of coronary angioplasty: Current implications, limitations and nursing considerations. Heart Lung 18(5):507–513.
45. Hillis, LD, et al: Manual of Clinical Problems in Cardiology, ed 3. Little, Brown & Co, Boston, 1988, pp 126–132, 368–369.
46. Kudota, LT: Angioplasty. In Underhill, SL, et al: Cardiac Nursing, ed 2. JB Lippincott, Philadelphia, 1989, p 532.
47. Conti, CR and Roberts, AJ: Current Surgery of the Heart. JB Lippincott, Philadelphia, 1987.
48. Galan, KM and Hollman, JL: Recurrence of stenosis after coronary angioplasty. Heart Lung 15(6):585–587.
49. Hurst, JW, et al: The Heart, Arteries and Veins, ed 7. McGraw-Hill, New York, 1990.

50. Murdock, DK, et al: Rejection of the transplanted heart. Heart Lung 16(3):237–245.
51. Futterman, LG: Cardiac transplantation: A comprehensive nursing perspective, part 2. Heart Lung 17(6):631–638.
52. Hall, LT: Cardiovascular lasers: A look into the future. Am J Nurs 90(9):27–30.
53. Stoy, DB: Controlling cholesterol with drugs. Am J Nurs 89(12):1628–1633.
54. Zadai, C: Pulmonary pharmacology. In Malone, T (ed): Physical and Occupational Therapy: Drug Implications for Practice. JB Lippincott, Philadelphia, 1989.
55. Yee, A, Connors, G and Cress, D: Pharmacology and the respiratory patient. In Hodgkin, J, Zorn, E, and Connors, G: Pulmonary Rehabilitation: Guidelines to Success. Butterworth Publishers, Boston, 1984.
56. Lehnert, B and Schachter, E: The Pharmacology of Respiratory Care. CV Mosby, St. Louis, 1980, pp 117–171.
57. Ziment, I: Pharmacologic therapy of COPD. In Hodgkin, J, and Petty, T (eds): Chronic Obstructive Pulmonary Disease: Current Concepts. WB Saunders, Philadelphia, 1987.
58. Benson, D and Conte, R: 89/90 Nursing Meds. Appleton & Lange, Norwalk, CT, 1989.
59. Ciccone, C: Pharmacology in Rehabilitation. FA Davis, Philadelphia, 1990, pp 290–307.
60. Sertl, K, Clark, T and Kaliner, M: Inflammation and airway function: The asthma syndrome. Am Rev Respir Dis (Suppl)141:1–2, 1990. (Editorial.)
61. Svedmyr, N: Action of corticosteroids on beta adrenergic receptors. Am Rev Respir Dis (Suppl)141:31–38.
62. Check, W and Kaliner, M: Pharmacology and pharmacokinetics of topical corticosteroid derivatives used for asthma therapy. Am Rev Respir Dis (Suppl)141:44–51, 1990.
63. Berte, J: Critical Care: The Lung, ed 2. Appleton-Century-Crofts, Norwalk, CT, 1986, p 127.
64. Becker, DM, Larosa, JH and Watson, JE: Interpreting the new guidelines. Am J Nurs 89(12):1622–1624, 1990.

CHAPTER **8**

The Electrocardiogram

An electrocardiogram (ECG) is a graphic representation of the electrical activity generated by the atria and ventricles. Impulse formation and conduction in the cardiac muscle generate weak electrical currents throughout the body.[7] The electrical impulses progressively depolarize the cardiac muscle and cause cardiac contraction.[1] By means of a galvanometer, the difference in potential between a positive and a negative area in the body is detected, amplified, and recorded. The electrocardiogram allows for indirect observation of the sequence of cardiac muscle excitation over any given period of time.

As electrical activity passes through the myocardium, it is detected by external skin electrodes placed at specific points on the body surface and recorded as a series of deflections on the ECG. The deflections, or waves, are known arbitrarily as P, Q, R, S, and T (Fig. 8–1). The upward deflections are positive; they represent an electrical current moving toward the skin electrode. The downward deflections are negative; they represent an electrical current moving away from the skin electrode. In both instances, the magnitude of the deflection represents the thickness of the muscle mass through which the current is being conducted (see the section on waves, complexes, and intervals).

Each deflection, or wave, represents an aspect of the depolarization or repolarization of the cardiac muscle cells. Although the progressive wave of electrical current is infinitesimal, it can be detected by the skin electrodes as it passes through the heart. The wave of depolarization flows from the base of the heart to the apex. Depolarization, the change of the internal electrical potential of the cell from negative to positive, causes almost immediate myocardial contraction. Depolarization is followed by repolarization. During repolarization, the cells regain their electronegative state, and the heart is in a physically "quiet" state. Although the change in electrical potential during repolarization is seen on the ECG, no physical activity accompanies this electrical activity.

It is important to note that the ECG is a recording of the electrical activity of the heart (depolarization and repolarization of the muscle cells) and not a recording of the actual contraction and relaxation of the myocardium that should occur a split second after a deflection is observed. The ECG is a composite of the total electrical activity of the heart at any given moment; therefore, not every aspect of electrical activity is discernible. Most notably, atrial repolarization, occurring in conjunction with ventricular depolarization, is "lost" in the QRS complex because of the greater voltage of the latter.

152

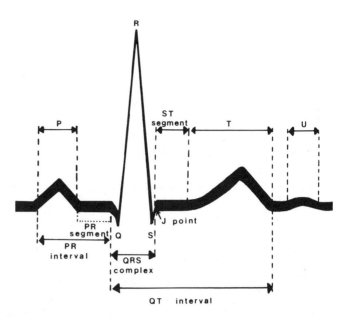

FIGURE 8–1. Normal PQRST wave configuration. ECG waves, complexes, and intervals. (From Underhill, SL, et al: Cardiac Nursing. JB Lippincott, Philadelphia, 1983, p. 204, with permission.)

THE CARDIAC CYCLE AND IMPULSE CONDUCTION

The cardiac cycle is one complete period of depolarization and repolarization of the cardiac muscle cells. Because of the heart cells' unique properties of automaticity, rhythmicity, and conductivity, the heart may regularly initiate and propagate an impulse along its conduction pathway without nervous system influence (Chapter 2). Every myocardial cell can initiate and propagate an impulse, but the sinoatrial node (SA node) is the "natural pacemaker" of the heart. It serves this function because the SA node cells maintain the lowest resting membrane potential in the heart's conduction system. They depolarize first and thereby initiate the impulse (at a rate of 60 to 100 beats per minute [bpm]) that is propagated throughout the conduction system by the heart's "all or nothing" conduction property. If the SA node does not initiate an impulse at appropriate intervals (60 to 100 bpm), another ectopic focus in the atria may initiate the heart beat. An ectopic focus is a site outside the SA node that initiates an impulse. In the normal sequence of events, once the impulse leaves the SA node, it traverses the atria and ventricles in a progressive wave of depolarization. The atria have not been determined to have any specialized conduction pathways; therefore, the impulse is propagated from cell to cell within the muscle. Almost immediately, simultaneous contraction of the left and right atria occur. The impulse is relayed from the atria to the ventricles via a specialized conduction pathway known as the atrioventricular node (AV node).

The AV node also has the capacity to perform the pacemaker function (at a rate of 40 to 70 bpm) if it does not receive any stimulation from the SA node. In normal conduction, the impulse is slowed as it passes through the AV node. Ventricular depolarization rapidly proceeds as the impulse moves via the bundle of His to the left and right bundle branches and through the Purkinje fibers, terminating in the subendocardium. The ventricular septum is depolarized first, followed by almost simultaneous depolarization of the left and right ventricles. Despite the fact that the left ventricle is depolarized just a fraction of a second before the right, the ECG records all of the electrical activity of the ventricles as a composite, the QRS complex (see Fig. 8–1). Contraction of the ventricles normally occurs within a split second of depolarization of the myocardium and then ventricular recovery (cellular repolarization) begins immediately. The repolarization of the atrium occurs simultaneously with ventricular depolarization. After ventricular repolarization occurs, the entire myocardium is returned to its electronegative state, and one cardiac cycle is completed.

WAVES, COMPLEXES, AND INTERVALS

The ECG is composed of a series of waves, complexes, and intervals, including the P wave, QRS complex, T wave, ST segment, and PR interval (see Fig. 8–1).

P Wave

The P wave is the first positive deflection on the ECG. It represents the depolarization of the atrial muscle cells following the release of an impulse from the SA node or some other focus in the atrium. The wave is symmetrical in appearance, usually 2.5 mm or less in height, and of 0.08 to 0.11 second duration (Fig. 8–2).

PR Interval

The PR interval is measured from the beginning of the P wave to the beginning of the QRS complex. It represents the time required for the impulse to travel from the atrium through the conduction system to the Purkinje fibers. The pause of the impulse

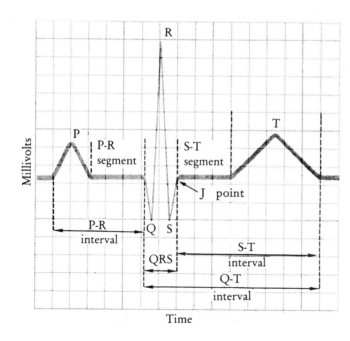

FIGURE 8–2. Normal electrocardiography and timing. Graphic representation of the normal electrocardiogram. Vertical lines represent time, each square represents 0.04 second, and every five squares (set off by heavy black lines) represents 0.2 second. The normal PR interval is less than 0.2 second; the average is 0.16 second. The average duration of the P wave is 0.08 second; the QRS complex is 0.08 second; the ST segment is 0.12 second; the T wave is 0.16 second; and the QT interval is 1.36 seconds. Each horizontal line represents voltage; every five squares equals 0.5 millivolt (mV). (From McHenry and Salerno,[28] p. 445, with permission.)

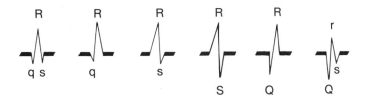

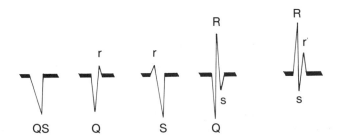

FIGURE 8–3. Variations in the QRS complex. Note that capital letters are assigned to large waves and that lowercase letters are assigned to small waves. (From Bernreiter, M: Electrocardiography. JB Lippincott, Philadelphia, 1963, p. 15, with permission.)

at the AV node is within the PR interval. The entire atrial-AV node activity is 0.12 to 0.20 second in duration (see Fig. 8–2).

QRS Complex

The first negative deflection of the QRS complex is known as the Q wave; it is followed by the upward R wave. Small Q waves seen in leads I, II, V^4, and V^5 are usually insignificant. A large Q wave is not often present, and it may indicate a recent infarction. A diagnostically significant Q wave is usually 0.04 second in duration and one third the size of the QRS complex. The R wave is the first upward deflection followed by a downward deflection, the S wave. There are several variations of the QRS complex, but despite the variations, all represent ventricular depolarization (Fig. 8–3) and are collectively known as the QRS complex.[12] The QRS complex has an amplitude of 20 to 30 mm and a duration of 0.06 to 0.10 second. An increase in duration is a sign of delayed conduction through the ventricle. An amplitude greater than 35 mm indicates ventricular hypertrophy. An amplitude less than 5 mm may indicate coronary artery disease (CAD), emphysema, marked obesity, generalized edema, or pericardial effusion.

ST Segment

The ST segment begins at the end of the QRS complex and represents the beginning of ventricular muscle repolarization. It is generally isoelectric (returns to the baseline), but it may rise above the isoelectric line 1 mm in normal individuals. (In healthy black males, the ST segment may be elevated as much as 2 mm.) The point at which the ST segment begins is known as the J (junction) point (Fig. 8–4). In evaluation of the cardiac patient, the J point is significant, because an ST-segment depression greater than 1 mm occurring 0.08 second after the J point is indicative of ischemia and diagnostic of CAD (see Fig. 8–4).[21,22]

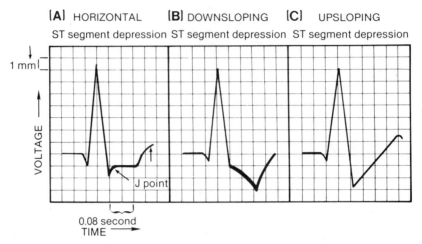

FIGURE 8–4. ST segment patterns: *A*, Horizontal ST segment depression; *B*, downsloping ST segment depression; *C*, upsloping ST segment depression. (From Vinsant and Spence,[10] p. 231, with permission.)

In an acute infarction, the ST segment is elevated, suggesting myocardial injury. Over time, weeks to months, the ST segment returns to the baseline. Prolonged ST-segment elevation suggests ventricular aneurysm. Generally, the ST segment is an average of 0.12 second in duration and slopes gently upward to the isoelectric line and the beginning of the T wave.

T Wave

Representing ventricular repolarization, the T wave is slightly rounded and slightly asymmetric. The deflection is in the same direction as the QRS, and the duration is about 0.16 second.

The time elapsed during the ST segment through the first half of the T wave is known as the absolute refractory period of the cardiac cycle. During that time, no impulse, no matter how strong, will be propagated through the ventricles. The second half of the T wave is referred to as the relative refractory period. During the relative refractory period, the vulnerable period of the cardiac cycle, a "stronger than normal" stimulus may initiate depolarization of the heart earlier than would normally be expected. A contraction resulting from this early impulse is said to be premature. When premature ventricular depolarization occurs on the second half of the T wave, a lethal arrhythmia could be precipitated. This phenomenon is known as the R-on-T phenomenon.

QT Interval

The QT interval represents electrical systole; it extends from the beginning of the QRS complex to the end of the T wave.

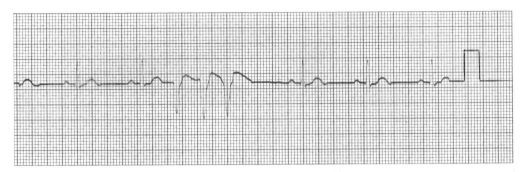

FIGURE 8–5. Standard ECG paper with standardization mark.

Standard Electrocardiogram Paper

ECG paper is standardized. It usually progresses through the cardiograph at a rate of 25 mm per second. Time is measured horizontally, with each small block equal to 0.04 second and each bold block 0.2 second (Fig. 8–5). Amplitude is measured vertically. Each small block equals 0.1 mV and is equivalent to 1 mm.

Standardization

Each electrocardiograph machine contains a 1-mV standard for calibration purposes that should appear on every ECG recording. The standard mark provides a manual check on the instrument's calibration. One millivolt of cardiac impulse should deflect the stylus exactly 1 cm (10 mm). The standard mark that appears on the ECG should be precisely 10 mm (1 cm) high, with a sharp upper left-hand corner. A slight sloping downward toward the right is normal. The shape and size of the standardization mark are significant, because lack of calibration may distort the ECG recording.

Electrocardiogram Leads

Measurement of the normal ECG requires the use of 12 leads or reference points from which the electrical activity of the heart can be detected and subsequently viewed. Six leads are known as the limb leads (I, II, III, aVR, aVL, aVF) and six are known as the precordial or chest leads (V_1 through V_6). Leads I, II, and III are formed by three sides of a triangle connecting the right arm, left arm, and left foot. The heart is located approximately at the center of the triangle (Einthoven's triangle) formed by those three points (Fig. 8–6). An 80 to 90 percent accuracy in diagnosis can be ensured by correct interpretation of those three leads alone.

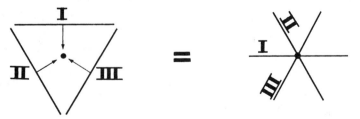

FIGURE 8–6. Vectors of leads I, II, and III. When these three lines are pushed to the center of the triangle, there are three intersecting lines of reference. (From Dubin,[2] p. 33, with permission.)

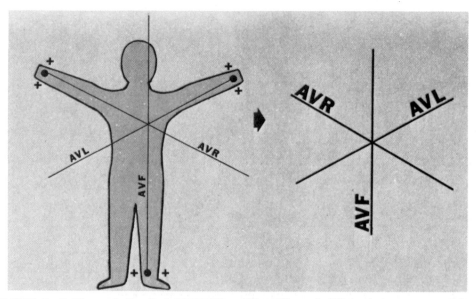

FIGURE 8–7. The unipolar limb leads. The aVR, aVL, and aVF leads intersect at different angles and produce three other intersecting lines of reference. (From Dubin,[2] p. 36, with permission.)

The limb leads I, II, and III are bipolar. They represent the difference in electrical potential between two specific points in the body. Lead I is the difference of potential between the left arm (LA) and the right (RA). Lead II is the difference in potential between the left leg (LL) and the right arm. Lead III is the difference in potential between the left leg and the left arm. The unipolar leads, aVF, aVL, and aVR, represent a difference in electrical potential between one positive lead and the average of the potential between the other two leads. Lead aVR (augmented voltage right) is the difference in potential between the right arm and the average of the potential of the left arm and left leg (Fig. 8–7). Lead aVL (augmented voltage left) is the difference in potential between the left arm and the average of the potential between the left leg and

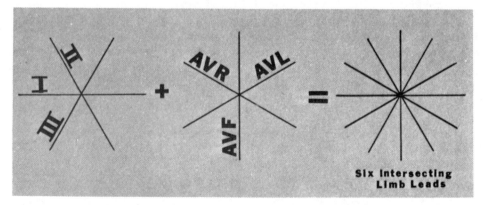

FIGURE 8–8. The limb leads. All six leads, I, II, III, aVR, aVL, and aVF, meet to form six neatly intersecting reference lines that lie in a flat plane on the patient's chest. (From Dubin,[2] p. 37, with permission.)

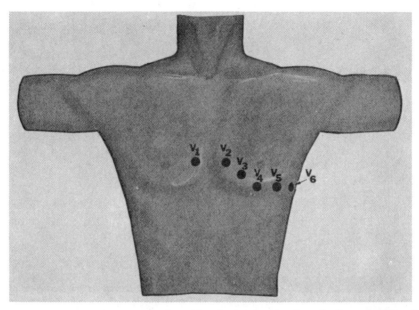

FIGURE 8-9. Chest lead reference sites. To obtain the six chest leads, a positive electrode is placed at six different positions around the chest. (From Dubin,[2] p. 41, with permission.)

the right arm. Lead aVF (augmented voltage foot) is the difference in potential between the left leg and the average of the potential between the left arm and right arm (see Fig. 8-7).[2] The waveforms of the aV leads are augmented (increased in size) in order to get waveforms of ample magnitude for evaluation.

The six limb leads intersect at 30° angles to form six intersecting reference lines in the frontal plane of the heart (Fig. 8-8). The six chest, or precordial, leads (V_1, V_2, V_3, V_4, V_5, and V_6) reflect the limb leads and are marked at six different positions, right to left, across the chest (Fig. 8-9); all the leads are positive. Normally on an ECG, the QRS will become progressively more positive from V_1 to V_6 (right to left across the chest) because the chest leads follow the same vectors as the electrical activity of the heart (Fig. 8-10). The chest leads record the electrical potential under each electrode compared to the central terminal connection, or V, that is made by connecting wires from the right arm, left arm, and left leg. The electrical potential of the V does not vary significantly throughout the cardiac cycle. Therefore, the recordings made with the V connections show the electrical activity that is occurring under each precordial electrode. In all 12 leads, the right leg serves as the ground or indifferent lead. Extraneous electrical activity is minimized by utilizing a ground lead.

Lead Placement

ECGs of the highest quality are necessary for meaningful interpretation. The quality of an ECG depends on both equipment and proper technique in recording the electrical events. Proper skin preparation (cleansing the skin with acetone or alcohol to reduce skin resistance and shaving the electrode site to ensure secure lead placement), as well as the selection of appropriate lead sites, ensures a definitive tracing. The limb leads

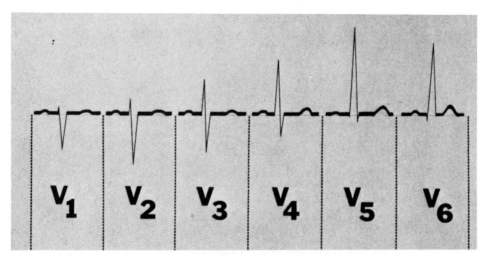

FIGURE 8–10. Progression of positive amplitude, from V_1 to V_6. The ECG tracing will thus show progressive changes from V_1 to V_6. (From Dubin,[2] p. 43, with permission.)

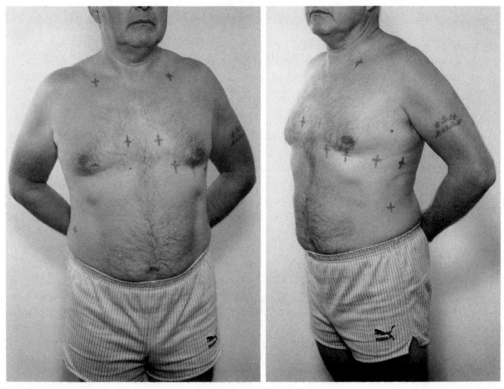

FIGURE 8–11. Electrode placement for a 12-lead exercise ECG recording. Electrode location and identification is as follows: (1) RL (right leg): just above the right iliac crest on the midaxillary line. (2) LL (left leg): just above the left iliac crest on the midaxillary line. (3) RA (right arm): just below the right clavicle medial to the deltoid muscle. (4) LA (left arm): just below the left clavicle medial to the deltoid muscle. (5) V_1: fourth interspace at the right sternal margin. (6) V_2: fourth interspace at the left sternal margin. (7) V_3: midway between V_2 and V_4. (8) V_4: fifth interspace at the midclavicular line just below the nipple. (9) V_5: midway between V_4 and V_6 on the anterior axillary line. (10) V_6: same transverse line as V_4 at the midaxillary line. (From Brannon, FJ: Experiments and Instrumentation in Exercise Physiology, Kendall-Hunt, Dubuque, IA, 1978, p. 101, with permission.)

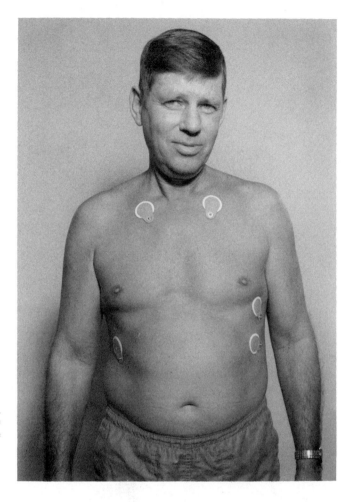

FIGURE 8-12. A modified chest lead V_5 (CMV$_5$). RL = right leg; LL = left leg; RA = right arm; LA = left arm; V_5 = left fifth intercostal space on anterior axillary line.

are placed on the extremities. To ensure maintenance of good contact, they may be placed proximally when doing ECGs or monitoring during exercise testing and therapy (Fig. 8-11).

Although the 12-lead ECG gives the most complete view of the heart, it may be inappropriate during exercise therapy. Modified lead placement for exercise is effective. It is not cumbersome to the individual and will not impede activity. In most cases, one lead alone will be sufficient to observe for arrhythmias.

A modified chest lead V_5 (CMV$_5$) may be recommended for exercise monitoring. It minimizes interference and permits ease of defibrillation should an emergency arise (Fig. 8-12). Of all arrhythmia disturbances, 98 percent are thought to be detected by CMV$_5$ during exercise testing and therapy.[10,14]

The 12-Lead Electrocardiogram

The interpreter of the ECG can gain a great deal of information from the 12-lead composite. Particular alterations in the depolarization and repolarization patterns reflect

TABLE 8–1 Normal Ranges and Variations in the Adult 12-Lead Electrocardiogram.

Lead	P	Q	R	S	T	ST
I	Upright deflection	Small. <0.04 s & <25% of R.	Dominant. Largest deflection of the QRS complex.	<R, or none	Upright deflection	Usually isoelectric; may vary from +1 to −0.5 mm.
II	Upright deflection	Small or none	Dominant	<R, or none	Upright deflection	Usually isoelectric; may vary from +1 to −0.5 mm.
III	Upright, flat, diphasic, or inverted, depending on frontal plane axis	Small or none, depending on frontal plane axis; or large (0.04 − 0.05 s or >25% of R).	None to dominant depending on frontal plane axis	None to dominant depending on frontal plane axis	Upright, flat, diphasic, or inverted depending on frontal plane axis.	Usually isoelectric; may vary from +1 to −0.5 mm.
aVR	Inverted deflection	Small, none, or large	Small or none depending on frontal plane axis.	Dominant (may be QS)	Inverted deflection	Usually isoelectric; may vary from +1 to −0.5 mm.
aVL	Upright, flat, diphasic, or inverted depending on frontal plane axis	Small, none, or large depending on frontal plane axis	Small, none, or dominant depending on frontal plane axis	None to dominant depending on frontal plane axis	Upright, flat, diphasic, or inverted depending on frontal plane axis	Usually isoelectric; may vary from +1 to −0.5 mm.

	Upright deflection					
aVF		Small or none	Small, none, or dominant depending on frontal plane axis.	None to dominant depending on frontal plane axis	Upright, flat, diphasic, or inverted depending on frontal plane axis	Usually isoelectric; may vary from +1 to −0.5 mm.
V_1	Inverted, flat, upright, or diphasic	None (may be QS)	$<S$ or none (QS); small r' may be present.	Dominant (may be QS)	Upright, flat, diphasic, or inverted*	0 to +3 mm
V_2	Upright; less commonly, diphasic or inverted	None (may be QS)	$<S$, or none (QS); small r' may be present.	Dominant (may be QS)	Upright; less commonly flat, diphasic, or inverted*	0 to +3 mm
V_3	Upright	Small or none	$R <, >,$ or $= S$	$S >, <,$ or $= R$	Upright*	0 to +3mm
V_4	Upright	Small or none	$R>S$	$S<R$	Upright*	Usually isoelectric; may vary from +1 to −0.5 mm
V_5	Upright	Small	Dominant (<26 mm)	$S<SV_4$	Upright	
V_6	Upright	Small	Dominant (<26 mm)	$S<SV_5$	Upright	

*Inverted in infants, children, and occasionally in young adults.

Source: From Goldman, MJ: Principles of Clinical Electrocardiography, ed 12. Lange Medical Publications, Los Altos, California, 1986, with permission.

myocardial pathology. By carefully reviewing the 12 different views of the heart, the pathological problem can be localized. Of course, the ECG must always be interpreted in conjunction with other clinical data, including laboratory results and the individual's activity tolerance and state of well-being.

Table 8–1 describes the characteristics of wave configuration for each lead of a normal 12-lead ECG, and Figure 8–13 represents a normal ECG. The reader is referred to any of the many excellent ECG interpretation texts for more in-depth interpretation of the ECG.[5-7] In this text, the information reviewed will be in regard to the basic interpretation of the most commonly occurring cardiac arrhythmias.

A standard 12-lead ECG tracing is normally used for diagnostic purposes. Arrhythmia detection in both the hospital and the outpatient cardiac rehabilitation settings can be accomplished easily and accurately by monitoring a single lead. (Lead I, II, or CMV_5 may be used.) In cardiac rehabilitation settings, telemetry systems, in which the individual's ECG is transmitted via radio waves to a remote observer, are most often used to free the patient from the hard-wire connection of the oscilloscope and to allow for unencumbered exercise.

A true understanding of the normal range and normal variation of the ECG depends on a basic understanding of both normal and abnormal cardiac electrophysiology. It must be remembered that many of the configurations tabulated below may represent cardiac abnormalities when interpreted in the context of the entire tracing and in light of the clinical history and physical examination. Therefore, the information contained in Table 8–1 is intended to be used only as a rough preliminary guide to the interpretation of ambiguous and borderline tracings.

INTERPRETING THE ELECTROCARDIOGRAM

Learning to interpret the 12-lead ECG takes a great deal of time and practice. In this text the primary focus is the basic interpretation of single-lead ECGs, or rhythm strips. Evaluation of the rate, rhythm, and individual waveform and their relations to one another will prepare the reader for basic interpretation. This skill is necessary for safely monitoring patients during exercise testing and exercise therapy. Individuals involved in cardiac rehabilitation programs most frequently have atherosclerosis of the coronary arteries. This condition interferes with the heart's normal response to exercise and increased myocardial oxygen demand. Such an individual most likely has a lower ischemic threshold and a more limited activity tolerance than one with healthy coronary arteries. Therefore, the clinician must be alert to the possibility of rate-dependent blocks and rhythm disturbances at low levels of activity.

In order to interpret an ECG strip properly, the clinician must answer five questions:

1. What is the rate?
2. What is the rhythm? Is it regular or irregular?
3. Are there P waves?
4. What is the QRS duration?
5. By evaluating the PR interval, what is the relation between the P waves and the QRS complexes?

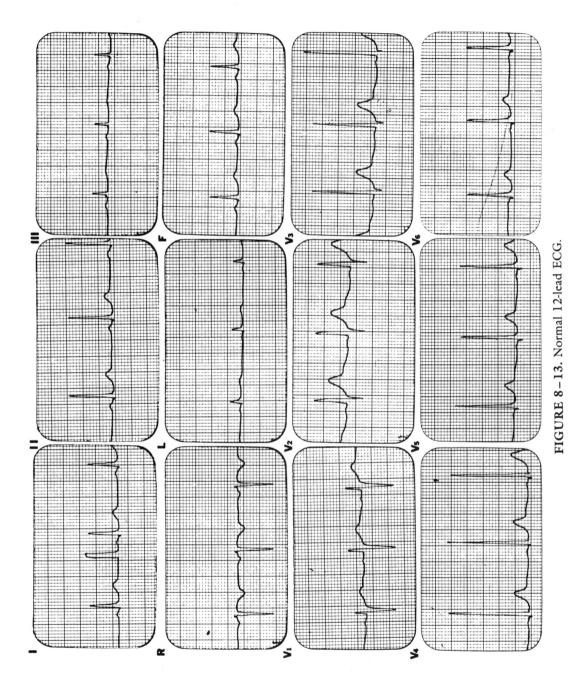

FIGURE 8–13. Normal 12-lead ECG.

165

The following sections describe how to answer those five questions, and they will enable the reader to identify common cardiac arrhythmias.

Calculating the Rate

As already noted, the SA node is the natural pacemaker of the heart. It has an intrinsic rate of 60 to 100 bpm. When, for some reason, the SA node does not fire, there are other pacemakers in the atria, ectopic foci, that can take over the pacemaker function. (An ectopic focus is a potential pacemaker site somewhere outside the SA node that can take over as the pacemaker if the SA node is not effective.[2]) Ectopic atrial pacemakers discharge at a rate of approximately 75 bpm, but that rate may increase to 150 to 250 bpm in pathologic situations. The intrinsic rate of the AV node is approximately 60 bpm, and the AV node may assume pacemaker activity when no impulse is received from the atria. Pathologic conditions may cause an ectopic focus in the ventricle to fire at a rate of 150 to 250 bpm, although the intrinsic rate of the ventricle is 20 to 40 bpm.

The heart rate is the first determination to be made in interpreting an ECG. One of the simplest methods used is to count the number of QRS complexes in a 6-second strip and multiply by 10 (chart speed = 25 mm per second). (Standard ECG paper has 3-second marks across the top of the paper; see Fig. 8–15.) A second method is looking at consecutive R waves. Find an R wave that falls on a heavy black vertical line on the ECG paper. Count off 300, 150, 100 on each of the heavy black lines that follow in succession. (Do not count the initial R wave that was selected.) Continue to count off 75, 60, 50 on the next three successive dark lines. (These numbers must be memorized.) Now, look for the next R wave by scanning to the right of the initial R wave identified. Where the next R wave falls will estimate the rate. If the second R wave falls between two heavy black lines, the location of its position between the two lines will affect the estimation of the rate (Fig. 8–14). This method allows the reader to quickly look at an ECG strip and roughly estimate the heart rate.[2,10] The two methods can be used to calculate the rate of regular rhythms, a rhythm in which there is a constant interval between similar waves. Irregularly occurring rhythms are best estimated by counting the R waves that occur within a minute. Rates greater than 100 bpm are, by definition, tachycardias, and rates below 60 bpm are bradycardias.

Determining the Rhythm

In regular rhythm, there is a consistent distance between similar waves. The normal sinus rhythm (NSR) of the heart is a regular rhythm occurring at a rate of 60 to 100 bpm. Irregular rhythms may be regularly irregular, in which patterns of irregularity are identified and repeated, or they may be completely chaotic and termed irregularly irregular (Fig. 8–15). Disturbances in rhythm, cardiac arrhythmias, are caused by an abnormality in automaticity (initiation of the impulse), an abnormality in conduction (propagation of the impulse), or both. Disturbances in automaticity may be either decreased automaticity of the SA node, which may force an ectopic focus to take over or "escape," or enhanced automaticity of an ectopic focus, in which the ectopic focus may

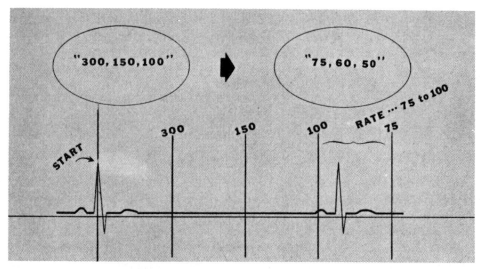

FIGURE 8–14. Calculating the heart rate. Note that the series of numbers assigned to the successive heavy black lines must be memorized: 300, 150, 100, 75, 60, 50. This figure represents an approximate rate of 90 bpm. (From Dubin,[2] p. 62, with permission.)

actively "usurp" or override the sinus pacemaker. The ectopic focus may be a point anywhere in the atria, AV node, or ventricles. Disturbances in conduction are the result of a block at some point in the conduction system that may be a result of ischemia to that area. Identification of arrhythmias is based on the location of the origins of the arrhythmias in the conduction system and by the characteristics of the particular rhythm.

Characteristics of Rhythms

NORMAL SINUS RHYTHM

Definition and Cause

NSR is the conventional rhythm of the healthy heart (Fig. 8–16, Table 8–2). Arising from the SA node, the impulse follows normal conduction pathways. It is a regular rhythm, although there may be some phasic variation with respiration that

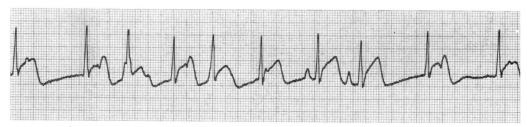

FIGURE 8–15. Ventricular response is irregularly irregular. There is no pattern to the occurrence of the R waves. Note the 3-second marks across the ECG paper.

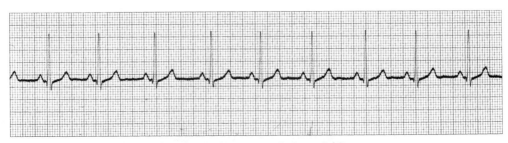

FIGURE 8–16. Normal sinus rhythm.

increases with inspiration and decreases with expiration. This is frequently seen in young adults. The rate may also be influenced by exercise, emotions, environmental and body temperature, drugs, and various disease states.

Hemodynamic Implications
   None.

Treatment
   No treatment is necessary.

SINUS BRADYCARDIA

Definition and Cause
   A sinus bradycardia is a slow rhythm of less than 60 bpm originating from a supraventricular source. It occurs normally during sleep and is commonly seen in individuals who are physically fit. It also occurs in response to increased vagal tone owing to gastrointestinal (GI) distress, pain, carotid sinus pressure, ocular pressure, increased intracranial pressure, and acute myocardial infarction (MI). Administration of digoxin, beta-adrenergic blocking agents, and calcium ion antagonists also may cause bradycardia.

ECG Appearance
   All waves (Fig. 8–17) are of normal configuration with a rate of less than 60 bpm.

Hemodynamic Implications
   Unless bradycardia is profound (less than 40 bpm), it is well tolerated. However, if cardiac output is not adequate, the individual is compromised hemodynamically and exhibits signs of decreased cardiac output (cold, clammy skin, low blood pressure, syncope).

TABLE 8–2 Normal Configuration of ECG Waves

	Duration	Amplitude
P wave	0.08–0.12 sec	1–3 mm
PR interval	0.12–0.20 sec	Isoelectric after the P wave deflection
QRS	0.06–0.10 sec	25–30 mm (maximum)
ST segment	0.12 sec	−½ to +1 mm
T wave	0.16 sec	5–10 mm

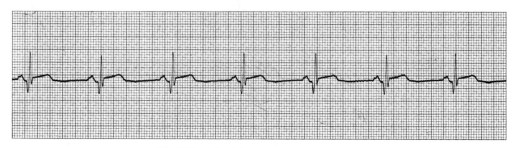

FIGURE 8–17. Sinus bradycardia.

Treatment

Uncomplicated bradycardia requires no treatment. If the individual is compromised by the slow rate, atropine administered intravenously rapidly and dramatically increases the heart rate. Temporary or permanent pacing may be necessary if there is profound, poorly tolerated bradycardia.

SINUS TACHYCARDIA

Definition and Cause

Tachycardia is a rapid sinus rhythm of greater than 100 bpm. A sinus rhythm originates in the SA node. Anything that increases sympathetic activity, such as excitement, pain, fever, hypovolemia, hypoxia, strenuous exercise, and the consumption of caffeine and/or nicotine, can frequently cause tachycardia. Cardiac failure, MI, and many other diseases of the heart are accompanied by sinus tachycardia. The tachycardia may also be induced by administration of drugs, including Isuprel, atropine, epinephrine, and alcohol.

ECG Appearance

Waveforms are normal (Fig. 8–18). The rate is greater than 100 bpm.

Hemodynamic Implications

Unless associated with a pathological state, sinus tachycardia is usually inconsequential and of brief duration. The rapid heart rate does, however, increase myocardial oxygen demand and may decrease coronary artery perfusion and result in angina in the individual with CAD. Symptoms of low cardiac output might also be exhibited when the decreased diastolic time prevents adequate ventricular filling.

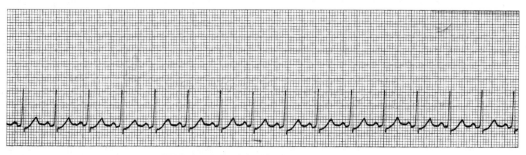

FIGURE 8–18. Sinus tachycardia.

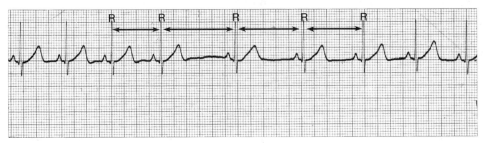

FIGURE 8–19. Sinus arrhythmia.

Treatment
Intervention should include rest and treatment of the underlying pathologic state. Oxygen and sublingual nitroglycerin may be necessary if the individual experiences angina. Digoxin may be administered to increase contractility, slow AV conduction, and decrease the heart rate if the patient is symptomatic.

SINUS ARRHYTHMIA

Definition and Cause
A sinus arrhythmia is a varying irregular rhythm with all impulses originating in the SA node. It may occur in the young and the elderly in response to enhanced vagal tone, digitalis, or morphine.[3] The arrhythmia may be related to respiration, with the rate increasing with inspiration and decreasing with expiration.

ECG Appearance
All waves are normal in size and shape (Fig. 8–19), but the timing of the cycles is irregular. The rate is usually between 60 and 100 bpm.

Hemodynamic Implications
There are usually no hemodynamic consequences of sinus arrhythmia.

Treatment
No treatment is necessary.

Atrial Arrhythmias

Atrial arrhythmias are caused by the rapid and repetitive firing of one or more foci in the atria outside the sinus node. They override the slower SA node pacemaker and take control of the rhythm of the heart. In atrial arrhythmias with rates of less than 200, every impulse may be conducted through the AV node to the ventricles (1:1 conduction). At rates greater than 200, the physiologic refractory period of the AV node introduces a block to conduction and therefore the conduction ratio (atrial:ventricular impulses) may be 2:1, 3:1, or greater. On the ECG, the P waves are variable in shape and rhythm, depending on the location of the ectopic focus. The configuration of the QRS may be normal because the conduction pathways below the AV node are normal. However, the rhythm may be very irregular because the atrial impulses are often conducted in an irregular pattern.

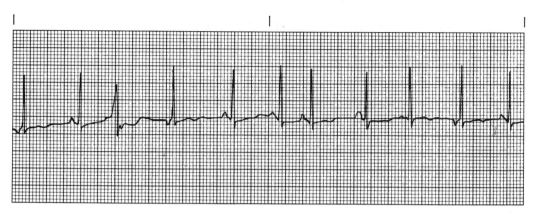

FIGURE 8-20. Wandering atrial pacemaker.

WANDERING ATRIAL PACEMAKERS

Definition and Cause

The wandering atrial pacemaker is a varying rhythm caused by the changing focus of the pacemaker. It occurs when there is a change in vagal tone or there are changes in sympathetic stimulation to the heart. It is not uncommon, and it is most likely to be observed in athletes, the young, and the elderly.

ECG Appearance

The atrial rate is very irregular. There is no consistent pattern to the rhythm (Fig. 8-20). The shape of the P waves and length of the PR intervals vary with the pacemaker firing and the proximity of the ectopic pacemaker to the AV node. When the pacemaker site is closer to the AV node, the PR interval is shorter and the P wave becomes flatter. The ventricular rate is equal in rate and rhythm to the atrial rate, because all atrial impulses are conducted to the ventricle. The QRS is normal in appearance, because ventricular conduction is normal.

Hemodynamic Implications

There are no hemodynamic consequences, because the rate is usually 60 to 100 bpm and cardiac output is maintained.

Treatment

No treatment is necessary unless there is a symptomatic bradycardia; in that event, a sympathomimetic drug (Isuprel) may be administered. (Sympathomimetic drugs are synthetic substances of similar chemical structure, and they have many effects similar to those of adrenergic neurohormones. They act on the alpha and beta receptors, increase heart rate and contractility, and accelerate conduction.) If the rate is over 100 bpm, treatment is directed toward eliminating the cause and decreasing the heart rate with a beta-blocker such as propranolol.

PREMATURE ATRIAL CONTRACTIONS

Definition and Cause

A premature atrial contraction (PAC) is an earlier than expected depolarization from an ectopic focus. The impulse travels through the atria by an unusual pathway and creates a P wave of different configuration. If the ventricle is not in absolute refractory at the time the impulse reaches the AV node, the impulse will be conducted normally through the ventricles and produce a normal QRS complex. PACs are seen in hearts that are healthy as well as in those with CAD. Many other pathological conditions may cause the development of PACs, including rheumatic heart disease, MI, hypertension, and hyperthyroidism. Stress, fatigue, and anxiety may cause PACs, as will the administration of epinephrine, digoxin, and/or the ingestion of stimulants (caffeine, nicotine).

ECG Appearance

NSR is present except for the PAC, which occurs earlier than expected (Fig. 8–21). The P wave of the PAC is abnormal, but all other waves are normal in configuration.

Hemodynamic Implications

PACs are usually well tolerated, because cardiac output is not altered.

Treatment

The only treatment is to omit the stimulus that may be precipitating the PACs (e.g., digoxin, caffeine, nicotine).

PAROXYSMAL ATRIAL TACHYCARDIA

Definition and Cause

Paroxysmal atrial tachycardia (PAT) is rapid atrial rhythm characterized by abrupt onset and abrupt cessation. It is triggered by emotions, tobacco, fatigue, caffeine, alcohol, or sympathomimetic drugs (Isuprel). It is not usually related to organic heart disease. The rhythm may be sustained for seconds, minutes, or hours, and the patient's tolerance for the arrhythmia may depend on the underlying pathology. The rate is usually 150 to 250 bpm, and there is a 1:1 atrial:ventricular conduction.

ECG Appearance

The P wave is slightly to grossly abnormal, and it may often be found in the preceding T wave (Fig. 8–22). The PR interval may be shortened (less than 0.12 second). QRS-complex and T-wave configurations are normal. In rapid rhythms, the T wave may not be discernible.

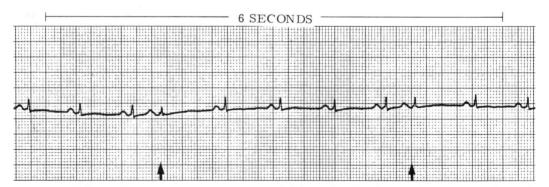

FIGURE 8–21. Normal sinus rhythm with a premature atrial contraction. Note that the fourth complex from the left and the third complex from the right occur early in the cycle; the P waves are of a slightly different configuration from the other P waves.

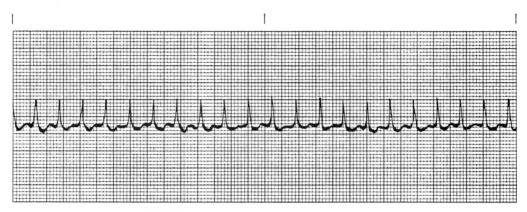

FIGURE 8-22. Paroxysmal atrial tachycardia.

Hemodynamic Implications

PAT of short duration is of little consequence to the healthy heart. However, in the presence of an impaired left ventricle, sustained PAT may precipitate left ventricular failure. Angina may also occur as a result of decreased coronary artery blood flow.

Treatment

Treatment is directed at both eliminating the cause of the tachycardia and decreasing the heart rate. Carotid sinus massage or Valsalva maneuvers are usually the first measures instituted. Pharmacologically, intravenous varapamil is the most effective agent for acute termination. PAT is also treated with digoxin, propranolol, or quinidine and in some cases beta-blocking agents or amiodarone.[33] If drug therapy is not successful in converting PAT to normal sinus rhythm, cardioversion may be used to terminate the rapid rhythm and restore NSR. (Cardioversion is the delivery of an electrical charge to the heart, synchronized with the R wave, that results in complete depolarization of the myocardium. The charge has the potential to interrupt certain arrhythmias, which allows the SA node, the normal pacemaker of the heart, to resume control of the rhythm.)

ATRIAL FLUTTER

Definition and Cause

Atrial flutter is a rapid, regular, atrial arrhythmia arising from one atrial focus with a rate of 250 to 350 bpm but most commonly 300 bpm. It is easily recognizable because of the regular, saw-toothed baseline (called F, or flutter, waves). The refractory time of the AV nodal tissue prevents conduction of more than 200 impulses per minute through the AV node. The rate of impulses conducted to the ventricles is normally an even-numbered ratio to the atrial impulses initiated (2:1 and 4:1). Seen less frequently than atrial fibrillation, atrial flutter may convert to atrial fibrillation spontaneously or during treatment. Individuals with normal hearts experience occasional atrial flutter precipitated by anxiety, caffeine, alcohol, or nicotine. Persistent atrial flutter is usually associated with rheumatic heart disease, valvular disease, CAD, or pulmonary emboli.

ECG Appearance

The rhythm is recognizable by the regular saw-toothed baseline (Fig. 8-23). The configuration of the QRS complex is normal. Ventricular conduction follows the normal

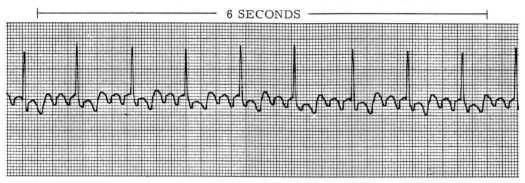

FIGURE 8–23. Atrial flutter (4:1 ratio). Note the saw-toothed baseline, known as F waves.

pathways. T waves are usually not identifiable because of the overriding F waves. When calculating the atrial rate, the F wave that falls within the QRS complex also is counted.

Hemodynamic Implications

The individual may experience a fluttering sensation in the chest or throat. If it is short-lived, there is probably minimal or no hemodynamic consequence. If the cardiac output is compromised by a rapid ventricular response, the individual will experience symptoms of decreased cardiac output.

Treatment

The goals of therapy are to terminate the rhythm or control ventricular response, as well as to identify and treat the cause. Verapamil or vagal stimulation may be used to slow the ventricular response temporarily and to permit clear identification of flutter waves. Digoxin is the drug of choice, and it may restore NSR within 24 hours. If digoxin alone does not control the ventricular rate, the addition of a beta-blocker, propranolol, will slow it. Long-term management may include the use of quinidine, procainamide, and disopyramide in conjunction with digitalis. Cardioversion is also effective in converting this rhythm. Many patients require atrial pacing or cardioversion, because chemical conversion is often unsuccessful.[33]

ATRIAL FIBRILLATION

Definition and Cause

Atrial fibrillation is a rapid, chaotic atrial arrhythmia caused by the firing of multiple ectopic foci in the atria. The atrial rate may be 350 to 600 bpm. The ventricular response may be very rapid or controlled, but it is usually irregularly irregular (Fig. 8–24) owing to the refractory period of AV nodal cells.[9] The atrial activity does not support complete atrial contraction and is out of sequence with ventricular activity. This causes a loss of the atrial "kick." The etiology of atrial fibrillation is not known. The fibrillation may occur paroxysmally (occurring and recurring suddenly) in the healthy heart. Chronic atrial fibrillation usually indicates heart disease and is seen in patients with congestive heart failure (CHF), CAD, and pulmonary embolism and following coronary artery bypass graft (CABG) surgery. Atrial fibrillation occurs frequently in the elderly with or without underlying cardiac disease. It is considered to be an arrhythmia of old age.

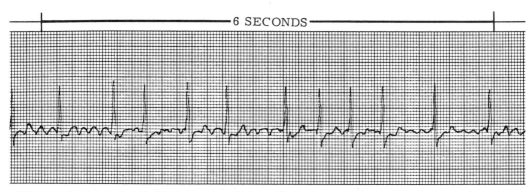

FIGURE 8–24. Atrial fibrillation with rapid ventricular response. (Note the irregular pattern of the ventricular response. There is no pattern to the irregularity, and therefore it is referred to as irregularly irregular.)

ECG Appearance

P waves are not identifiable. There is an undulating baseline, or a series of fine fibrillatory waves, representing the erratic atrial activity (Figs. 8–24 and 8–25). The ventricular response is irregularly irregular and occurs at a rate of 100 to 150 bpm in the untreated patient. The configuration of the QRS is normal. In atrial fibrillation with a controlled ventricular response, the ventricular rate is less than 100 bpm and, because of the irregular baseline, the T waves are usually unrecognizable.

Hemodynamic Implications

In atrial fibrillation with a controlled ventricular response (less than 100 bpm), the cardiac output is often adequate. However, at higher rates of ventricular response, there may be a decrease in cardiac output because ventricular fill time is decreased and coordination of atrial and ventricular systole is lost. There is a loss of the atrial kick that normally contributes as much as 30 to 35 percent to the left ventricular volume. Chaotic motion of the atria may also predispose the individual to the development of mural thrombi. This is frequently a concern during an attempt to convert atrial fibrillation to NSR, particularly when the atrial fibrillation has been present for longer than 6 months. The more vigorous motion of the myocardia in NSR may dislodge a thrombus, and pulmonary or cerebral emboli may result.

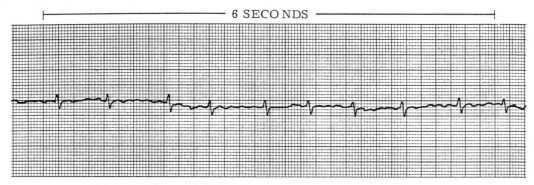

FIGURE 8–25. Atrial fibrillation with a controlled ventricular response.

Treatment

Atrial fibrillation may be chronic or occur paroxysmally. Drugs that block AV node conduction (i.e., digitalis, verapamil, and propranolol) are the treatment of choice to convert the rhythm to NSR. No treatment is indicated when the ventricular response is controlled and the individual is asymptomatic. Individuals with chronic atrial fibrillation may be placed on anticoagulant therapy, because the major concern is thrombus formation and subsequent embolization. Cardioversion may also be successfully used, especially when atrial fibrillation is new and the patient is hemodynamically compromised.

SUPRAVENTRICULAR TACHYCARDIA

Definition and Cause

Supraventricular tachycardia (SVT) is any tachycardia in which the impulse initiating the rhythm arises from a location above the ventricles. Examples include sinus, atrial, and junctional tachycardias. The extremely rapid rates often make it difficult to identify the origin of the rhythm. Differentiation from ventricular tachycardia may be difficult, especially if the impulse is aberrantly conducted (by other than normal pathways) and results in a QRS complex of greater than 0.12 second. In SVT, the ventricular rate is regular and is usually 150 to 200 bpm. SVT may be sustained rhythm or may last only a few seconds. SVT is most often observed in an individual with ischemic heart disease or as a complication of MI.

ECG Appearance

The origin of the arrhythmia determines the ECG appearance. If it is a sinus or atrial tachycardia, a P wave and PR interval should precede each QRS complex (Fig. 8–26). If it is junctional tachycardia, P waves may appear before or after or be buried within the QRS complex. The QRS complex either is a normal configuration or is widened and bizarre. A T wave is usually not observed.

Hemodynamic Implications

Usually the rapid rate is poorly tolerated. There is inadequate ventricular fill time, decreased cardiac output, and inadequate myocardial perfusion time.

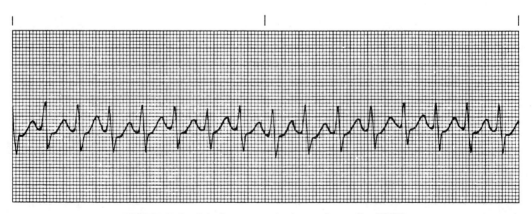

FIGURE 8–26. Supraventricular tachycardia (SVT).

Treatment

Treatment is aimed at controlling the ventricular rate and preventing CHF. The physician may apply carotid sinus massage or supraorbital pressure to stimulate a vagal response. Asking the patient to bear down (creating a Valsalva maneuver) may have the same response. The drugs of choice are verapamil, propranolol, and digoxin. Cardioversion may also prove effective in terminating SVT.

Atrioventricular Nodal Rhythms/Junctional Rhythms

AV nodal or junctional rhythms originate in the AV node when the SA node fails to initiate an impulse. The AV node fires intrinsically at a rate of 35 to 60 bpm. On ECG (Fig. 8–27), the P wave may be absent or inverted, and it may appear before or after or be buried within the QRS, because conduction in the atria occurs in a retrograde fashion. If the conduction pathways are healthy below the AV node, the QRS will be normal in configuration. With the loss of the synchronized cardiac contraction, the atrial contribution to the ventricular systolic volume (atrial kick) is lost and cardiac output may be decreased 30 to 35 percent.

PREMATURE NODAL/JUNCTIONAL CONTRACTIONS

Definition and Cause

Premature nodal contractions (PNCs) or premature junctional contractions (PJCs) are premature beats originating in the AV node. They occur in conditions that cause sinus bradycardia or in digitalis toxicity, in which there is increased automaticity of the AV node. The drugs Isuprel and atropine also may cause PNCs.

ECG Appearance

There is NSR or sinus bradycardia except for premature beats (Fig. 8–28). The P wave of the premature beat may precede, be buried in, or come after the QRS complex. If the PNC stimulates retrograde conduction through the atria, it will interrupt the sinus mechanism and produce a noncompensatory pause as the sinus mechanism is reset. If there is no retrograde conduction, the sinus mechanism is not interrupted and a compensatory pause will appear. (See the following section on premature ventricular contractions [PVCs] for definition of compensatory pause.)

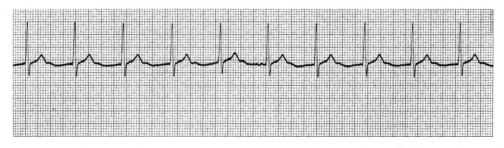

FIGURE 8–27. Junctional rhythm. Note the absence of P waves.

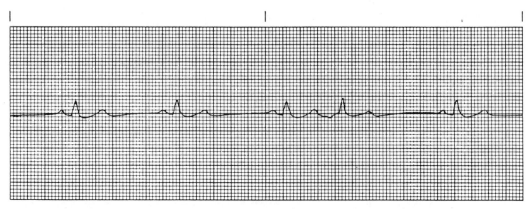

FIGURE 8–28. Normal sinus rhythm with one premature nodal contraction.

Hemodynamic Implications

The PNC may cause decreased stroke volume because the ventricle does not have sufficient time to fill prior to the premature contraction. The radial pulse palpated following the PNC may be much fuller, owing to the extra ventricular volume because the compensatory pause allows for extra fill time.

Treatment

No treatment is necessary unless the PNCs are related to digitalis toxicity. In that case, digoxin is withheld until the digoxin level is again within the therapeutic range.

Ventricular Arrhythmias

Ventricular arrhythmias originate from foci somewhere in the ventricles. Ventricular pacemakers are erratic, slow, and undependable. An effective cardiac output is rarely maintained, and a life-threatening situation is created. Ventricular arrhythmias constitute an emergency. Immediate intervention and conversion of the arrhythmia to a rhythm that produces effective circulation is essential. The goal of long-term maintenance therapy is the prevention of the arrhythmia and sudden cardiac death.[35]

PREMATURE VENTRICULAR CONTRACTIONS

Definition and Cause

The most common of all arrhythmias, the PVC is a premature beat arising from the ventricle.[14] Occurring occasionally in the majority of the normal population, PVCs may be precipitated by anxiety, tobacco use, alcohol, or caffeine consumption.

Any condition resulting in ischemia of the myocardium (MI, CAD, CHF) may cause PVCs. Hypokalemia (decreased serum potassium) also may precipitate PVCs.

ECG Appearance

The ECG may appear normal except for the premature beats (Fig. 8–29). Depolarization begins in the ventricle and follows an abnormal pathway that results in a tall and wide QRS complex (greater than 0.12 second). Such a complex is said to be bizarre. A compensatory pause follows the PVC. (A compensatory pause is longer than the regular

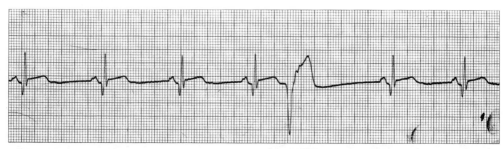

FIGURE 8–29. Normal sinus rhythm with unifocal premature ventricular contractions.

pause between beats and is a result of the PVC coming early in the cardiac cycle.) Most often, the sinus mechanism has not been interrupted, and the next impulse is initiated, from the SA node, at the regular interval in the existing sinus rhythm. The RR interval containing the PVC is two times the RR interval between the sinus beats (Fig. 8–30). If the PVC is conducted backward and interrupts the sinus mechanism, the sinus mechanism resets and a compensatory pause does not appear.[14] The T wave is opposite in deflection to the R wave of the PVC. PVCs that occur close to the vulnerable period of the preceding T wave are of concern because they may fall on the T wave and precipitate ventricular fibrillation (the R-on-T phenomenon).

Hemodynamic Implications

Occasional PVCs have minimal consequences. Increasingly frequent or multifocal PVCs suggest an increasingly irritable ventricle with potential for the development of life-threatening ventricular arrhythmias.

Patterns of Premature Ventricular Contractions

PVCs often occur in ratios to normal sinus beats. Bigeminy (Fig. 8–31) is a PVC coupled with each sinus beat. Trigeminy is a PVC every third beat. Quadrigeminy is a PVC every fourth beat, and a couplet (see Fig. 8–30) is two PVCs occurring together.

Treatment

The goal of treatment is elimination of the PVCs and their cause. The individual should rest, and oxygen should be administered if the PVCs continue at rest. A symptomatic individual will complain of feeling "skipped beats" or fluttering sensations in the

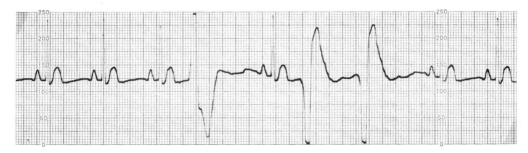

FIGURE 8–30. Premature ventricular contractions: single PVC, then a couplet. Note the compensatory pause. The RR interval containing the PVC is two times the RR interval between sinus beats.

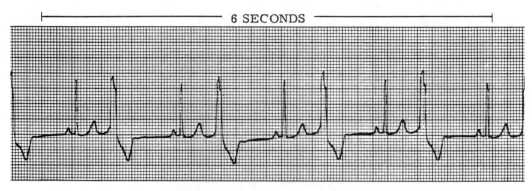

FIGURE 8–31. Ventricular bigeminy.

chest or throat. In the acute care setting, intravenous lidocaine may be administered when PVCs, couplets, or multifocal PVCs occur at rates greater than 6 per minute (a standard point for intervention). In the cardiac rehabilitation setting, some individuals may have chronic PVCs that do or do not change with exercise and do not require treatment even at rates greater than 6 PVCs per minute. Others may experience an expected increase in PVCs during some phase of their exercise or recovery period. In such individuals, the exercise prescription should include specific parameters delineating the circumstances under which the individual's exercise should be terminated and appropriate treatment should be initiated. Treatment of chronic PVCs is typically accomplished with procainamide or other antiarrhythmic medications such as propranolol, tocainamide, or mexiletine. Treatment of any underlying cause is continued concomitantly.

VENTRICULAR TACHYCARDIA

Definition and Cause

Three or more PVCs occurring sequentially at a rate of 150 to 200 bpm constitute a run of ventricular tachycardia (VT). VT is usually the result of an irritable, ischemic ventricle. In the healthy heart, VT may occur paroxysmally, produce no symptoms, and convert spontaneously to an effective cardiac rhythm. Sustained VT is life-threatening because a sufficient cardiac output is not maintained. As the ventricle becomes increasingly ischemic, VT degenerates to ventricular fibrillation. This progression of arrhythmias is believed to be responsible for sudden cardiac death unrelated to MI.

ECG Appearance

The QRS is wide, bizarre, and usually of high amplitude (Fig. 8–32). There is no P wave, and the RR intervals are usually regular.

Hemodynamic Implications

Coronary artery blood flow is estimated to decrease 60 percent in VT owing to ineffective cardiac output from a rapidly contracting ventricle. Syncopal episodes occur. (If the patient remains alert with no signs of decreased cardiac output, the arrhythmias may actually be supraventricular, a rhythm that may also begin paroxysmally and have large, regular QRS complexes. However, some patients do experience repeated VT episodes that are hemodynamically well tolerated.)

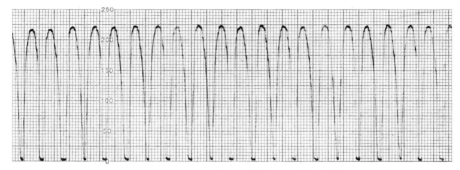

FIGURE 8–32. Ventricular tachycardia.

Treatment

Once the rhythm has been identified, treatment should begin immediately and without hesitation. Electrical cardioversion is the treatment of choice, with addition of lidocaine or procainamide to prevent recurrence of VT and to restore NSR. Bretylium also may be used.

Prophylactic drug therapy in patients with recurrent VT is highly individualized. Currently no single agent appears to stand out in its effectiveness. The Food and Drug Administration (FDA) has approved an automatic implantable cardioverter-defibrillator for use in patients who have chronic intractable VT or fibrillation that cannot be controlled by drug therapy (see page 193). When tachycardia or fibrillation is sensed by the implanted pulse generator, it sends an electrical shock to the heart. This shock depolarizes the entire myocardium and allows the sinus node to regain control of the rhythm.

VENTRICULAR FIBRILLATION

Definition and Cause

Ventricular fibrillation (VF) is chaotic activity of the ventricle originating when multiple foci in the ischemic ventricle fire simultaneously. Because of electrical disorganization, the ventricles do not contract as a unit. There is absolutely no effective cardiac output or coronary perfusion. VF is associated with severe myocardial ischemia; it may also be precipitated by drug overdose (digitalis, procainamide, potassium chloride, and others), anesthesia, electrical shock, or cardiac surgery. This is a life-threatening arrhythmia that usually results in death if not treated within 4 minutes.

ECG Appearance

There are no recognizable P waves, QRS complexes, or T waves. The erratic waveforms vary in size and may initially be unrecognizable waves of large amplitude (coarse VF) that quickly decrease in amplitude (fine VF) as myocardial death occurs. A flat baseline (asystole) indicates absolute electrical silence and death (Figs. 8–33 and 8–34).

Hemodynamic Implications

There is no systemic or coronary circulation. Clinical death occurs within 4 minutes.

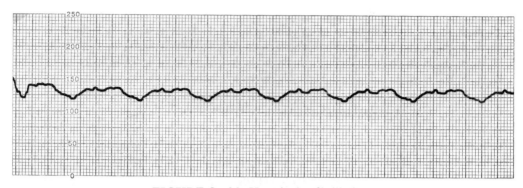

FIGURE 8–33. Ventricular fibrillation.

Treatment

Immediate defibrillation with 200 to 400 Watt-seconds. If unavailable or ineffective, cardiopulmonary resuscitation must be initiated immediately. Bretylium and lidocaine and many other drugs may be used during the resuscitation efforts to treat arrhythmias, hypoxia, acidosis, and hypokalemia.

Heart Blocks

Heart blocks are anatomical or functional interruptions in the normal conduction of an impulse through the heart's conductive pathways. This text briefly describes some of the more common blocks.

SINOATRIAL BLOCK

Definition and Cause

In sinoatrial block (SA node block), the impulse is discharged from the SA node but for some reason is unable to reach the surrounding atrial tissue. Although SA block is most frequently the result of drug therapy (digoxin or quinidine), it may occur in CAD.

ECG Appearance

The appearance of all waves is normal. There is an occasional or frequent interruption in the rhythm in which one or more cardiac cycles are missed. The rhythm is the

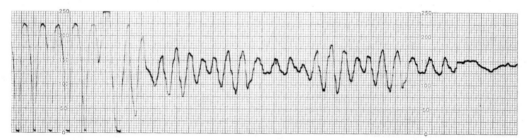

FIGURE 8–34. Progression of ventricular arrhythmias. Note that the rhythm rapidly changes from VT to coarse VF and then to fine VF.

same before and after the pause. If the pause is prolonged, an ectopic focus may fire. The sinus node usually continues to function as the pacemaker.

Hemodynamic Implications

There are hemodynamic implications only if the pause is prolonged. Prolonged pauses may be associated with signs of decreased cardiac output.

Treatment

Treatment is not necessary unless bradycardia is profound and the individual becomes symptomatic. Atropine, epinephrine, or isoproterenol may be administered to increase the heart rate if that occurs. Medications should be withdrawn if the block is the result of drug therapy.

Atrioventricular Blocks

AV conduction blocks are abnormal delays or failure of conduction through the AV node or bundle of His. The electrical impulse arises normally from the SA node and depolarizes the atria, but on reaching the AV node or bundle of His, the conduction is slowed to greater than 0.20 second or completely blocked. The block may be a result of CAD, rheumatic heart disease, or MI. Therapy with quinidine, digitalis, and/or procainamide also may delay AV conduction. Treatment is based on the symptomatology the patient demonstrates and on etiology of the block.

FIRST-DEGREE ATRIOVENTRICULAR BLOCK

Definition and Cause

In first-degree AV block, all impulses arise normally from the SA node. The impulse is, however, slowed for more than 0.20 second at the AV node or bundle of His and is then conducted to the ventricle. The delay may be as great as 0.8 second, and it usually remains constant. The most common causes of first-degree AV block include CHD, digitalis therapy or toxicity, MI, and complications of coronary artery bypass surgery.

ECG Appearance

The configuration of all waves is normal. The PR interval is, however, prolonged (Fig. 8-35).

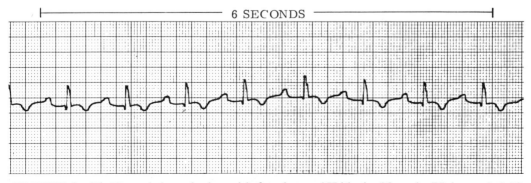

FIGURE 8-35. Normal sinus rhythm with first-degree AV block. (Note the PR interval, 0.28 second.)

Hemodynamic Implications

There are no hemodynamic implications. First-degree AV block must be observed for progression to further block, especially in acute onset.

Treatment

Correction of first-degree block requires treatment of the underlying cause. If it is pharmacologic, the benefits of treatment are weighed against the complication of heart block.

SECOND-DEGREE ATRIOVENTRICULAR BLOCK MOBITZ TYPE I (WENCKEBACH)

Definition and Cause

In the Wenckebach phenomenon, there is a repeated pattern of progressively lengthening PR intervals until finally an atrial impulse is completely blocked at the AV node. MI, electrolyte imbalance, or digoxin, quinidine, or procainamide therapy may bring on this unusual transient arrhythmia. The Wenckebach phenomenon rarely progresses to complete heart block.

ECG Appearance

The rate is usually slow because of AV conduction block. The PR interval is progressively lengthened until the P wave is completely blocked and there is no ventricular complex (Fig. 8–36). It is a cyclic phenomenon.

Hemodynamic Implications

The Wenckebach rhythm is fairly well tolerated unless profound bradycardia, a rate less than 40 bpm, results. If bradycardia is profound and the cardiac output is inadequate, the individual will exhibit signs of decreased cardiac output (cold, clammy skin, syncope, low blood pressure).

Treatment

Treatment is necessary only if the heart rate is slow and the individual exhibits symptoms of low cardiac output. Atropine may be utilized to increase the heart rate. Medications that slow AV conduction (digoxin, quinidine, calcium channel blockers, and procainamide) may be withheld. In rare instances, an artificial pacemaker may be necessary to establish a rate consistent with an adequate cardiac output.

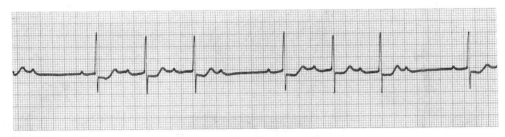

FIGURE 8–36. Second-degree AV block Mobitz type I (Wenckebach). (Note the progressively lengthening PR interval and then the absence of the QRS complex.)

SECOND-DEGREE ATRIOVENTRICULAR BLOCK MOBITZ TYPE II

Definition and Cause

Mobitz type II block is rare. It is clinically very significant; it indicates disease in the distal conduction system, and it may occur as the result of a large anterior MI. In Mobitz type II block, atrial impulses occur at a regular rate but are irregularly conducted to the ventricle. The P waves occur in a regular ratio to the QRS (i.e., 2:1 or 3:1). However, a progressive lengthening of the PR interval before the blocked P wave is absent. The site of the block is usually below the bundle of His and is a form of bilateral bundle branch block. This block usually progresses to complete heart block, and it therefore requires immediate therapeutic intervention.

ECG Appearance

The atrial rate is regular. P waves are normal in appearance. The ventricular rate is slow and irregular. Conduction of the atrial impulse to the ventricle is intermittent. The PR interval is consistent (Fig. 8–37). The QRS complex may either be normal in appearance or have a bundle branch pattern, depending on the level of the block.

Hemodynamic Implications

Symptoms experienced depend on the ventricular rate. When impulses are conducted from the atria to the ventricle, the normal atrioventricular sequence remains intact. If the ventricular rate is adequate, the individual will not experience symptoms of low cardiac output. Symptoms of low cardiac output appear as the ventricular rate slows.

Treatment

The insertion of a permanent pacemaker and the withdrawal of medications that may increase AV conduction time are the treatment of choice. Atropine may be administered initially in an attempt to increase the conduction of impulses across the AV node. That is usually not effective, however, because of the level of the block.

COMPLETE HEART BLOCK

Definition and Cause

In complete heart block, the atrial and ventricular rhythms are independent of one another and therefore the rhythm is termed AV dissociation. There is a failure of

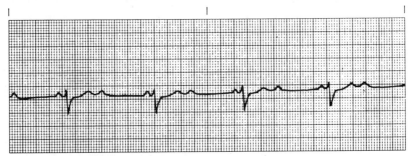

FIGURE 8–37. Second-degree AV block Mobitz type II. The AV node selectively conducts some beats while blocking others. Those that are not blocked are conducted through to the ventricles, although they may encounter a slight delay in the node. Once in the ventricles, conduction proceeds normally.

conduction of impulses from the atria to the ventricle. Any apparent sequence of those independent rhythms is coincidental. An escape rhythm from the junctional or ventricular area must take over as the pacemaker of the ventricle. The intrinsic ventricular rate is 20 to 40 bpm. Complete heart block is usually seen as a complication of acute MI or severe angina in which sustained ischemia of the AV node has occurred. It may also occur as a result of drug toxicity (class I antiarrhythmics, or digoxin).

ECG Appearance

The atrial and ventricular rhythms appear as independent regular rhythms. The P wave is of normal configuration. The appearance of the QRS depends on the location of the ventricular pacemaker: the lower the site of the escape focus, the wider and more bizarre the QRS complex. PP and RR intervals are regular. There is no relation between the P and R waves. Ventricular irritability may be seen as a result of the slow heart and the resulting myocardial ischemia (Fig. 8–38).

Hemodynamic Implications

A slow heart rate, low cardiac output, and compromised coronary perfusion may result in acute CHF. Individuals may also experience syncope, which, when a result of complete heart block, is known as the Stokes-Adams syndrome.

Treatment

Complete heart block is usually a life-threatening emergency because the ventricle is an unreliable pacemaker. However, some older individuals may be asymptomatic when the ventricular escape rhythm is 45 to 60 bpm, and they may tolerate it even with exertion.[34] Emergency treatment with intravenous atropine or isoproterenol may be used until a temporary pacemaker can be instituted. Determination of the need for permanent pacing will be based on the underlying cause of the block.

Bundle Branch Blocks

Bundle branch blocks (BBBs) are blocks in conduction along either the right or left bundle branch or both. ("Bundle branches" refers to the major branches of the intraventricular conduction system.) A block in the bundle of His or bundle branches slows the depolarization of the ventricle because the impulse must travel retrograde to the "blocked" ventricle from the ventricle with the "normal" conduction pathway. The depolarization, now occurring at separate times, is represented on the ECG by two

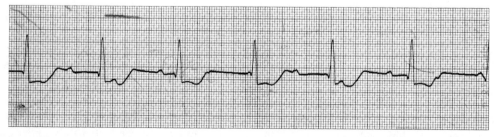

FIGURE 8–38. Complete heart block. (Note that the atrial and ventricular rates are independently occurring rhythms.)

joined QRS complexes. The QRS is wider than 0.10 second and has a notched configuration that represents two R waves: R and R'. The tracing reflects the nonsimultaneous depolarization and is diagnostic of BBB. There is usually no serious impairment to conduction as long as one branch remains intact.[34] A 12-lead ECG is necessary for diagnosis. BBB is best seen in leads V_1 and V_6.

RIGHT BUNDLE BRANCH BLOCK

Definition and Cause

Right bundle branch block (RBBB) is an anatomical or functional block in the right bundle branch that slows the depolarization and contraction of the right ventricle. Although seen in healthy hearts, RBBB is most frequently seen in anterior MI.

ECG Appearance

Atrial conduction is normal. The QRS is greater than 0.12 second and is notched (rSR') in lead V_1. There are large S waves in leads I and V_6. The T wave is opposite in deflection to the QRS (Fig. 8–39).

Hemodynamic Implications

There are no hemodynamic implications. Despite delayed conduction, diastolic fill time and cardiac output remain normal.

Treatment

No treatment is necessary.

LEFT BUNDLE BRANCH BLOCK

Definition and Cause

Left bundle branch block (LBBB) is caused by a block in the left bundle branch that delays conduction and contraction of the left ventricle. LBBB occurs in ischemic heart disease, MI, valvular heart disease, and in other cases of serious heart disease. In some instances, LBBB may be rate-dependent (i.e., it appears only when a "critical rate" is reached). The significance of this event is yet to be determined. The LBBB will disappear immediately when the individual's heart rate falls below the critical rate and can be immediately reproduced by raising the heart rate to the critical level.

ECG Appearance

The rate and rhythm are normal, with a widened QRS, greater than 0.12 second, that appears notched in the left chest leads (V_5 and V_6) (Fig. 8–40).

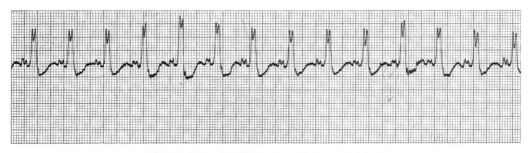

FIGURE 8–39. Right bundle branch block.

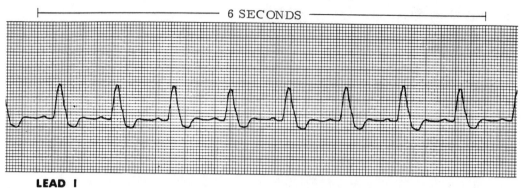

LEAD I

FIGURE 8-40. Normal sinus rhythm with complete left bundle branch block (lead I).

Hemodynamic Implications

There are no complications.

Treatment

No treatment is necessary for the block itself.

ARTIFICIAL PACEMAKERS

An artificial pacemaker is an electronic device that provides repetitive electrical stimuli to the heart muscle. These stimuli, like the heart's natural pacemaker, allow for the origin and conduction of an impulse through the heart. Pacemakers may be inserted on a temporary or permanent basis. They are generally used when an individual has an arrhythmia that has caused, or may potentially cause, a decreased cardiac output. This may occur with complete heart block, severe bradycardia, or tachycardia. Pacemakers are also used to control tachyarrhythmias. There has been only limited clinical applicability of the antitachycardic mode to date.[10,19,34]

Specific guidelines for the use of pacemakers have been developed by the American Medical Association. As pacemakers become increasingly complex in their functions and programmability, they also become increasingly expensive. The guidelines represent an effort to guard against overutilization.

Pacemaker Components

Pacemakers are composed of a pulse generator (a battery and electrical circuit) and a lead wire. The pulse generator initiates the electrical stimulus to the heart. It may also have a mechanism with which it senses the individual's heart beat.

Pacemaker generators have various types of power sources with varying lifespans including mercury-zinc (3 to 4 years), lithium (approximately 10 years), and plutonium nuclear (20 years to a lifetime). In addition, there are batteries that are externally rechargeable. In permanently implanted pacemakers, the pulse generator usually "fails" over a period of weeks to months. The symptoms exhibited depend on the patient's underlying rhythm. The failure of the battery is usually detected by a change in heart rate, either bradycardia or uncontrolled tachyarrhythmias and associated symptoms.

The lead is the conducting wire and electrode tip. It extends from the generator to the patient's heart and delivers the stimulus to the myocardium. The lead may be placed transvenously by threading it through the subclavian vein into the right atrium. When properly positioned, the electrode tip lies against the atrial or ventricular endocardium. It is held in place by a tinelike tip. If the pacemaker is placed during open heart surgery, the electrodes are sutured directly to the epicardium.

Types of Pacemakers

Pacemakers are classified as either temporary or permanent and as single- or dual-chamber. Temporary pacing, usually via the transvenous approach, is used when the arrhythmia is believed to be reversible, to evaluate the effects of a pacer-supported rhythm, or as an emergency intervention until the permanent pacer can be inserted. Single-chamber pacing is the system that stimulates either the atria *or* ventricle. Usually it is the ventricle that is paced. Dual-chamber pacing stimulates both the atria and the ventricle. Both modes may be used temporarily or permanently.

A permanent pacemaker is most commonly indicated in cases of complete heart block. It is also indicated in cases of symptomatic irreversible bradycardia, symptomatic sinus node dysfunction, bradycardia-tachycardia syndromes, and symptomatic Mobitz type I and type II blocks.

Pacemakers are also used diagnostically to assess SA and AV conduction in electrophysiologic studies, for hemodynamic evaluation of varying heart rates, and for the identification of the mechanisms of onset and termination of tachyarrhythmias.

Classification/ICHD Code

Pacemakers are classified according to five parameters: chamber-paced, chamber-sensed, mode of response, programmable features, and special tachyarrhythmia features.

"Chamber-paced" and "chamber-sensed" refer to the chamber of the heart in which the electrode lies (atrial, ventricular, or dual chamber). "Chamber-sensed" depends on the presence and function of the sensing mechanism. "Mode of pacing" refers to sensing function and how it relates to stimulus release. Programmable pacemakers have a variety of modes and specific functions that can be adjusted by external reprogramming. Special antitachycardia functions are available on only a few highly specialized pacemakers. With the antitachyarrhythmia function, the fixed-rate mode is activated by external application of a magnet or radio-frequency unit over the pulse generator during tachycardic episodes. Pacemaker signals are initiated, and they interrupt the tachycardic cycle.

To allow for uniform description of pacemaker function, a five-letter pacemaker code was developed in 1974 and revised in 1980 by the Intersociety Commission for Heart Disease (ICHD). This code is used universally. The first letter refers to the chamber paced. The second letter refers to the chamber sensed, and the third letter indicates how the pulse generator responds to the impulse. The fourth and fifth letters identify the programmability and the special tachyarrhythmia features of the pacemaker, respectively (Table 8–3). The reader should consult the references for further details.[10,27,34,38]

TABLE 8–3 ICHD Pacemaker Code

First letter Chamber-paced	
	A = atria V = ventricle D = dual O = none
Second letter Chamber-sensed	A = atria V = ventricle D = dual O = none
Third letter Mode of response	T = Triggered I = Inhibited D = Dual (T and I) O = No response R = Reverse

Fourth letter
  Programmability
	P = Simple external programming
	        possible
	O = No adjustment possible
	M = Multiple adjustment possible

Fifth letter Special features for treatment of arrhythmias	B = Bursts N = Normal rate competition S = Scanning E = External

Modes of Pacing

There are five pacing modes: fixed-rate or asynchronous, demand or inhibited, triggered or synchronous, dual, and reverse pacing.

Fixed-rate pacemakers fire continuously without regard to the patient's own rhythm. This preset firing may result in competition; that is, the ventricles may receive impulses simultaneously from both natural and artificial pacemakers, which compete for dominance. The competition may cause chaotic rhythm disturbances and is the primary disadvantage associated with fixed-rate pacemakers.

A demand or inhibited pacemaker senses the inherent rhythm of the heart and does not discharge an impulse if the heart initiates its own impulse. The pacemaker fires only when needed.

A triggered or synchronous pacemaker paces constantly when there is no intrinsic beat. When the pacemaker senses a ventricular depolarization owing to natural pacing, it releases its impulse. Because the ventricle is already depolarized and is refractory to another stimulus, the pacer impulse is ineffectual.

Dual-chamber pacemakers are capable of sensing and pacing both the atria and the ventricles. That enables each atrial contraction, whether spontaneous or paced, to be followed at a preset interval by a ventricular contraction. These are AV sequential pacemakers. Their primary advantage is that they preserve the normal sequence of cardiac events. The atrial contribution to ventricular filling is maintained. Dual-chamber pacemakers are more versatile than single-chamber units. AV sequential pacemakers can be reprogrammed to either single-chamber (atrial or ventricular) or dual-chamber function as needed.

Reverse pacemakers fire oppositely to what is normally expected. They sense tachyarrhythmias and interrupt the rhythm disturbance.

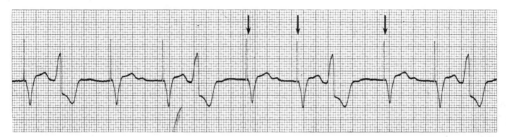

FIGURE 8–41. Ventricular pacemaker rhythm. (Note the spike preceding each ventricular complex. The ventricular complex is wide and bizarre because the ventricle is where the impulse is initiated.)

Electrocardiogram Appearance

On the ECG, the pacemaker impulse is recorded as a spike immediately preceding the depolarization of the atria and/or ventricles (Figs. 8–41 and 8–42). The spike may be of varying amplitude. It is instantaneous and has no real duration. When a pacemaker is stimulating adequately, each pacing spike produces a cardiac response. If the electrode is in the atria, each spike should produce a P wave. If the electrode is in the ventricles, each spike should produce a QRS complex. When a pacing spike fails to produce a response, the pacemaker is said to be out of "capture." Frequent causes of failure to capture are a loss of contact between the electrode and the chamber wall, depletion of the power source, and a fracture in the electrode (Fig. 8–43).

In appearance, the waves of the cardiac cycle differ from those of the individual's natural rhythm because the pacemaker impulses arise from a different site in the myocardium. Conduction does not follow normal pathways. In a ventricularly paced rhythm, the QRS will often be wide and bizarre in appearance.

Occasionally, the patient's intrinsic stimulus occurs at the same time as the pacemaker-generated stimulus. Both stimuli initiate depolarization of the ventricle at the same time from different directions and result in a shared or "fusion" beat appearing on the ECG. The QRS follows the pacing spike, and it is a distorted blend of the two contributing waveforms (Fig. 8–44).

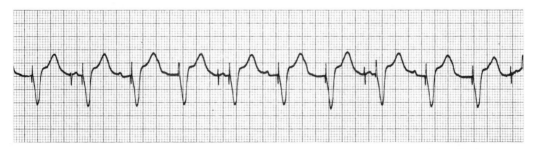

FIGURE 8–42. Atrioventricular pacemaker rhythm. (Note that the atrial pacing is intermittant. The individual's intrinsic P wave can be identified on those complexes that do not have an atrial pacing spike. Every QRS is paced.)

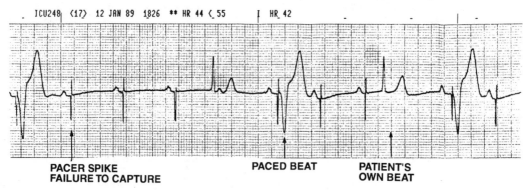

PACER SPIKE
FAILURE TO CAPTURE   **PACED BEAT**   **PATIENT'S**
                                                    OWN BEAT

FIGURE 8–43. Failure to capture. (Note the pacing spikes that are not followed by any waveform.)

Complications

Complications associated with pacemaker function include local infection or hematoma formation at the lead or pulse generator insertion site, arrhythmias from irritation of the ventricle, perforation of the right ventricle by the catheter, and loss of capture. The individual is treated symptomatically for each complication, and appropriate adjustments are made to the pacemaker to ensure optimal functioning.

Response to Exercise

The response to exercise of an individual who has a pacemaker depends on his or her underlying cardiac disease, level of fitness prior to the implanting of the pacemaker, degree of dependence on the pacemaker, and type of pacemaker implanted. Individuals with normal SA node function and dual-chamber pacers often have a "normal" cardiovascular response to exercise because they maintain the normal sequence of cardiac events. Those with ventricularly paced rhythms may not tolerate exercise as well because they may not have the benefit of the atrial kick (which contributes up to 30 percent of the cardiac output).[38]

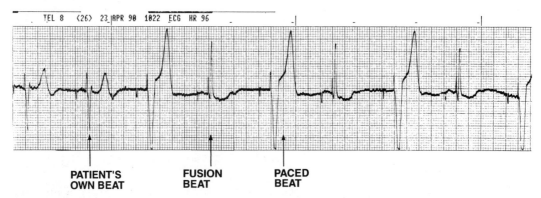

PATIENT'S   **FUSION**   **PACED**
OWN BEAT   **BEAT**   **BEAT**

FIGURE 8–44. Fusion beat. (Note the unusual configuration of the fusion beat in comparison to the paced beats and the patient's intrinsic heart beats.)

Individuals with pacemakers should be taught to recognize such symptoms as shortness of breath and fatigue to determine their tolerance for exercise. With proper cardiac monitoring, exercise can be undertaken safely and confidently. It is possible for these individuals to achieve training effects and relatively high levels of fitness.[38,40]

ELECTROPHYSIOLOGIC STUDIES

An electrophysiologic (EP) study is an invasive technique used to detect abnormalities in impulse origination and conduction in the heart. Via electrode catheters passed transvenously into the heart, the electrical potential of specific areas of the heart can be observed and evaluated. The procedure is used for diagnosis and to determine treatment of specific arrhythmias, for treatment of arrhythmias in some cases, and to establish prognosis in relation to a specific arrhythmia.

Diagnosis of a particular arrhythmia is made by observing the intracardiac ECG or by electrically stimulating the heart and deliberately inducing sustained ventricular tachycardia or supraventricular tachycardia. The rhythm is promptly terminated by pacing or electrical cardioversion, but it allows the physician to observe potentially lethal tachyarrhythmias. Drug therapies may be elevated based on repeat EP studies. If the particular arrhythmia is not able to be reinduced following the initiation of a particular drug, the antiarrhythmic drug is effective.[35] If it is ineffective, other drug therapies may be tested in this manner; if effective, it appears to correlate well with long-term prognosis for that patient in regard to that arrhythmia.[34] It may be used for direct treatment of cardiac arrhythmias by mapping ventricular conductions so that surgical or catheter ablation of an ectopic focus may be performed. It is also used to predict the efficacy of an antiarrhythmic device or pacemaker.

The major drawbacks are the risks inherent to cardiac catheterization and the psychologic impact of repeat studies, should they become necessary.

The biggest indications for EP studies are ventricular arrhythmias unresponsive to routine drug therapy, especially in individuals experiencing sudden cardiac death, symptomatic supraventricular arrhythmias, and syncope of undetermined origin.

AUTOMATIC IMPLANTABLE CARDIOVERTER-DEFIBRILLATOR

The automatic implantable cardioverter-defibrillator (AICD) is a battery-powered electrical device implanted to detect and correct life-threatening ventricular arrhythmias. A little larger than a permanent pacemaker, the AICD monitors the heart through epicardial leads and discharges an R wave–synchronized shock up to 33 J when it senses VT or VF.[35] The device is able to monitor rate only or rate and QRS morphology and deliver a shock sufficient to convert the arrhythmia to normal sinus rhythm.

Indications for an AICD include individuals who have survived an episode of sudden cardiac death unrelated to MI or who have experienced recurrent tachyarrhythmias despite conventional drug therapy.[41]

The AICD has been well tolerated and has significantly decreased the mortality rate to approximately 1.8 percent in the first year from recurrent cardiac arrest in that high-risk population.[35] Its safety record so far represents a promising approach to the management of individuals at particularly high risk for recurrent lethal arrhythmias.[38]

Such individuals can benefit significantly from cardiac rehabilitation, but it is definitely very important for both the patient and the cardiac rehabilitation specialist to be well aware of the patient's exercise tolerance evaluation indicating any exercise-induced arrhythmias and to be aware of the rate cutoff (the rate at which the AICD is activated). There should be an adequate safety margin between the individual's target heart rate and the rate cutoff so the individual may exercise safely and confidently.

ELECTROCARDIOGRAM CHANGES SEEN WITH EXERCISE

Individuals with healthy hearts demonstrate a number of expected and insignificant ECG changes during exercise (Table 8–4). Most notable is the significant tachycardia that occurs with moderate to heavy physical exertion accompanied by a rapid return to the preexercise heart rate following cessation of the exercise (during recovery). The healthy individual may experience single or rare premature atrial, junctional, or ventricular contractions during exercise. These arrhythmias are without hemodynamic consequences.[23] Individuals with CAD should demonstrate the same changes during exercise, but they may be at a much lower level of exercise. Beneficial ECG changes and a low heart rate (at rest and during submaximal exercise) that occur as a result of physical conditioning are demonstrated by both healthy individuals and those with CAD. Individuals with CAD also develop the ability to engage in more vigorous activity before reaching ischemic threshold (training effect).

Abnormal ECG responses observed during exercise reflect an imbalance between myocardial oxygen supply and demand. Usually they are either exertional arrhythmias or alterations in the ST segment and T wave (see Table 8–2).[10,21] Exertional arrhythmias occur during both exercise and the recovery period. They are significant in their rela-

TABLE 8–4 ECG Changes during Exercise*

Healthy Individual†	Individual with CAD‡
1. Slight increase in amplitude of P wave 2. Shortening of PR interval 3. Slight shift to right of QRS axis 4. ST-segment depression of less than 1 mm 5. Decreased amplitude of the T wave 6. Single or rare PVCs during exercise and recovery 7. Single or rare PJCs or PACs	1. ppearance of a BBB at a "critical heart rate" 2. Recurrent or multifocal PVCs during exercise and/or recovery 3. VT (three or more consecutive ventricular beats) 4. Appearance of bradyarrhythmias/tachyarrhythmias—rapid rate abruptly slowing or vice versa, not related to exercise 5. ST-segment depression/elevation of greater than 1 mm, 0.08 second after the J point 6. Bradycardia in response to exercise 7. Tachycardia that results in an HR greater than the individual's upper limit 8. Increase in frequency or severity of any arrhythmia the individual is known to have

*Decreases in the resting heart rate and the submaximal heart rate are observed in both groups with physical conditioning.

†All these ECG changes are normal in response to exercise.

‡Occurrence of any one of these changes should result in cessation of exercise and thorough evaluation of the ECG change and related symptoms.

tions to an individual's cardiac output. If the arrhythmia causes inadequate cardiac output, it may induce syncope, angina, or CHF. Alterations in the ST segment and T wave (see Fig. 8–5) fall into three categories: horizontal, downsloping, and upsloping. ST-segment depression or elevation of 1 mm or greater measured at 0.08 second from the J point indicates ischemia of the myocardium. It is an abnormal response to exercise. When exercise in cardiac rehabilitation is monitored, this parameter should be assessed carefully in relation to other clinical symptoms to determine intervention. There is little or no agreement concerning the significance of the varying shapes of both the ST segment and T wave that occur with exercise.[21]

Many pathophysiologic conditions, including anemia, hypoxemia, and ventricular aneurysm, as well as cardioactive drugs, cause the same ST segment and T wave changes commonly induced by exercise. In determining the significance of ST-segment depression during exercise, it is important not only to observe and evaluate the associated symptoms but also to observe and evaluate how quickly the individual's ECG returns to normal upon cessation of the exercise. Table 8–4 lists other abnormal ECG changes that may be observed. For all these abnormalities and any other new and potentially significant clinical symptoms reported by the patient, including fatigue, chest discomfort, dizziness, and palpitations, exercise should be terminated. Observation of the arrhythmia and assessment of the patient, including vital signs and objective and subjective symptoms, should be done immediately, and appropriate treatment should be instituted. If the situation is nonemergency, the individual should remain at the cardiac rehabilitation site under observation until symptoms have completely abated. The patient should be instructed to seek prompt evaluation by a physician. Information regarding the episode should be forwarded to the physician by the cardiac rehabilitation staff. Appropriate results should be forwarded to the cardiac rehabilitation staff before the individual exercises again. In addition, new arrhythmias or other new symptoms observed *prior* to exercise should always be evaluated before the individual is permitted to exercise. Exercise is contraindicated in any individual who is found to be in complete heart block or is demonstrating CHF symptoms. Such an individual should seek immediate medical attention.

EFFECTS OF DRUGS ON ELECTROCARDIOGRAM

Drugs that affect the heart rate may have some effect on the ECG pattern. Cardiac glycosides, antiarrhythmics, and beta-blockers all have varying effects on the cardiac cycle. Beta-blockers, in particular, may cause bradycardia. They may produce heart rates in the range of 40 to 50 bpm. Digitalis preparations and calcium ion antagonists increase AV conduction time. The most prominent characteristic of digitalis toxicity is AV block. Digitalis may also produce sagging in the ST segment (Fig. 8–45) and shortening of the QT interval (measured from the Q wave through the T wave). In digitalis toxicity, arrhythmias of all types (atrial, junctional, and ventricular) have been documented[1] (Table 8–5). (See Chapter 7.)

Quinidine and procainamide may prolong the AV conduction time and result in a prolonged PR interval. A wide QRS complex and a wide, notched T wave or even an inverted T may also be seen. In toxicity, patients will frequently demonstrate an AV block, widening of the QRS (to as much as one and a half normal duration), or ventricular arrhythmias.[12]

Drugs used in the treatment of concurrent illnesses also may cause changes in the

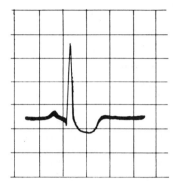

FIGURE 8–45. Digitalis effect. Note the rounded sagging appearance of the ST segment. (From Brunner, LS and Suddarth, DS: Textbook of Medical Surgical Nursing, ed 5. JB Lippincott, Philadelphia, 1984, p. 571, with permission.)

ECG. Phenothiazines (Phenergan, Thorazine) and tricyclic antidepressants (Elavil, Sinequan) cause T wave changes, PR and QT prolongation, conduction disorders, and supraventricular and ventricular arrhythmias.[16] It is therefore important to keep current records of patients' complete medical and pharmacologic regimens. Patients should be encouraged repeatedly to keep the cardiac rehabilitation team aware of any changes in their medications, because changes could have a dramatic effect on their exercise prescription and their response to exercise.[12]

TABLE 8–5 Effects of Selected Drugs on the ECG[8,16]

Drug	ECG Effect
Digitalis	1. Shortens ventricular activation time
	2. Increases AV conduction time
	3. Shortens QT interval
	4. Depresses ST segments and makes them sag
	5. In large doses:
	Decreases T wave amplitude
	Prolongs PR interval
	Sinus bradycardia, PACs, PVCs, and bigeminy
	Multiple conduction abnormalities
	6. Toxicity: AV block
Quinidine and procainamide	1. Prolonged PR interval
	2. Wide QRS complex; lengthened QT interval
	3. Depressed, widened, or notched T wave
	4. Toxicity:
	SA or AV block
	Ventricular arrhythmias
	Up to 50% increase in QRS duration
Phenothiazines (Phenergan, Thorazine)	1. Nonspecific T wave changes
	2. Decreased T wave amplitude
	3. Intraventricular conduction disturbances
	4. Supraventricular and ventricular arrhythmias
Tricyclic antidepressants (Elavil, Sinequan)	1. T wave changes
	2. PR interval, QT interval, and QRS complex prolongation
	3. Conduction disturbances
	4. Supraventricular and ventricular arrhythmias

SUMMARY

Electrocardiography is discussed in this chapter. Information regarding the significance of electrocardiograms in the diagnosis and treatment of cardiac pathology is presented. The individual waveforms are identified and are related to the heart's corresponding electrical and muscular activity. Lead placements for proper ECG recording at rest and during exercise are identified and illustrated.

In addition, the basic concepts of rate, rhythm, and waveform configuration for the interpretation of ECGs most commonly encountered in a cardiac rehabilitation setting are presented. Arrhythmias as well as abnormalities in initiation and/or conduction of the heart beat, are described, with sample electrocardiographic strips for the purpose of illustration. Information outlining each arrhythmia's specific etiology, hemodynamic implication, and treatment is included for common arrhythmias and conduction blocks. Brief discussions of pacemakers, electrophysiologic studies, AICD, and the effects of drug therapy on the ECG conclude the chapter.

Review questions and ECG rhythm strips in workbook fashion are given after the references for the purpose of providing an opportunity for evaluation of basic arrhythmia identification skills.

REFERENCES

1. Kniesl, CR and Ames, SW: Adult Health Nursing. Addison-Wesley, Reading, MA, 1986.
2. Dubin, D: Rapid Interpretation of EKGs, ed 4. Cover Publishing, Tampa, FL, 1988
3. Woods, SL and Underhill, SL: Cardiac arrhythmias and conduction abnormalities. In Patrick, ML, et al (eds): Medical-Surgical Nursing: Pathophysiological Concepts. JB Lippincott, Philadelphia, 1986.
4. Littman, D: The Electrocardiogram: Examination of the Heart, Part 5. American Heart Association, Dallas, TX, 1973.
5. Marriott, HJL: Practical Electrocardiography, ed 8. Williams & Wilkins, Baltimore, 1988.
6. Conover, M: Understanding Electrocardiography: Physiological and Interpretive Concepts, ed 5. CV Mosby, St. Louis, 1988.
7. Goldman, MJ: Principles of Electrocardiography, ed 11. Lange Medical Publications, Los Altos, CA, 1982.
8. Woods, SL: Electrocardiograms and Heart Arrhythmias. In Brunner, LS and Suddarth, DS: Textbook of Medical-Surgical Nursing, ed 6. JB Lippincott, Philadelphia, 1987.
9. Norsen, L, Telfair, M, and Wagner, AL: Detecting dysrhythmias. Nursing '86 16:11, 1986.
10. Vinsant, MO and Spence, MI: Commonsense Approach to Coronary Care, ed 5. CV Mosby, St Louis, 1989.
11. Sumner, SM and Grau, PA: Guidelines for running a 12-lead EKG. Nursing '85 15:12, 1985.
12. Liss, JP (ed): Reference Guide: Preventative Rehabilitative Exercise Specialist Workshop/Certification. American College of Sports Medicine, Madison, WI, 1981.
13. Introduction to Arrhythmia Recognition. California Heart Association, San Francisco, 1968.
14. Pearl, MJ: Electrocardiography. In Amundsen, LA (ed): Cardiac Rehabilitation. Churchill Livingstone, New York, 1981, pp 61–81.
15. Brannon, FJ: Experiments and Instrumentation in Exercise Physiology. Kendall-Hunt, Dubuque, IA, 1978.
16. Woods, SL: Electrocardiography, vectocardiography and polarcardiography. In Underhill, SL, et al (eds): Cardiac Nursing, ed 2. JB Lippincott, Philadelphia, 1989.
17. Poyatos, ME, et al: Predictive value of changes in R-wave amplitude after exercise in CHD. Am J Cardiol 54:10, 1984.
18. Lipman, BS, Dunn, M, and Massic, E: Clinical Electrocardiology, ed 8. Year Book Medical Publishers, Chicago, 1989.
19. Braunwald, E (ed): Heart Disease: A Textbook of Cardiovascular Medicine, ed 3. WB Saunders, Philadelphia, 1989.
20. Sokolow, M and McIlroy, MB: Clinical Cardiology. Lange Medical Publications, Los Altos, CA, 1986.
21. Sivarajan, ES: Exercise testing. In Underhill, LS, et al (eds): Cardiac Nursing, ed 2. JB Lippincott, Philadelphia, 1989.
22. Wenger, NK: Exercise therapy for patients with coronary artery disease. Consultant, 24:150–159, 1984.
23. Dehn, MM: Rehabilitation of the cardiac patient: The effects of exercise. Am J Nurs 80:5, 1980.

24. Shephard, RJ: The value of exercise in ischemic heart disease: A cumulative analysis. J Cardiac Rehabil 3:294, 1983.
25. Berkovits, BV: AV sequential demand pacemakers for treatment of cardiac arrhythmias. Journal of Cardiovascular and Pulmonary Technology, Feb/March, 1980.
26. Cardiovascular Disorders: Nursing '84 Books. Springhouse, Springhouse, PA, 1984.
27. Feldman, MS and Helfant, RH: Cardiac pacing. In S Bellet (ed): Essentials of Cardiac Arrhythmias, ed 2. WB Saunders, Philadelphia, 1980.
28. McKenry, LM, and Salerno, E: Pharmacology in Nursing, ed 17. CV Mosby, St. Louis, 1989.
29. Mangiola, S and Ritota, MC: Cardiac Arrhythmias, ed 2. WB Saunders, Philadelphia, 1980.
30. Phillips, RE and Feeney, MK: The Cardiac Rhythms, ed 2. WB Saunders, Philadelphia, 1980.
31. Purcell, JA and Haynes, L: Using the ECG to detect MI. Am J Nurs 84:5, 1984.
32. Stapleton, JF: Essentials of Clinical Cardiology. FA Davis, Philadelphia, 1983.
33. Charnow, B (ed): Essentials of Critical Care Pharmacology. Abridged from The Pharmacologic Approach to the Critically Ill Patient, ed 2. Williams & Wilkins, Baltimore, 1989.
34. Vlay, SC (ed): Manual of Cardiac Arrhythmias. Little, Brown & Co, Boston, 1988.
35. Lehman, MH and Steinman, RT: Preventing Sudden Cardiac Death. Post Grad Med 82:7, 1989.
36. Brooks, R, et al: The Automatic Implantable Cardioverter Defibrillator (AICD): Early development, current utilization and future directions. In Braunwald, E (ed): Heart Disease Update, No 9. WB Saunders, Philadelphia, 1990, pp 193–205.
37. King, SC and Sivarajan Froelicher, ES: Cardiac rehabilitation: Activity and exercise program. In SL Underhill, et al (eds): Cardiac Nursing, ed 2. JB Lippincott, Philadelphia, 1989.
38. Riegel, B, et al: Dreifus Pacemaker Therapy: An Interprofessional approach. FA Davis, Philadelphia, 1986, pp 180–187.
39. Tamarisk, NK: Enhancing activity levels with permanent cardiac pacemakers. Heart Lung 17(part 1):698–705, 1988.
40. Superko, HR: Effects of cardiac rehabilitation in permanently paced patients with third degree heart block. J Cardiac Rehabil 3:561–568, 1983.
41. Moser, SA, Crawford, D, and Thomas, A: Caring for Patients with Implantable Cardioverter Defibrillators. Critical Care Nurse 8(2):52–65, 1988.
42. Lehman, M, et al: The AICD as antiarrhythmic treatment modality of choice for survivors of cardiac arrest unrelated to myocardial infarction. Am J Cardiol 62:803–805, 1988.
43. Cooper, DK, Valladeres, BK and Futterman, LG: Care of the patient with the automatic implantable cardioverter-defibrillator: A guide for nurses. Heart Lung 16(part 1):640–648, 1987.
44. Hillis, LD, et al: Manual of Clinical Problems in Cardiology, ed 3. Little, Brown & Co, Boston, 1988, pp 53–58.

CHAPTER 8 REVIEW QUESTIONS

Instructions: Briefly answer the following questions as they apply to electrocardiography as discussed in Chapter 8. (Answers follow.)

1. ECG interpretation is based on _____,

   _____, _____, and

   _____.

2. _____ is the hallmark ECG sign of myocardial ischemia.
3. Disturbances in cardiac rhythm, cardiac arrhythmias, are caused by abnormalities

   in either _____ or _____ or in both.

4. The _____, the "natural pacemaker of the heart," fires

   intrinsically at a rate of _____ times per minute.

5. _____ leads and _____ leads make up

   the 12 standard ECG leads. _____ is often used as a single
   monitoring lead during exercise.

6. Match the wave or waves of the ECG in Figure 8-46 that are described by one of the
   following definitions or phrases.

   a. _____ ventricular depolarization

   b. _____ the cardiac cycle

   c. _____ absolute and relative refractory period

   d. _____ ventricular repolarization

   e. _____ atrial depolarization

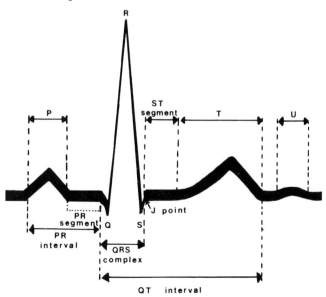

FIGURE 8–46. ECG wave configuration. (From Underhill, SL et al: Cardiac Nursing. JB Lippincott, Philadelphia, 1983, p. 204, with permission.)

7. Identify the most common heart blocks.

   a.

   b.

   c.

   d.

   e.

8. All are characteristics of NSR *except*:
   a. The rhythm is essentially regular.
   b. The impulse arises from the sinoatrial node at a rate of 60 to 100 bpm.
   c. The appearance of the QRS complex is variable.
   d. The rate may increase slightly with deep inspiration and decrease with expiration.

9. In individuals with coronary artery disease and angina, sinus tachycardia:
   a. increases myocardial oxygen demand.
   b. may significantly decrease coronary artery perfusion because of the decrease in the duration of diastole.
   c. may result in an anginal episode if the underlying cause is not identified and treated to decrease the heart rate.
   d. all of the above.

10. Regularly occurring premature ventricular contractions (PVCs) may be identified

    as _____ when a PVC is coupled with every normal beat and

    as _____ when the PVC occurs every third beat.

11. Briefly explain the mechanism by which the heart meets the increased oxygen demand of exercise.

    How does this differ in the individual with atherosclerosis?

12. Sinus bradycardia:
    a. may be well tolerated.
    b. is often seen in individuals who are physically fit and in many individuals during sleep.
    c. may be profound (less than 40 bpm) and lead to signs and symptoms of low cardiac output.
    d. may be seen in individuals on digoxin therapy.
    e. all of the above.

13. Identify the average duration of the:

    a. P wave _____

    b. PR interval _____

    c. QRS complex _____

    d. ST segment _____

    e. T wave _____

14. When an abnormal ECG change is detected and persists or increases in frequency with exercise, the health professional should do all of the following *except*:
    a. terminate the exercise with the appropriate monitored cool-down period.
    b. check and record the individual's vital signs and associated symptoms.
    c. allow the individual to resume exercise as soon as the abnormality disappears.
    d. notify the client's physician of the ECG change.
    e. caution the client against exercise until the ECG change is evaluated.
    f. none of the above.
15. All of the following are *normal* ECG changes seen with exercise except:
    a. depression of the ST segment of less than 1 mm.
    b. tachycardia.
    c. recurrent and/or multifocal PVCs during exercise or in the recovery phase.
    d. decreased amplitude of T wave.
16. An anatomic or functional interruption to conduction of an impulse through the normal conductive pathway is:
    a. atrial fibrillation.
    b. heart block.
    c. heart failure.
    d. ventricular muscle depolarization.
17. Identify four characteristics of PVCs.

    a.

    b.

    c.

    d.
18. Premature ventricular contractions may be precipitated by:

    a.

    b.

    c.
19. Briefly describe why arrhythmias arising in the ventricles (other than occasional PVCs) require immediate treatment.

20. Atrial flutter is characterized by all of the following *except*:
    a. ventricular response may be irregular or regular and stated in a ratio of atrial to ventricular activity.
    b. the atrial activity has a saw-toothed configuration on ECG and is known as F or flutter waves.
    c. there is an abnormal configuration to the QRS waves.
21. List the categories of cardiac drugs that will most commonly affect the ECG and give their effects.

    a.

    b.

    c.

    d.

22. Atrial arrhythmias
    a. include atrial fibrillation, atrial flutter, and premature atrial contractions as the most common.
    b. arise from ectopic foci in the atria.
    c. have P waves of abnormal or various configurations, or there may be an absence of identifiable P waves.
    d. may have normal QRS configurations.
    e. all of the above.
23. Why is it essential to maintain up-to-date medication profiles on all patients in a cardiac rehabilitation program?

24. What is the biggest advantage of atrioventricular sequential pacemakers?

25. How is a pacemaker detected on ECG?

ANSWERS TO REVIEW QUESTIONS

1. Rate, rhythm, regularity, and the individual wave configurations.
2. ST-segment depression/elevation of greater than 1 mm occurring 0.08 second after the J point.
3. Automaticity, conduction.
4. Sinoatrial node, 60 to 100.
5. Six limb, six chest, modified chest lead V_5 (CMV_5).
6. a. QRS complex.
   b. the entire PQRST complex.
   c. ST segment and T wave.
   d. T wave.
   e. P wave.
7. a. sinoatrial node block (SA node block).
   b. first-degree AV block (Mobitz type I).
   c. second-degree AV block (Mobitz type II).
   d. complete heart block.
   e. bundle branch block.
8. c.
9. d.
10. bigeminy, trigeminy (in that order).
11. Because the heart is extremely efficient in extracting oxygen from the blood at normal rates, the healthy heart meets increased oxygen demand brought on by exercise by increasing the heart rate (and consequently, increasing the coronary artery blood flow) and through dilation of the coronary arteries.

    In CAD there are changes in the vessel walls that inhibit dilation, and therefore the increase in heart rate is the only mechanism that increases oxygen supply to the myocardium during exercise.
12. e.
13. a. P wave: 0.08 to 0.12 second.
    b. PR interval: less than 0.20 second.
    c. QRS complex: 0.06 to 0.12 second.
    d. ST segment: 0.12 second.
    e. T wave: 0.16 second.
14. c.
15. c.
16. b.
17. Any four of these answers:
    a. QRS is prolonged owing to the abnormal pathway of myocardial conduction and depolarization.
    b. A compensatory pause follows the PVC.
    c. Often occurs in the cool-down or recovery phase following exercise.
    d. If untreated, may degenerate into life-threatening arrhythmias of ventricular tachycardia or ventricular fibrillation.
    e. The T wave is opposite in deflection to the R wave of the PVC.

18. Premature ventricular contractions may be precipitated by any three of these answers:
    a. caffeine.
    b. alcohol.
    c. anxiety.
    d. tobacco.
    e. any ischemia-producing event.
19. With the exception of occasional PVCs, arrhythmias that have their origin in the ventricles are life-threatening because the ventricular pacemakers are undependable, and chaotic rhythms may result in a cardiac output that may be well below what is necessary to meet the body's metabolic demands.
20. c.
21. a. Cardiac glycosides. *Effect*: Increased AV conduction time; sagging ST segment; shortened QT interval.
    b. Beta-blockers. *Effect*: Bradycardia at rest; slower heart rate than may be predicted with exercise.
    c. Calcium antagonists. *Effect*: Increased AV conduction time; slowing of heart rate.
    d. Antiarrhythmics. *Effect*: Varies with the drug and the arrhythmia it is being used to treat.
22. e.
23. Different medications have various effects on patients when they exercise and may cause some complications or ECG changes. Knowledge of a patient's medication profile allows for more appropriate interpretation of a change in the ECG or a new symptom brought on by exertion.
24. The atrioventricular pacemaker mimics the normal conduction system of the heart, the atria, and ventricle pump in sequence. The atrial kick is maintained.
25. The properly functioning pacemaker is detected by the appearance of a spike (a deflection with no duration) just prior to the atrial and/or the ventricular depolarization wave.

RHYTHM STRIP REVIEW

Interpret each of the following rhythm strips by answering the following questions:
1. What is the rate?
2. What is the rhythm? regular or irregular?
3. Are there P waves?
4. What is the QRS duration?
5. By evaluating the PR interval, what is the relationship between the P waves and the QRS complexes? (Answers follow.)

RHYTHM STRIP REVIEW NOTES

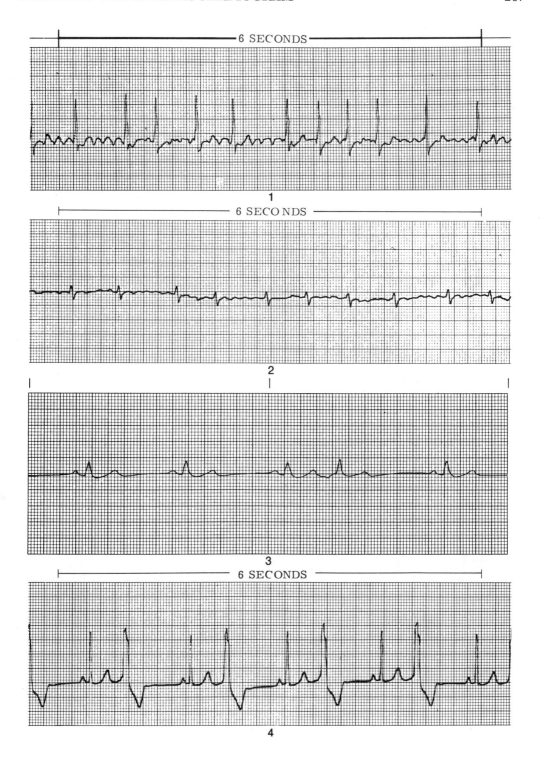

RHYTHM STRIP REVIEW NOTES

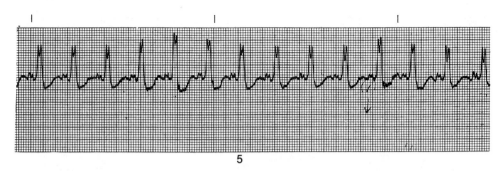

5

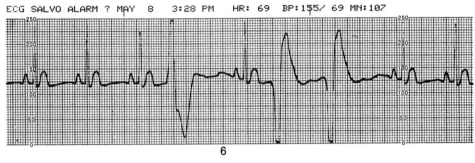

ECG SALVO ALARM ? MAY 8 3:28 PM HR: 69 BP:155/ 69 MN:107

6

6 SECONDS

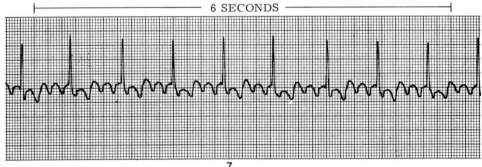

7

6 SECONDS

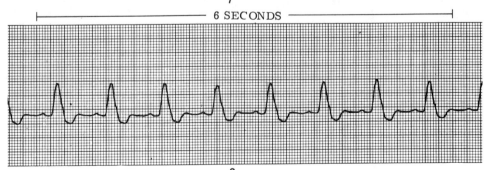

LEAD I 8

RHYTHM STRIP REVIEW NOTES

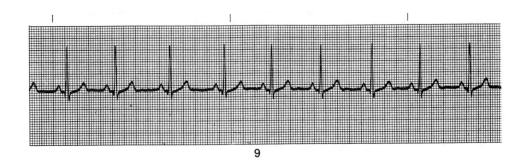

9

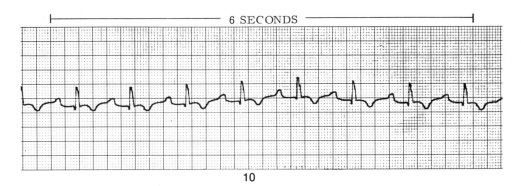

6 SECONDS

10

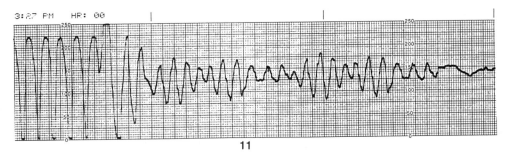

3:27 PM   HR: 00

11

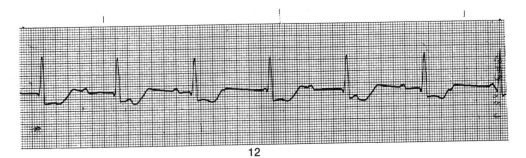

12

RHYTHM STRIP REVIEW NOTES

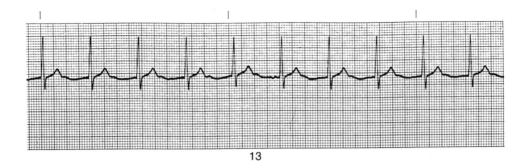

13

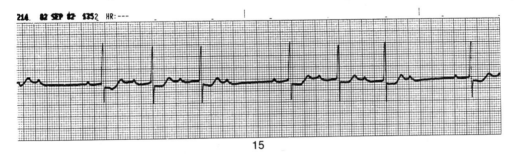

atrial

ventricular

Ventricular pacemaker spikes

(atrial pacemaker spike)

14

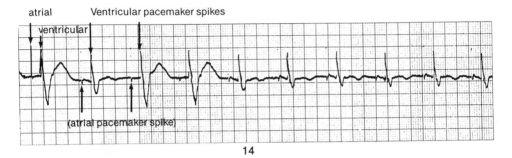

15

PATIENT 1   TELEMETRY ECG X2 RATE LIMIT ALARM MAY

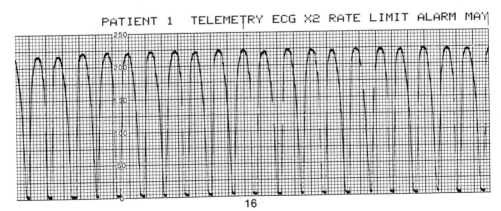

16

RHYTHM STRIP REVIEW NOTES

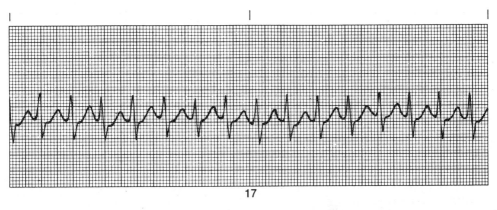

17

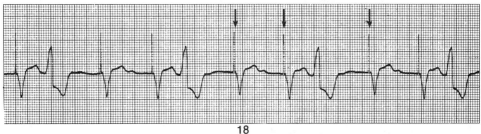

18

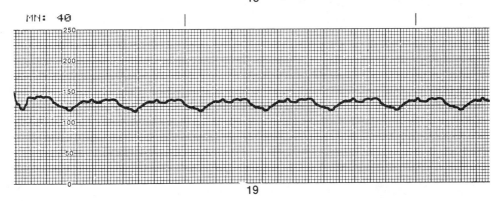

19

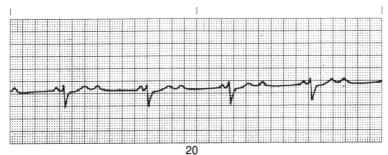

20

RHYTHM STRIP REVIEW ANSWERS

1. Atrial fibrillation with rapid ventricular response.
2. Atrial fibrillation with controlled ventricular response.
3. Sinus bradycardia with one premature nodal contraction.
4. Ventricular bigeminy.
5. Normal sinus rhythm with right bundle branch block (RBBB).
6. Normal sinus rhythm with multifocal PVCs (single PVC and a couplet).
7. Atrial flutter.
8. Normal sinus rhythm with left bundle branch block (LBBB).
9. Normal sinus rhythm.
10. Normal sinus rhythm with first-degree AV block.
11. Progression of ventricular arrythmias. Ventricular tachycardia degenerates to coarse ventricular fibrillation and then fine ventricular fibrillation.
12. Complete heart block or third-degree heart block.
13. Junctional rhythm.
14. Atrioventricular sequentially paced rhythm.
15. Second-degree AV block, type I (Wenckebach).
16. Ventricular tachycardia.
17. Supraventricular tachycardia (SVT).
18. Ventricular paced rhythm.
19. Ventricular fibrillation.
20. Second-degree AV block, type II.

CHAPTER **9**

Assessment of the Cardiac Patient

This text is not intended to discuss the many more technical diagnostic tests that can be employed by the referring physician to determine a cardiac patient's medical status accurately. Many of those tests will have been performed prior to the referral of a patient for outpatient cardiac rehabilitation. The purpose of the more technical tests is to determine the etiology and the severity of the cardiac disease. They are, therefore, necessary for the classification of patients according to diagnosis(es), cardiac function, and risk and thereby determine whether a particular patient is a candidate for cardiac rehabilitation. For information on risk stratification to identify patients who may be at risk for developing new clinical manifestations of coronary artery disease (CAD), see Chapters 11 to 13. Ideally, these tests should be comprehensive and, in addition to screening for cardiac disease, should evaluate the patient for concomitant vascular, pulmonary, and/or metabolic disorders.

The technical diagnostic tests, which may include echocardiography, coronary angiography, thallium stress testing, and Doppler screening for peripheral vascular disease in symptomatic patients, have been extensively described from a clinical standpoint in various texts.[1-5] Therefore, the following discussion of laboratory assessment and procedures focuses not on the more technically sophisticated tests but rather on the basic assessment procedures most commonly employed in the outpatient cardiac rehabilitation setting. The basic tests provide the necessary information for writing and executing an accurate, effective exercise prescription: (1) a physical examination (if not performed by the referring physician), (2) a medical history and risk factor analysis, (3) miscellaneous physical measurements, including body composition analysis, (4) blood and urine analysis (if not performed by the referring physician), (5) electrocardiography, including a monitored graded exercise tolerance test (GXTT), and (6) functional heart classification based on the results of the GXTT. In this section, the administrative forms required to perform the laboratory assessment also are discussed, and examples are provided.

217

INFORMATION REGARDING PATIENT MEDICAL STATUS

Prior to scheduling assessments, specific information regarding a patient's medical status must be obtained. It is gathered from two primary sources: the patient and the referring physician. Tests performed by the referring physician do not have to be repeated if they were performed within a reasonable length of time prior to the initiation of therapy and if a full report of the results is made available to the cardiac rehabilitation staff. The "reasonable" length of time that may elapse from the test date to the initiation of therapy varies with each test but, in most cases, 8 weeks is considered reasonable.[2,3,5] In some cases, however, because of recurring cardiovascular complications, medication changes, or illness, the GXTT may have to be repeated just prior to the initiation of exercise therapy.

The information required to determine medical status prior to assessment should be inclusive because it will assist not only in the determination of the testing procedures and techniques, for example, the exercise test modality and protocol, but also in the exercise prescription and the strategies used to modify risk factors.

Information Provided by the Patient

Specific forms have been developed to obtain information from, as well as to provide information for, the patient. In most cases, these forms are mailed to the prospective patient after the patient makes the initial request for information. Although the packet of application forms can be expensive to mail, properly completed forms in advance of the laboratory assessment can save considerable staff time and expense. Five separate forms should be included in the patient program application packet: the patient information letter, the medical history form (including the risk factor questionnaire), an insurance information form, a medical release authorization form, and an exercise evaluation instruction sheet (for examples, see Appendix A).

The patient information letter, which should be individually addressed and signed by the program director, contains general information about the purpose and goals of the cardiac rehabilitation program. The staff facilities and geographic location of the rehabilitation center may also be mentioned. The primary purpose, however, is to inform the prospective patient of the appropriate entry procedures, that is, the accurate completion of the enclosed forms, the information to be supplied by the referring physician, and the scheduling of the laboratory assessment. Information regarding the cost of the program and insurance reimbursement may also be included. To be most effective, this letter should be clear and concise.

The medical history and risk factor analysis forms are included in the packet of patient application forms and should be reviewed for accuracy in a later interview. The interview is an essential part of the laboratory assessment conducted by the cardiac rehabilitation staff. The laboratory procedures essentially begin with the interview.

There are many ways to administer a medical history. Medical histories may be patient- (self-) administered, computer-administered, obtained through interviews by physicians or paramedical personnel, or obtained by a combination of those methods. There are advantages and disadvantages to each method,[6] but the self-administered history in combination with a patient interview conducted by trained paramedical staff or the physician is generally the most effective in a variety of situations.[2,6] The effectiveness of the interview is maximized by the skill of the interviewer. A well-trained interviewer familiar with the medical history form and skilled in the use of the technique of active listening is needed.[7,8] Active listening is a technique developed by Rogers[7] that helps clarify the patient's response and thereby prevent misinterpretation of the question and a faulty response.[8]

Although the cardiovascular history (including symptoms and medications) is the most significant part of the medical history for cardiac patients, the medical history should also include information pertaining to the major systems of the body. It can be divided into three categories: past history, family history, and present symptoms. In addition, information regarding allergies, medications, injuries, operations, and hospitalizations should be reviewed and documented. The self-administered history may take various forms, but it is most effective with clear and precise questions and a short-answer format. (For an example, see Appendix A.)

Information regarding the patient's lifestyle and health habits should be included as part of the comprehensive medical history. This information can be regarded as "social" history, and it should include a risk factor appraisal. The appraisal should include assessments of an individual's smoking and drinking habits, physical activity (occupational and leisure time), dietary habits, and a stress profile. The information is helpful in planning counseling and patient education and in enhancing modification of habits that are detrimental to the cardiac patient.

In addition to the aforementioned information, a social history may review the following items:[2]

Job description
Job satisfaction
Family responsibilities
Family socioeconomic history
Marital status
Socioeconomic background
Sexual activity
Geographic history

However, the most useful information gleaned from the social history is data about the patient's lifestyle, health habits, and risk factors. This information may be included in the medical and personal history form or may be obtained separately (Chapter 13).

Much of the optional information may be reviewed informally with the patient after the rehabilitation program has been initiated. Patients feel more comfortable discussing personal information when they understand the relevance of the information to the rehabilitative process.[7] Also, after working with patients for a short period of time, it is easier for the health-care team to identify patients for whom the information may be more important. All information about a patient's social history should be documented and placed in the patient's permanent file, which should be available to all rehabilitation professionals working with the patient.

There are many examples of medical history and risk factor appraisal forms,[2,5,6,9-13] but it is best to develop the required forms in accordance with individual needs. Forms should be adapted to specific needs before being accepted for use.

Information Provided by the Referring Physician

The information that is requested on the referring physician's form influences the testing procedures performed in the physical examination. An example of a referring physician's form is given in Appendix B.

Although various suggestions have been made regarding when the physical examination should take place in relation to the initiation of cardiac exercise therapy,[1,2,6] patients with known coronary heart disease (CHD) should have a physical examination immediately prior to the exercise test.[1] As previously mentioned, tests performed within 8 weeks of the initiation of therapy in most cases need not be repeated.

Information requested of the referring physician may include the following.[2,6]

1. Specific etiology of the disease
2. Findings of cardiovascular evaluation
   a. Coronary angiography
   b. Thallium stress test
   c. Echocardiography
   d. Chest x-ray
   e. A copy of a 12-lead electrocardiogram (ECG) with interpretation (special note of rhythm and/or other abnormalities)
   f. Additional tests for peripheral vascular disease, etc. (as needed)
3. Diagnosis(es) (including those other than cardiac, for example, diabetes or musculoskeletal)
4. Medications
5. Dated results of urinalysis: albumin, glucose, micro.
6. Dated results of blood analysis: complete blood count (Hbg, Hct, WBC, differentials) and lipid profile (triglycerides, cholesterol, HDL, LDL, HDL/cholesterol)
7. Blood pressure
8. Results of the GXTT

Often the referring physician does not have current data regarding the urinalysis, blood analysis, electrocardiogram, or GXTT findings. These tests may then be performed as a part of the cardiac rehabilitation center's laboratory assessment. If necessary, the center may perform the physical examination, but from a practical standpoint it is often better for the referring physician to perform the examination.

The referring physician's form must be completed by the referring physician for each patient and returned to the rehabilitation center prior to the initiation of treatment. The referring physician's form clarifies the objectives and procedures of the rehabilitation program, requests specific information regarding the physician's physical examination of the patient (Appendix B), and requests the physician's signature on the STAT and PRN emergency orders as well as a prescription for cardiac rehabilitation.

The referring physician's form also establishes a line of communication between the cardiac rehabilitation staff and the patient's primary care physician. This initial contact should lead to the good rapport that is important in maintaining a high standard of patient care and may also increase the likelihood of future referrals.

If, during the course of treatment, a patient experiences a medically significant cardiac episode at the rehabilitation center, he or she must again be referred to the program by the primary care physician. (See the physician re-referral form in Appendix B.) The primary care physician must be informed of medically significant episodes directly and in the patient's monthly progress report. Such episodes may include the onset of new symptoms such as dysrhythmias, angina, or atypical blood pressure or heart rate responses to exercise; syncopal episodes; and episodes requiring transportation of the patient for inhospital emergency care. The decision regarding which episodes require the immediate attention of and response from the referring physician should be made by the medical director.

Like all the forms previously discussed, the referring physician's forms must be adapted to specific needs and properly evaluated before they are adopted for use.

The referring physician's form should always be accompanied by the patient's medical information release authorization form (Appendix A). The form must be signed by the prospective patient (or other legally authorized individual), witnessed (usually by the spouse), and dated in order to request information from the patient's referring physician. This form should be retained in the referring physician's file for that patient. The form gives the rehabilitation center the legal right to request information regarding the results of the physical examination and various diagnostic tests performed on the patient.

Once the information is gathered from the patient and the referring physician, the therapist can determine the battery of tests that will comprise the patient's laboratory assessment at the rehabilitation center. Because the physical examination, blood and urine analyses, electrocardiogram (12-lead), and more technical cardiovascular screening tests have been performed prior to the rehabilitation center's laboratory assessment, the center is involved primarily in pulmonary function testing, physical measurements including body composition analysis, GXTT (if current data are unavailable or the referring physician requests that the GXTT be performed by the rehabilitation center), and functional heart classification based on the results of the GXTT. The exercise prescription also is formulated by the rehabilitation center's staff as a part of the assessment procedures. The prescription is thoroughly discussed in Chapter 11.

LABORATORY ASSESSMENT AT THE CARDIAC REHABILITATION CENTER

When a patient comes to the rehabilitation center for a scheduled assessment, he or she is interviewed and the medical history and risk factor appraisal forms are confirmed for accuracy. At that time, the patient signs informed consent and release forms prior to the conduct of any laboratory assessments.

Informed Consent

Specific policies for the protection of the legal rights and safety of patients must be developed. Obtaining informed consent assures preservation of the patient's rights and documents his or her voluntary assumption of risk. All staff members must understand the document as well as the importance of obtaining the informed consent.

Informed consent forms should be developed through careful study of national and local practices relating to this area and adopted only after approval by medical and legal advisors. Because not all situations are similar, following these guidelines will help to assure the best standard of reasonable and prudent care.

Rehabilitation centers that provide diagnostic services for patients who may not subsequently participate in rehabilitation therapy should have two separate informed consent forms: one for use prior to exercise testing and another for use prior to beginning the cardiac rehabilitation program. (For an example, see Appendix C.)

INFORMED CONSENT/EXERCISE TESTING FORM

Prior to administration of the exercise test, the patient must receive an explanation of the testing procedures, which is contained in the written informed consent form. The form should explain the possible risks and discomforts involved in the testing, as well as the possible benefits to be expected. If the patient is unable to read the form, the form must be read to the patient. Following the explanation, the patient, other legally authorized individual, or both must be asked if there are any questions that have not been answered. The questions and the replies must be documented. The patient (or legally authorized individual) and the individual responsible for the test administration must sign and date the informed consent form.[1] (For an example, see Appendix C.)

INFORMED CONSENT/REHABILITATION PROGRAM FORM

All forms of the consent/rehabilitation nature must suit the needs of the individual rehabilitation center. Again, this form should be adopted only after the approval of medical and legal advisors. However, the following nine concepts are standard to all forms and should be included.[1]

1. The form should explain the intent of the program, the scheduling of the exercise therapy and other counseling, the re-evaluation process, and the progress reports and other forms of communication with the referring physician.
2. The method by which the patient will be monitored should be discussed, as well as the possibility of other tests that may be recommended if needed.
3. The risks and discomforts associated with exercise therapy must be fully disclosed, including the possibility of a heart attack. This information should be balanced with reassuring statements related to the screening process, professional staff, and emergency procedures.
4. The benefits resulting from exercise therapy and rehabilitation programs, which have been demonstrated by research, should be explained. A statement that indicates the rehabilitation center in no way "guarantees" that these benefits will be derived from participation should be included.
5. The concept of patient responsibility should be fully explained, and lists of behavioral objectives, including specific do's and don'ts, are helpful in reinforcing proper conduct.
6. Policy regarding the use of medical records for statistical analysis or scientific purpose as well as the confidentiality of medical records should be explained.
7. Inquiries regarding any aspect of the rehabilitation program should be encouraged, and an opportunity for questions and further explanation should be provided. Questions and replies should be documented.
8. A statement of freedom of consent should be included, as well as a statement indicating the patient's comprehension of the form and willingness to accept the policies described. (For an example, see Appendix C.)
9. A clause that legally releases the rehabilitation center from liability is optional but, in many cases, desirable. This clause must also include a description of the services rendered by the rehabilitation center to the patient.

The informed consent form must be signed and dated by the patient (or other legally authorized individual) and the program director. It should also be witnessed by either another staff member or the patient's spouse. (For an example, see Appendix C.)

After all preliminary forms have been completed and the procedures described thus far have been performed, all information required to perform the cardiorespiratory exercise evaluation should be in the possession of the rehabilitation center's test administrators. In the next section, various modalities and protocols utilized in the administration of laboratory tests, including the GXTT, are presented.

Pulmonary Function Testing

Pulmonary function testing is indicated for the cardiac patient primarily to determine (1) the presence of lung disease or abnormal lung function, (2) the extent of the abnormality, should one exist, (3) the disabling effect of the abnormality, and (4) the appropriate exercise prescription for the patient with abnormal lung function.[14-16] For information on pulmonary assessment, see Chapter 10.

Physical Measurements

Physical measurements also are important in assessing the patient. They may be performed on a separate visit to the rehabilitation center either prior to or after the scheduling of the GXTT or on the same day the GXTT is performed. They can be made quickly and do not require extensive equipment. The information provided by them is useful in planning, evaluation, and motivational aspects of the program. Usually, they are obtained at the rehabilitation center by any of the trained staff, that is, a nurse, laboratory technician, or exercise specialist. Although most of the procedures are simple, adequate time and training must be provided to ensure that the measurements are properly taken. They generally include height, body weight, body girth measurements, and percentage body fat (estimated by skinfolds and anthropometric measurements), and may include various measurements for strength and range of joint motion as needed. Instructions for obtaining physical measurements follow.

HEIGHT

Accurate height is desirable for utilizing height-weight charts[17] and for use in various formulas for the prediction of percentage body fat[18,19] or metabolic equivalents. Use of a stadiometer is recommended for measurement (Fig. 9–1). The patient should remove both socks and shoes prior to measurement and stand with his or her back to the measuring device with feet together and arms relaxed at the sides of the body. Eyes should be directed straight ahead. The measuring square should be adjusted to rest lightly on the scalp, and the measurement should be recorded to the nearest quarter inch or centimeter.

BODY WEIGHT

A standard balance scale is preferred to a spring-balance or digital scale because it is more easily calibrated. All weighings should be performed with the same scale. The scale should be checked in the zero position before each weighing, the balance should be returned to zero after each weighing, and the scale should be recalibrated periodically. The patient can be weighed at the same time that the height measurement is obtained. Weight recorded during the patient's participation in the rehabilitation program may be measured with or without socks and shoes as long as the measurement technique is consistent.

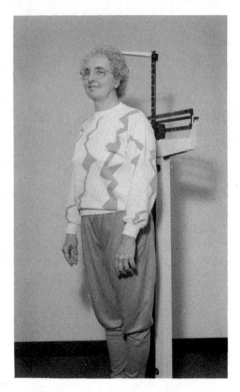

FIGURE 9-1. Use of the stadiometer to measure height.

PERCENTAGE BODY FAT

Body composition can be divided into two components: lean body mass and body fat. The lean body mass encompasses all the body's nonfat tissues including the skeleton, water, muscle, connective tissue, organ tissues, and teeth. The body fat component includes both the essential and the nonessential lipid stores. Essential fat includes fat that is a part of organs and tissues such as nerves, brain, heart, lungs, liver, and mammary glands.[19,20] The storage of nonessential fat is primarily within the adipose tissue. Average values for nonessential body fat have been established for men and women (Chapter 11).

Various methods (e.g., hydrostatic or underwater weighing) can provide precise estimations of body composition, but are not practical for use in most cardiac rehabilitation centers. Therefore, the indirect methods of anthropometry and skinfold measurement are commonly used.

Wilmore and Behnke Method

The Wilmore and Behnke method of estimating percentage body fat from lean body weight is a technique that uses anthropometric data and requires only a measuring tape[18] (Fig. 9-2).

Equation for men:
Waistline girth (WG) _____ inches
Body weight (BW) _____ lb (substract 2 to 3 lb for clothing)
LBW = 98.42 + [(1.082 × BW) − (4.15 × WG)] = _____

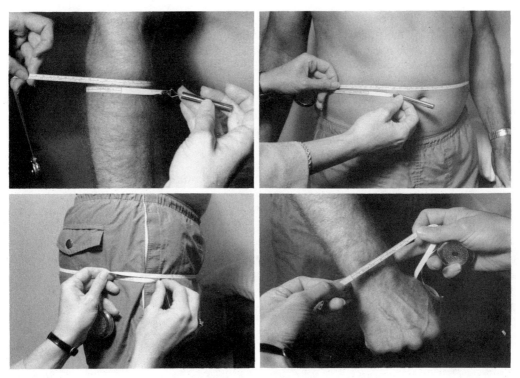

FIGURE 9–2. Measurement of circumference at three body sites and of diameter at one site, for use in estimating body fat percentage.

To calculate percent fat:

$$\text{Percent fat} = \frac{\text{BW (lb)} - \text{LBW (lb)}}{\text{BW (lb)}} \times 100 = \underline{\hspace{1cm}}$$

Equation for women:
Body weight (BW) _____ kg (weight in lb ÷ 2.2)
Wrist diameter (WD) _____ cm
Maximum abdominal circumference (MAC) _____ cm
Hip circumference (HC) _____ cm
Forearm circumference (FC) _____ cm
LBW = 8.987 + [(0.732 × BW) + (3.786 × WD) − (0.157 × AC) −
    (0.249 × HC) + (0.434 × FC)] = _____ kg
LBW (kg) × 2.2 = LBW _____ lb
To calculate percent fat:

$$\text{Percent fat} = \frac{\text{BW (lb)} - \text{LBW (lb)}}{\text{BW (lb)}} \times 100 = \underline{\hspace{1cm}}$$

Instructions for the Wilmore and Behnke method of measuring body girth are as follows (see Fig. 9–2):[18,19]

1. Upper arm circumference. Measure the maximum girth of the dominant limb midpoint between the head of the humerus and the elbow with the arm extended in the sagittal plane, hand supinated.

2. Forearm circumference. Measure the maximum girth of the dominant arm just below the elbow with the elbow extended and hand supinated.
3. Maximum abdominal circumference. Measure the maximum abdominal protrusion at the level of the navel following a normal exhalation.
4. Hip circumference. Measure around the fullest part of the hips with the patient's heels together.
5. Wrist diameter. Measure the dominant limb between the styloid processes by using a small sliding caliper or small metric ruler.

Skinfold Method

Skinfold measurements are probably the most common method of assessing body composition. The skinfold equations are derived by using multiple regressions that predict the result of hydrostatic weighing (the most accurate indirect means of measuring body composition) from the measurement of various skinfold sites.[20,21] Hydrostatic weighing equations have been developed from the direct chemical analysis of human cadavers; the two most widely used equations are derived by Brozek and associates[22] and by Siri.[23]

Several models of skinfold calipers are available. The ideal caliper should have parallel jaw surfaces and a constant spring tension, regardless of the degree of opening (Fig. 9–3).

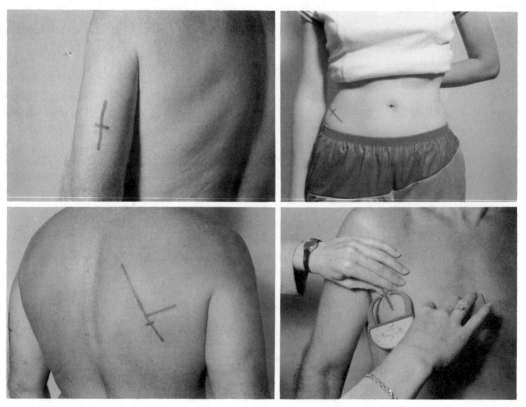

FIGURE 9–3. Lange skinfold calipers and location of skinfold measurement sites.

The skinfold method of assessing body composition has the potential for considerable error, even when employed by skilled evaluators. Dehydration can decrease a skinfold thickness by as much as 15 percent; therefore, an attempt must be made to schedule re-evaluations at the same time of day. The accuracy of the method can be increased by the use of multiple measurements performed by the same experienced evaluator.

In obtaining the skinfold measurement, a fold of skin and subcutaneous tissue is pinched between the thumb and forefinger and lifted firmly away from the underlying muscle. (Active contraction of the muscle in the skinfold site prior to measurement helps the test administrator to discriminate between the muscle and the subcutaneous tissue.) The fold should be held between the finger and thumb when the measurement is being made, and the calipers should be applied to the fold at a point approximately 1 cm below the finger. The measurement should be recorded to the nearest millimeter. Most skinfolds are measured in the vertical plane except where the natural skinfold lines distort the skinfold, for example, the suprailiac skinfold, in which case the skinfold is taken along the natural line. Skinfolds should be measured on the dominant side of the body (Table 9-1).

Tables 9-2 and 9-3 provide an estimation for the prediction of percentage body fat from the sum of three skinfold measurements for men and for women, respectively.[24] The three skinfold sites and instructions for measurement of men are as follows:

1. Triceps skinfold. Measure at the midpoint between the acromion and the olecranon process on the posterior aspect of the upper arm. Pinch the skinfold in the vertical plane with the arm relaxed and extended (Fig. 9-3).
2. Chest skinfold. Measure between the anterior axillary line and the nipple on a diagonal fold.
3. Subscapular skinfold. Measure on a diagonal line from the vertebral border of the scapula to within 1 to 2 cm from the inferior angle of the scapula.

Those measurements of women are as follows:

1. Triceps skinfold. Measure the same as for men.
2. Abdominal skinfold. Measure approximately 2 cm laterally from the umbilicus in a vertical plane.
3. Suprailiac skinfold. Measure a diagonal fold above the iliac crest at the anterior axillary line.

TABLE 9-1 Summary of Instructions for Skinfold Measurement

1. Pinch the fold of skin and subcutaneous tissue between thumb and forefinger.
2. Lift the fold of tissue away from underlying muscle and hold while measurement is taken.
3. Apply calipers approximately 1 cm below the finger.
4. Measure:
   In the vertical plane (except where natural skinfolds distort the line).
   The dominant side.
   To the nearest millimeter.

TABLE 9–2 Percent Fat Estimate for Men: Sum of Triceps, Chest, and Subscapular Skinfolds

Sum of Skinfolds (mm)	Age to Last Year								
	Under 22	23–27	28–32	33–37	38–42	43–47	48–52	53–57	Over 57
8–10	1.5	2.0	2.5	3.1	3.6	4.1	4.6	5.1	5.6
11–13	3.0	3.5	4.0	4.5	5.1	5.6	6.1	6.6	7.1
14–16	4.5	5.0	5.5	6.0	6.5	7.0	7.6	8.1	8.6
17–19	5.9	6.4	6.9	7.4	8.0	8.5	9.0	9.5	10.0
20–22	7.3	7.8	8.3	8.8	9.4	9.9	10.4	10.9	11.4
23–25	8.6	9.2	9.7	10.2	10.7	11.2	11.8	12.3	12.8
26–28	10.0	10.5	11.0	11.5	12.1	12.6	13.1	13.6	14.2
29–31	11.2	11.8	12.3	12.8	13.4	13.9	14.4	14.9	15.5
32–34	12.5	13.0	13.5	14.1	14.6	15.1	15.7	16.2	16.7
35–37	13.7	14.2	14.8	15.3	15.8	16.4	16.9	17.4	18.0
38–40	14.9	15.4	15.9	16.5	17.0	17.6	18.1	18.6	19.2
41–43	16.0	16.6	17.1	17.6	18.2	18.7	19.3	19.8	20.3
44–46	17.1	17.7	18.2	18.7	19.3	19.8	20.4	20.9	21.5
47–49	18.2	18.7	19.3	19.8	20.4	20.9	21.4	22.0	22.5
50–52	19.2	19.7	20.3	20.8	21.4	21.9	22.5	23.0	23.6
53–55	20.2	20.7	21.3	21.8	22.4	22.9	23.5	24.0	24.6
56–58	21.1	21.7	22.2	22.8	23.3	23.9	24.4	25.0	25.5
59–61	22.0	22.6	23.1	23.7	24.2	24.8	25.3	25.9	26.5
62–64	22.9	23.4	24.0	24.5	25.1	25.7	26.2	26.8	27.3
65–67	23.7	24.3	24.8	25.4	25.9	26.5	27.1	27.6	28.2
68–70	24.5	25.0	25.6	26.2	26.7	27.3	27.8	28.4	29.0
71–73	25.2	25.8	26.3	26.9	27.5	28.0	28.6	29.1	29.7
74–76	25.9	26.5	27.0	27.6	28.2	28.7	29.3	29.9	30.4
77–79	26.6	27.1	27.7	28.2	28.8	29.4	29.9	30.5	31.1
80–82	27.2	27.7	28.3	28.9	29.4	30.0	30.6	31.1	31.7
83–85	27.7	28.3	28.8	29.4	30.0	30.5	31.1	31.7	32.3
86–88	28.2	28.8	29.4	29.9	30.5	31.1	31.6	32.2	32.8
89–91	28.7	29.3	29.8	30.4	31.0	31.5	32.1	32.7	33.3
92–94	29.1	29.7	30.3	30.8	31.4	32.0	32.6	33.1	33.4
95–97	29.5	30.1	30.6	31.2	31.8	32.4	32.9	33.5	34.1
98–100	29.8	30.4	31.0	31.6	32.1	32.7	33.3	33.9	34.4
101–103	30.1	30.7	31.3	31.8	32.4	33.0	33.6	34.1	34.7
104–106	30.4	30.9	31.5	32.1	32.7	33.2	33.8	34.4	35.0
107–109	30.6	31.1	31.7	32.3	32.9	33.4	34.0	34.6	35.2
110–112	30.7	31.3	31.9	32.4	33.0	33.6	34.2	34.7	35.3
113–115	30.8	31.4	32.0	32.5	33.1	33.7	34.3	34.9	35.4
116–118	30.9	31.5	32.0	32.6	33.2	33.8	34.3	34.9	35.5

Source: From Jackson, AS and Pollock, ML: Practical assessment of body composition. Phys Sportsmed 13(5):87, 1985, with permission of McGraw-Hill, Inc.

Graded Exercise Tolerance Test

THE EXERCISE ELECTROCARDIOGRAM

Equipment basic to the gathering of ECG data during exercise includes a cardiograph with multilead capabilities and a monitor to continuously view the ECG. Although individual preferences vary, most practitioners require a 12-lead cardiogram at rest (supine, sitting, standing, or hyperventilating), during, and after the stress test has been completed. Some experts feel that the standard 12-lead system is impractical in

TABLE 9–3 Percent Fat Estimate for Women: Sum of Triceps, Abdomen, and Suprailiac Skinfolds

Sum of Skinfolds (mm)	18–22	23–27	28–32	33–37	38–42	43–47	48–52	53–57	Over 57
8–12	8.8	9.0	9.2	9.4	9.5	9.7	9.9	10.1	10.3
13–17	10.8	10.9	11.1	11.3	11.5	11.7	11.8	12.0	12.2
18–22	12.6	12.8	13.0	13.2	13.4	13.5	13.7	13.9	14.1
23–27	14.5	14.6	14.8	15.0	15.2	15.4	15.6	15.7	15.9
28–32	16.2	16.4	16.6	16.8	17.0	17.1	17.3	17.5	17.7
33–37	17.9	18.1	18.3	18.5	18.7	18.9	19.0	19.2	19.4
38–42	19.6	19.8	20.0	20.2	20.3	20.5	20.7	20.9	21.1
43–47	21.2	21.4	21.6	21.8	21.9	22.1	22.3	22.5	22.7
48–52	22.8	22.9	23.1	23.3	23.5	23.7	23.8	24.0	24.2
53–57	24.2	24.4	24.6	24.8	25.0	25.2	25.3	25.5	25.7
58–62	25.7	25.9	26.0	26.2	26.4	26.6	26.8	27.0	27.1
63–67	27.1	27.2	27.4	27.6	27.8	28.0	28.2	28.3	28.5
68–72	28.4	28.6	28.7	28.9	29.1	29.3	29.5	29.7	29.8
73–77	29.6	29.8	30.0	30.2	30.4	30.6	30.7	30.9	31.1
78–82	30.9	31.0	31.2	31.4	31.6	31.8	31.9	32.1	32.3
83–87	32.0	32.2	32.4	32.6	32.7	32.9	33.1	33.3	33.5
88–92	33.1	33.3	33.5	33.7	33.8	34.0	34.2	34.4	34.6
93–97	34.1	34.3	34.5	34.7	34.9	35.1	35.2	35.4	35.6
98–102	35.1	35.3	35.5	35.7	35.9	36.0	36.2	36.4	36.6
103–107	36.1	36.2	36.4	36.6	36.8	37.0	37.2	37.3	37.5
108–112	36.9	37.1	37.3	37.5	37.7	37.9	38.0	38.2	38.4
113–117	37.8	37.9	38.1	38.3	39.2	39.4	39.6	39.8	39.2
118–122	38.5	38.7	38.9	39.1	39.4	39.6	39.8	40.0	40.0
123–127	39.2	39.4	39.6	39.8	40.0	40.1	40.3	40.5	40.7
128–132	39.9	40.1	40.2	40.4	40.6	40.8	41.0	41.2	41.3
133–137	40.5	40.7	40.8	41.0	41.2	41.4	41.6	41.7	41.9
138–142	41.0	41.2	41.4	41.6	41.7	41.9	42.1	42.3	42.5
143–147	41.5	41.7	41.9	42.0	42.2	42.4	42.6	42.8	43.0
148–152	41.9	42.1	42.3	42.8	42.6	42.8	43.0	43.2	43.4
153–157	42.3	42.5	42.6	42.8	43.0	43.2	43.4	43.6	43.7
158–162	42.6	42.8	43.0	43.1	43.3	43.5	43.7	43.9	44.1
163–167	42.9	43.0	43.2	43.4	43.6	43.8	44.0	44.1	44.3
168–172	43.1	43.2	43.4	43.6	43.8	44.0	44.2	44.3	44.5
173–177	43.2	43.4	43.6	43.8	43.9	44.1	44.3	44.5	44.7
178–182	43.3	43.5	43.7	43.8	44.0	44.2	44.4	44.6	44.8

Source: From Jackson, AS and Pollock, ML: Practical assessment of body composition. Phys Sportsmed 13(5):87, 1985, with permission of McGraw-Hill, Inc.

emergency situations, because the electrodes covering the chest impede defibrillation procedures. As a result, a lead system referred to as CMV_5 (Chapter 8) is frequently used, and it has been reported to be 98 percent accurate in detecting cardiac problems during exercise testing.[18]

Some practitioners prefer to record a variety of ECG leads during the stress-testing process. Assuming the electrocardiograph has that capability, an example of one format might be:

Preexercise: 12-lead sitting
12-lead standing
12-lead hyperventilating

TABLE 9-4 Troubleshooting Poor ECG Tracings

Troublesome ECG Lead	Electrode and Lead-Wire Check
II and III	LL
I and II	RA
I and III	LA
I, II, and III	RL
aVR, aVL, aVF	I, II, III (as above)
V_1, V_2, V_3, etc.	V_1, V_2, V_3, etc.

Exercise: 3-lead (II, aVF, V_5) during last 10 seconds of each minute
Postexercise: 12-lead cool-down each minute
               12-lead recovery each minute

When necessary, 12 leads and/or rhythm strips are obtained, or individual leads can be selected for recording.

The Electrocardiogram Recording

Good ECG recordings during exercise are more difficult to obtain than those at rest, even when the practitioner has followed proper procedures for patient preparation in applying the electrodes. ECG tracings can be poor owing to such electromagnetic interference as AC interference and static electricity created by the patient wearing nylon or other synthetic clothing. (Cotton clothing should be recommended prior to testing.) Other reasons for poor ECG tracings include loose electrodes, movement artifact, and large amounts of fatty tissue present at electrode sites. Methods for checking poor tracings in any lead recording are outlined in Table 9-4.

COMPARISON OF MODALITIES

The modalities available for stress testing generally include a treadmill, a bicycle ergometer, and a bench for stepping. Each modality has advantages and disadvantages, and the personnel who decide which modality is to be used must do so with the specific needs and situations in mind. Some patients may be too deconditioned or too uncoordinated to perform quantitative testing on either the treadmill or bicycle ergometer. Although there are a variety of tests and modalities for stress testing populations with specific needs (e.g., arm egometric testing of orthopedically impaired patients), this text will describe the most commonly used modalities and tests.

The treadmill has become the first choice among these three testing modalities. Walking on a treadmill requires little skill, is a more accurate predictor of $\dot{V}o_2$max, and uses more leg muscles, thus reducing leg fatigue, one of the most common reasons for premature test termination. The main disadvantages of the treadmill are its expense, its incapacity to test persons with balance problems, the difficulty in obtaining good ECG tracings, and the difficulty in determining accurate blood pressure measurements because of treadmill noise and patient movement. Equipment manufacturers have attempted to solve those problems by minimizing the noise on newer model treadmills and increasing the accuracy of electronic sphygmomanometers.

Use of the bicycle ergometer for testing is particularly attractive because of its relatively low cost and ease of calibration. It is also the modality to use when testing patients with poor balance, poor vision (as in diabetics), or limited range of motion in the joints of the lower extremities (as in arthritic patients). Blood pressure measurements are more accurate during bicycle tests, and ECG recordings are usually good because upper body movement is minimal in comparison with other modalities. It should be noted that some patients find the bicycle seat uncomfortable and have difficulty keeping their feet on the pedals or maintaining a regular pace. In addition, localized muscle (quadricep) fatigue may prevent maximal testing of the cardiovascular system.

Bench stepping is the least expensive of the three modalities utilized for stress testing. The major disadvantages of bench stepping include leg fatigue, lack of allowance for different stepping heights when considering differences in individual body heights, and the coordination required to step properly. Blood pressure measurements made with standard equipment are almost impossible to obtain. Bench stepping can, however, be modified successfully for use when testing individuals with low physical and functional capacities. (See the section on bench-stepping tests.)

ESTIMATION OF $\dot{V}O_2$max

Data gathered from stress tests are usually reported in terms of metabolic equivalent (MET). A MET is the amount of oxygen consumed at rest (sitting) and is equal to approximately 3.5 milliliter per Kg per minute.[1,25] Thus, MET levels (multiples of resting $\dot{V}O_2$) attained during maximal stress testing are determined by dividing the estimated $\dot{V}O_2$max achieved during the test by the resting $\dot{V}O_2$. Fortunately, various experiments of actual $\dot{V}O_2$max measurements have been conducted, and tables of MET equivalents have been devised to save time and avoid error in computing the actual METs achieved.

In using a standardized GXTT to predict $\dot{V}O_2$max, one must remember that MET equivalents for specific protocols have been based on the exercise responses of specific populations; for example, the Bruce treadmill protocol used data from apparently healthy young men to formulate the MET values. Therefore, using those values to predict $\dot{V}O_2$max for a cardiac patient may result in a considerable error (overestimate).[26] Some population-specific equations are available for patients with cardiac disease and for other populations.[26] The use of such equations results in estimated $\dot{V}O_2$max values that are more accurate and reliable than values calculated without the equations. For practical purposes, however, the estimated $\dot{V}O_2$max values calculated in METs for specific work loads on the treadmill, bicycle ergometer, or bench step may be used as guidelines for the purpose of exercise prescription.

A maximal stress test is generally defined in terms of a specific end-point target heart rate (since heart rate and $\dot{V}O_2$max are linearly related and are based on the patient's age (Chapter 4). This is usually referred to as the age-adjusted maximum heart rate (AAMHR), and it can be estimated by subtracting the individual's age from 220. In most cases, tests that do not elicit a heart rate equal to 100 percent of the AAMHR are considered submaximal. However, use of the AAMHR method to predict maximal heart rate is inherently inaccurate because of the wide variation in actual maximal heart rates. Shephard[27] indicates that the heart rate formula (220 − age, in years) underpredicts maximum heart rates for most older adults by 10 to 15 beats per minute (bpm). In addition, some cardiovascular medications lower the heart rate and thereby render inaccurate the AAMHR as a predictor of maximal effort. Therefore, the clinician must remember that the heart rate formula should be used as a guideline only when predicting maximal responses to a GXTT.

For the cardiac patient or otherwise physically impaired individual, the GXTT end point may not be based on AAMHR; instead, it should be based on such symptoms as the onset of angina, ECG changes, and dysrhythmias. Therefore, the classification of the GXTT as "maximal" or "submaximal" is determined not by heart rate, but by the onset of symptoms. This type of GXTT is described as "symptom-limited." The heart rate achieved at the end point of the GXTT is generally expressed as a percent of the predicted AAMHR. If a GXTT is terminated because of localized muscle fatigue or at the patient's request, the test is described as a "maximal volitional" test, and the end-point heart rate also is expressed as a percent of AAMHR. Although studies indicate that estimates of Vo_2max derived from submaximal performance on a GXTT may vary by $\pm$ 10 to 15 percent from actual Vo_2max,[28] the estimated Vo_2max in METs achieved at the end point of the symptom-limited or maximal volitional test is considered the "maximal" capacity for that individual for the purpose of exercise prescription.

At this point, it should be apparent that METs must be used carefully in prescribing exercise. For patients with cardiovascular disease, heart rate is a much better indicator of the myocardial oxygen status than the estimated MET level. Therefore, the GXTT end-point heart rate is more practical for determining the exercise prescription than the MET level attained. Patients also relate more easily to the concept of heart rate than to METs.

BLOOD PRESSURE RESPONSE TO GXTT

During the stress test, ECGs as well as blood pressure measurements must be frequently recorded. Record blood pressure measurements at rest; at least every 3 minutes during exercise (more if conditions warrant) (Fig. 9–4); and during recovery from the test. During the exercise test, systolic blood pressure should rise with increasing work loads and the diastolic pressure should remain about the same. The highest systolic blood pressure should be achieved at the maximal work load. Blood pressure should be taken in the supine, sitting, and standing positions prior to exercise.[1,28] After exercise, systolic blood pressure is elevated in the supine position, gradually returns to normal during recovery, and may drop below normal for several hours after the test. In

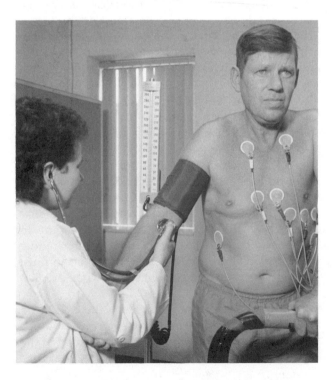

FIGURE 9–4. Blood pressure measurement technique.

response to exercise testing, a decline in diastolic pressure is encouraging, particularly if it has been over 86 mm Hg at rest or during the test.[29] Also, if the test administrator hears an extension of sounds toward or to zero with no cuff or stethoscope pressure on the artery, this response indicates both cardiodynamic and peripheral adaptive competence.[29]

RATE-PRESSURE PRODUCT (DOUBLE PRODUCT)

The rate-pressure product (RPP) is the product of the heart rate and the systolic blood pressure.[29,30] It is usually a five-digit number, the last two digits of which are dropped.[29,30] The product is an excellent indicator of aerobic conditioning, because the RPP decreases for a given work load as the patient becomes more conditioned. Cardiac and deconditioned subjects generally have higher RPPs for a given work load than physically trained individuals. The RPP relates well to measured myocardial oxygen consumption,[31,32] and it is possible to precipitate a patient's angina pectoris repeatedly at the same RPP when a standardized work load or exercise test is performed.[33] The RPP illustrates the importance of considering both heart rate and blood pressure responses when writing an appropriate exercise prescription.

Test Protocols

Regardless of the modality selected for the stress test, a variety of standard protocols are available for the practitioner's use. This text presents only the most common protocols, and stress test administrators should keep in mind that standard protocols may have to be adapted for individuals with low functional capacity or orthopedic limitations such as arthritis.

Adequate warm-up periods as well as provisions for a cool-down should be included as standard procedure in any test protocol. A major criticism of some stress-testing situations is that there is no allowance for warm-up and cool-down because of the extra time required. Proper warm-up allows the heart to adjust gradually to increased demands and reduces the incidence of ST-segment depression during exercise.[34] Although this may not be the goal of some test administrators who are interested in detecting clinical abnormalities, when the test administrator is primarily interested in determining functional work capacity, the warm-up not only decreases the incidence of muscular injuries but also decreases patient anxiety.[35] The decision to include proper warm-up and cool-down must be made by the test administrator, although some test protocols (Table 9–5; see also Table 9–10) begin at such a low level that adequate warm-up is an inherent part of the test. Most protocols do not specifically state what the cool-down should be, but the minimal length of time directed to cool-down should be 3 minutes. The cool-down helps to prevent pooling of the peripheral circulation (Chapter 4). When exercise is stopped, a number of patients (approximately 10 percent)[29] will demonstrate significant decreases in systolic pressure that are due to peripheral pooling. To avoid fainting, allow the patient to be seated after cool-down.

TREADMILL TESTS

The Bruce treadmill protocol (Table 9–6) is the test of choice for most physicians because of its ease of administration and economy of time. In many cases, however, it may be too strenuous to use for the initial evaluation of a deconditioned cardiac patient.

TABLE 9–5 Adapted Bruce Treadmill Protocol

Stage No.	Speed (mph)	Grade (%)	Time (min)	METs
1	1.7	0	3	2
2	1.7	5	3	3
3	1.7	10	3	5
4	2.5	12	3	7
5	3.4	14	3	10
6	4.2	16	3	13
7	5.0	18	3	16
8	5.5	20	3	19
9	6.0	22	3	22

Source: From Computer Assisted Exercise System. Marquette Electronics, Milwaukee, 1980, with permission.

In such cases, protocols with more gradually increasing intensities may be used, for example, the adapted Bruce.

The adapted Bruce treadmill protocol is a GXTT in which the speed or the grade of the treadmill is increased every 3 minutes (Table 9–5). The adapted Bruce is particularly good for use with cardiac patients because it begins at a very low level and the initial stage allows an adequate warm-up for most persons.

BICYCLE ERGOMETER TESTS

The bicycle tests also are graded (GXTT). The rate of pedaling is usually 50 to 60 rpm, but the resistance to pedaling usually increases every 3 or 6 minutes. Because treadmill tests are used more frequently than bicycle tests, analyses of data in terms of MET levels achieved are lacking. In the bicycle test utilized by the YMCA[36] and the Astrand-Rhyming bicycle test[28,37] the norms are based on predictions of maximal oxygen uptake in liters per minute, and Vo_2max predictions, along with age, determine an individual's score. In order to convert the liters per minute to METs, the appropriate mathematical calculations have to be made. An example of a bicycle ergometer protocol for multistage stress testing is given in Table 9–7.

A number of ergometers are currently utilized for conducting stress tests. Some work loads are set in terms of kiloponds, others in kilograms per minute, and still others in watts. These variances create some difficulty in standardizing tests. Although interpolations will probably have to be made, Tables 9–8 and 9–9 should help in converting the stress test data into MET levels achieved.

TABLE 9–6 Bruce Treadmill Protocol

Stage No.	Speed (mph)	Grade (%)	Time (min)	METs
1	1.7	10	3	5
2	2.5	12	3	7
3	3.4	14	3	10
4	4.2	16	3	13
5	5.0	18	3	16
6	5.5	20	3	19
7	6.0	22	3	22

Source: From Computer Assisted Exercise System. Marquette Electronics, Milwaukee, 1980, with permission.

TABLE 9-7 A Protocol for Multistage Stress Testing with the
Bicycle Ergometer

Stage	Speed (rpm)	Work Load	Time (min)
Warm-up	50	0	2-3
1	50	.5 KP	3
2	50	1.0 KP	3
3	50	1.5 KP	3
4	50	2.0 KP	3
5	50	2.5 KP	3
6	50	3.0 KP	3
7	50	3.5 KP	3
8	50	4.0 KP	3
Cool-down	50	0	3

Source: Adapted from American College of Sports Medicine,[1] p. 17.

BENCH-STEPPING TESTS

The Master's step test, or some variation thereof,[37] has been used most frequently in the past by the physician as a feasible test to administer in the office to assess cardiovascular function. Currently, however, it is being replaced by the treadmill or bicycle and therefore is not included in this text. When older individuals are unable to tolerate the treadmill or bicycle as a means of assessing cardiorespiratory function, it may be advisable to use a sitting-chair step test.[38] During the test, the patient sits in a straight-backed chair facing a step (which can be a bench or a pile of books). The step is placed a distance from the patient that is equal to the length of his or her leg when it is extended. Prior to the beginning of the test, the patient is sitting with both feet flat on the floor. A metronome should be set at 120, and at the count of 1, the arch of one foot is brought up to touch the edge of the step; on the count of 2, the foot is returned to the floor. On the next count of 1, the other foot touches the step edge and, on 2, returns to the floor. The process is continued, alternating right and left feet, so that 60 steps per minute are completed. The performances of stages 1, 2, and 3 are the same.

The heart rate is monitored continuously and is recorded after 2 minutes. If the patient is able to complete the 2 minutes without symptoms, the test is repeated at the same level for 5 minutes. The heart rate should be recorded after both the 2- and 5-minute intervals. If the heart rate at the 5-minute end point is less than 75 percent of AAMHR, the patient should be advanced to the next stage of the test.

The first stage uses a 6-inch-high step, the second a 12-inch-high step, and the third an 18-inch-high step, with the same testing procedure (see Fig. 9-5). The fourth stage also uses an 18-inch-high step. If a patient can continue the test to stage 4, the touching of the step with the foot remains as in stages 1 to 3. In addition, the patient should be instructed to raise the arm (on the same side as the leg with which he or she is touching the step) and extend it over the leg. As the touching foot returns to the floor, the arm should be lowered so that the hand rests on the knee (Table 9-10).

TEST AND EXERCISE TERMINATION

In most cases, the guidelines for terminating the stress test are followed during the exercise therapy sessions also. The guidelines for test and exercise therapy termination should be in accord with the particular situation and must be developed by the person-

TABLE 9–8 Conversion of Work Load in Kiloponds (KP) to METs for Bicycle Ergometry

Body Weight (lb)	Work Loads (KP*)								
	0.5	1	1.5	2	2.5	3	3.5	4	5
110	3.6	5.1	6.9	8.6	10.3	12.0	13.7	15.4	16.3
132	3.3	4.3	5.7	7.1	8.6	10.0	11.4	12.9	14.0
154	3.1	3.7	4.9	6.1	7.3	8.6	9.8	11.0	13.5
176	3.0	3.2	4.3	5.4	6.4	7.5	8.6	9.6	11.0
198	2.9	2.9	3.8	4.8	5.7	6.7	7.6	8.6	10.0
220	2.8	2.6	3.4	4.3	5.1	6.0	6.9	7.7	9.2

*0.5 KP = 150 kg/min = 25 watts
1.0 KP = 300 kg/min = 50 watts
1.5 KP = 450 kg/min = 75 watts, etc.

Source: Adapted from American College of Sports Medicine,[1] p. 171.

TABLE 9-9 Oxygen Requirements of Bicycle Ergometric Work Loads

		Work Load									
Watts		25	50	75	100	125	150	175	200	250	300
kg/min		150	300	450	600	750	900	1050	1200	1500	1800
Oxygen Used Total		600	900	1200	1500	1800	2100	2400	2700	3300	3900
kcal/min		3.0	4.5	6.0	7.5	9.0	10.5	12.0	13.5	16.5	19.5
Body Weight		Oxygen Used (ml/kg/min of body weight)									
(lb)	(kg)										
88	40	15.0	22.5	30.0	37.5	45.0	52.5	60.0	67.5	82.5	97.5
110	50	12.0	18.0	24.0	30.0	36.0	42.0	48.0	54.0	66.0	78.9
132	60	10.0	15.0	20.0	25.0	30.0	35.0	40.0	45.0	55.0	65.0
154	70	8.5	13.0	17.0	21.5	25.5	30.0	34.5	38.5	47.0	55.5
176	80	7.5	11.0	15.0	19.0	22.5	26.0	30.0	34.0	41.0	49.0
198	90	6.7	10.0	13.3	16.7	20.0	23.3	26.7	30.0	36.7	43.3
220	100	6.0	9.0	12.0	15.0	18.0	21.0	24.0	27.0	33.0	39.0
242	110	5.5	8.0	11.0	13.5	16.5	19.0	22.0	24.5	30.0	35.5
264	120	5.0	7.5	10.0	12.5	15.0	17.5	20.0	22.5	27.5	32.5

Source: From Ellestad,[41] p. 161, with permission.

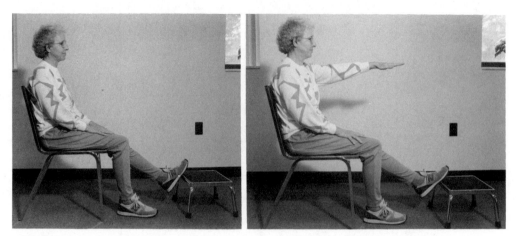

FIGURE 9–5. Proper technique for step-touching: stages 1–3 (*left*) and stage 4 (*right*).

nel in charge of the rehabilitation program. Some indications for exercise and test termination are given in Table 9–11 and later in Tables 9–16 to 9–24 in the section on case histories.

INTERPRETATION OF GXTT TEST RESULTS

Interpretation of test results and their application to exercise therapy require knowledge of physiology, pathophysiology, and exercise and should always be supervised by the medical director. Exercise prescription (according to heart rate) begins at a percent of the maximum heart rate attained during the stress test (Chapter 11). The end point for test termination may be related to the subject's age but may also be related to the point at which such symptoms as angina, dysrhythmias, adverse blood pressure responses, and the like occur. Occasionally, patients may be too unstable to participate in exercise therapy. If so, the decision must be made on an individual basis and with the medical and legal consequences in mind.

The GXTT results enable the therapist to classify a patient according to functional capacity (Tables 9–12 and 9–13). The functional classification is helpful in predicting subsequent cardiac events and determining prognosis for survival,[39,40] and it assists in the determination of maintenance levels for cardiac exercise therapy. Classification also aids in advising patients about recreational and occupational activities. That a patient achieves a maximal aerobic capacity of 8 METs as measured by performance on a GXTT does not indicate the level at which he or she can safely exercise. (See calculation of target zone in Chapter 11.) A patient must achieve a maximal aerobic capacity in the

TABLE 9–10 Chair Step Test Protocol

Stage	Time (min)	Step Height (in)	METs
1	5	6	2.3
2	5	12	2.9
3	5	18	3.5
4	5	18	3.9

Source: From Smith, EL and Gilligan, C: Physical activity prescription for the older adult. Phys Sportsmed 11:91–101, 1983, with permission of McGraw-Hill, Inc.

TABLE 9–11 Indications for Test and Exercise Therapy Termination

1. Subject requests to stop.
2. Failure of the monitoring system.
3. Progressive angina (stop at 3+ level or earlier on a scale of 1+ to 4+).
4. Two millimeters horizontal or downsloping ST depression or elevation.
5. Sustained supraventricular tachycardia.
6. Ventricular tachycardia.
7. Exercise-induced left or right bundle branch block.
8. Any significant drop (10 mm Hg) of systolic blood pressure, or failure of the systolic blood pressure to rise with an increase in exercise load after the initial adjustment period.
9. Light-headedness, confusion, ataxia, pallor, cyanosis, nausea, or signs of severe peripheral circulatory insufficiency.
10. Excessive blood pressure rise: systolic greater than 250 mm Hg; diastolic greater than 120 mm Hg.
11. R-on-T premature ventricular complexes.
12. Unexplained inappropriate bradycardia — pulse rise slower than two standard deviations below age-adjusted normals.
13. Onset of second- or third-degree heart block.
14. Multifocal PVCs.
15. Increasing ventricular ectopy (>30%).

Source: Adapted from American College of Sports Medicine,[1] p. 21, with permission.

TABLE 9–12 Establishing Functional Classification Based on GXTT Results in METS

FUNCTIONAL CLASS	CLINICAL STATUS	O₂ REQUIREMENTS ml O₂/kg/min	STEP TEST — NAGLE, BALKE, NAUGHTON* (2 min stages 30 steps/min)	TREADMILL TESTS — BRUCE† (3-min stages) mph	%gr	KATTUS‡ (3-min stages) mph	%gr	BALKE** % grade at 3.4 mph	BALKE** % grade at 3 mph	BICYCLE ERGOMETER** (For 70 kg body weight) kgm/min
NORMAL AND I	PHYSICALLY ACTIVE SUBJECTS	56.0	(Step height increased 4 cm q 2 min)					26		
		52.5						24		
		49.0		mph	%gr	4	22	22		1500
		45.5	Height (cm)	4.2	16			20		
		42.0	40			4	18	18	22.5	1350
		38.5	36					16	20.0	1200
	SEDENTARY HEALTHY	35.0	32	3.4	14	4	14	14	17.5	1050
		31.5	28					12	15.0	900
		28.0	24			4	10	10	12.5	750
	DISEASED, RECOVERED	24.5	20	2.5	12	3	10	8	10.0	
II		21.0	16					6	7.5	600
	SYMPTOMATIC PATIENTS	17.5	12	1.7	10	2	10	4	5.0	450
		14.0	8					2	2.5	300
III		10.5	4						0.0	
		7.0								150
IV		3.5								

Source: From Wells et al,[30] p. 104, with permission.

**TABLE 9–13 Metabolic Measurements during GXTT
for Functional Classification of the Cardiac Patient**

Functional class A (corresponds to I and II, Table 9–12)
   Max. V_{O_2} > ml/min per kilogram
   Little or no impairment in aerobic capacity
Functional class B (corresponds to II, Table 9–12)
   Max. V_{O_2} 16–20 ml/min per kilogram
   (4.6–5.7 METs)
   Mild to moderate impairment in aerobic capacity
Functional class C (corresponds to III, Table 9–12)
   Max. V_{O_2} 10–15 ml/min per kilogram
   (2.9–4.3 METs)
   Moderate to severe impairment in aerobic capacity
Functional class D (corresponds to III and IV, Table 9–12)
   Max. V_{O_2} <10 ml/min per kilogram
   (<2.9 METs)
   Severe impairment in aerobic capacity

Source: From Weber and Janick,[45] p. 22A, with permission.

area of 12 METs in order to perform cardiorespiratory exercise for an extended period of time (see steady state in Chapter 4) at the 8-MET level. This distinction in the interpretation of functional classification must be made clear to patients in order to avoid misinterpretation of test results.

To interpret the results of a GXTT correctly, one must also be aware of the specificity and sensitivity of the test. An exercise test that is interpreted as abnormal in a person who is not found to have disease is called a false-positive test; conversely, a test interpreted as normal in a person who is found to have disease is called a false-negative test.[1] The probability of a false-positive test is related to the specificity of a test; in this case, if 100 normal persons (free of disease) are tested and 90 percent of those tested are normal and 10 percent are abnormal (false-positive), the test specificity is 90 percent for prediction of CAD. The specificity of the GXTT is reported to be in the range of 80 to 90 percent for men and 70 percent for women.[1,41] On the other hand, false-negative test results are related to the sensitivity of the test; in this instance, if 100 diseased persons are tested and 90 percent of those tested are found to be diseased and 10 percent are not identified as having disease (false-negatives), the sensitivity of the test is 90 percent for prediction of CAD. Sensitivity for exercise testing is reported to be in the range of 60 to 80 percent. However, many of the studies that reported low sensitivity for exercise testing were not conducted under standardized conditions, and thus the true sensitivity of this type of testing may be higher than previously reported. Conditions that contribute to increased incidence of false-positive and false-negative tests are listed in Tables 9–14 and 9–15, respectively.

Interpretation of GXTT results is strongly influenced by an individual's age, sex, risk factors, and symptoms. An abnormal response must be interpreted in light of those factors.

EMERGENCY PROCEDURES, MEDICATIONS, AND BASIC EQUIPMENT

Written emergency procedures should be established and signed by the appropriate medical authorities. Equipment and medications for emergencies must be available

TABLE 9–14 Conditions Contributing to Increased Incidence of False-Positive Tests

1. A preexisting abnormal resting ECG (e.g., ST-T abnormalities)
2. Cardiac hypertrophy
3. Wolff-Parkinson-White syndrome and other conduction defects
4. Hypertension
5. Drugs (e.g., digitalis)
6. Cardiomyopathy
7. Hypokalemia
8. Vasoregulatory abnormalities
9. Sudden intense exercise
10. Mitral valve prolapse syndrome
11. Pericardial disorders
12. Pectus excavatum
13. Technical or observer error

Source: Adapted from American College of Sports Medicine,[1] p. 28.

during all testing and exercise sessions. An example of emergency procedures and a list of standard emergency medications and equipment[42-45] is given in Appendix D. Emergency procedures must be updated to keep pace with changes in technology and research in emergency medicine. Because situations and the laws that govern them are different, personnel in charge of such programs would be prudent to have a carefully documented plan for dealing with emergency situations. The plan should include specific instructions for the administration of basic and advanced life support, the periodic review of emergency procedures, and the plans for emergency drills for all members of the staff. All plans should be approved by the appropriate medical and legal advisors. The safety of patients involved in rehabilitation programs is the highest priority.

STRESS-TESTING CASE HISTORIES

One of the most difficult decisions an inexperienced practitioner may have to make is that of determining precisely when the stress test is of adequate duration for diagnostic and/or exercise prescription purposes to warrant test termination. The case histories presented in this section may provide some insight into this decision-making process, because they illustrate that test termination most often is a result of factors other than those attributed to age-related maximum heart rates.

TABLE 9–15 Conditions Contributing to Increased Incidence of False-Negative Tests

1. Failure to reach an adequate exercise work load
2. Insufficient number of leads to detect ECG changes
3. Failure to use other information, such as systolic blood pressure drop, symptoms, dysrhythmias, heart rate response, etc., in test interpretation
4. Single vessel disease
5. Good collateral circulation
6. Musculoskeletal limitations before cardiac abnormalities occur
7. Technical or observer error

Source: Adapted from American College of Sports Medicine,[1] p. 28.

CASE STUDIES

CASE STUDY 1

The patient is a 57-year-old woman with a history of CAD and coronary artery bypass grafts (CABG), and angina. Her medications are Persantine and Synthroid; her body fat is 32 percent; and her AAMHR is 163 bpm. Table 9–16 gives a summary of the results of her GXTT.

TABLE 9–16 Raw Data—Case Study 1

AGE: 57	SEX: F	AAMHR: 163 bpm		80% AAMHR: 130 bpm
BRIEF HISTORY:	CAD, CABG, Angina			
MEDICATIONS:	Persantine, Synthroid			
RESTING EKG:	Slight ST-T flattening, No PVCs or other dysrhythmias			
RESTING HR:	65 bpm	RESTING BP: 128/84		
PROTOCOL:	Adapted Bruce (Treadmill)			

STAGE:	HR (bpm)	BP (3-min)	METs	COMMENTS AND REASON FOR TEST TERMINATION:
1	80			
	82			
	80	. . . . 146/84	2	
2	84			
	84			
	86	. . . . 150/86	3	
3	96			
	92			
	96	. . . . 158/86	5	
4	112			
	118			
	118	. . . . 168/86	7	Dyspnea, fatigue; ECG showed ST-T sagging increasing to −2 mm. RPP = 198.

ENDPOINT HR: 118 bpm   ENDPOINT BP: 168/86

CONCLUSION: A mildly positive treadmill test with no dysrhythmias: heart rate and blood pressure responses were good. The test was terminated at the end of stage 4, which was considered adequate for prescription purposes.

CASE STUDY 2

The patient is a 60-year-old woman with a history of CAD, angina, and post-MI. Her medications are Inderal, Lanoxin, Lasix, and Isordil; her body fat is 28 percent; and her AAMHR is 160 bpm. Table 9–17 gives a summary of her GXTT.

TABLE 9–17 Raw Data—Case Study 2

AGE: 60	SEX: F	AAMHR: 160 bpm	80% AAMHR: 128 bpm

BRIEF HISTORY: CAD, Angina, Post-MI

MEDICATIONS: Inderal, Lanoxin, Lasix, Isordil

RESTING EKG: ST-T depression of −1 mm, No dysrhythmias

RESTING HR: 52 bpm   RESTING BP: 140/80

PROTOCOL: Adapted Bruce (Treadmill)

STAGE:	HR (bpm)	BP (3-min)	METs	COMMENTS AND REASON FOR TEST TERMINATION:
1	63			
	68			
	68	. . . . 140/88	2	
2	72			
	74			
	75	. . . . 168/88	3	
3	80			
	82	. . . . 176/90 (2-min)	~4	Throat dryness, chest pain and burning. RPP = 144.

ENDPOINT HR: 82 bpm   ENDPOINT BP: 176/90

CONCLUSION: The test was terminated after 2 minutes into Stage 3 owing to chest pain and chest burning and is positive for angina. The ST-T changes are mild and difficult to interpret because the patient is taking Lanoxin. The blood pressure responses were fairly normal, although somewhat hypertensive in view of the mild workload the patient was able to achieve.

CASE STUDY 3

The patient is an 81-year-old man with ASHD, post-MI, hypertension, arthritis, and a pacemaker implant. His body fat is 28 percent; his AAMHR is 139; and his medications are Pronestyl, Lanoxin, Cardizem, Dyazide, Clinoril, and Transderm-Nitro 10. Table 9–18 summarizes the results of his GXTT.

TABLE 9–18 Raw Data—Case Study 3

AGE: 81	SEX: M	AAMHR: 139 bpm	80% AAMHR: 112 bpm

BRIEF HISTORY: ASHD, Post-MI, Arthritis (knees), Pacemaker implant

MEDICATIONS: Pronestyl, Lanoxin, Cardizem, Dyazide, Transderm-Nitro 10, Clinoril

RESTING EKG: Frequent pacer beats, ST-T sagging, 1½ mm

RESTING HR: 74 bpm   RESTING BP: 110/70

PROTOCOL: Adapted Bruce

STAGE:	HR (bpm)	BP (3-min)	METs	COMMENTS AND REASON FOR TEST TERMINATION:
1	84			
	84			
	82	.... 112/70	2	
2	86			
	86			
	88	.... 120/70	3	
3	88			
	86			
	88	.... 124/72	5	
4	90			
	92			
	92	.... 132/78	7	Patient exhibits dyspnea, is fatigued. T-wave inversion noted. RPP = 121.

ENDPOINT HR: 92 bpm   ENDPOINT BP: 132/78

CONCLUSION: Pacer beats were not apparent during last stage of GXTT, but T waves were inverted. Inverted T waves indicate possible ischemia, but as the patient was asymptomatic, the inversion was most likely due to an old MI or post-pacemaker activity — difficult to interpret due to medications.

CASE STUDY 4

The patient is a 52-year-old man whose body fat is estimated to be 38 percent. He is a smoker with a history of hypertension and a pacemaker implant. His medications are quinidine, Minipress, and HydroDIURIL. Table 9–19 summarizes the results of his GXTT.

TABLE 9–19 Raw Data—Case Study 4

AGE: 52	SEX: M	AAMHR: 168 bpm	80% AAMHR: 134 bpm

BRIEF HISTORY: Hypertension, Pacemaker, Obesity

MEDICATIONS: Quinidine, Minipress, HydroDIURIL

RESTING EKG: Pacer spikes evident with occasional PVCs (<10 min) and 1 episode of coupling noted.

RESTING HR: 72 bpm   RESTING BP: 120/80

PROTOCOL: Adapted Bruce

STAGE:	HR (bpm)	BP (3-min)	METs	COMMENTS AND REASON FOR TEST TERMINATION:
1	82			2 episodes of coupling,
	85			frequent (>10 min) PVCs
	82	.... 140/82	2	with some bigeminy, asymptomatic
2	85			
	86			1 episode of coupling,
	86	.... 140/90	3	occasional PVCs, asymptomatic.
3	86			
	90			1 episode of coupling,
	96	.... 140/92	5	occasional PVCs, asymptomatic
4	102			
	102			
	102	.... 142/92	7	Dyspnea, Leg fatigue. RPP = 144.

ENDPOINT HR: 102 bpm   ENDPOINT BP: 142/92

CONCLUSION: Fairly frequent ventricular coupling and episodes of bigeminy that decreased in frequency during Stages 3 and 4. Pacer firings were intermittent with no ST-T changes noted. Treadmill test was negative for angina and positive for ventricular dysrhythmia.

CASE STUDY 5

The patient is a 70-year old woman with an estimated body fat of 44 percent. She is hypertensive, obese, and arthritic, and her medications are HydroDIURIL and Aldomet. Owing to the limitations imposed by her arthritis, she is being tested on a bicycle ergometer. A summary of the test results is shown in Table 9-20.

TABLE 9-20 Raw Data—Case Study 5

AGE: 70	SEX: F	AAMHR: 150 bpm	80% AAMHR: 120 bpm

BRIEF HISTORY: Hypertension, Obesity, Arthritis (knees, wrists, spine)

MEDICATION:　HydroDIURIL, Aldomet

RESTING EKG:　Normal

RESTING HR:　62 bpm　　　　　　　　　RESTING BP: 146/92

PROTOCOL:　Adapted Astrand-Rhyming Bicycle Test

STAGE:	HR (bpm)	BP (3-min)	METs	COMMENTS AND REASON FOR TEST TERMINATION:
1 (at one-half workload)	88			Headache with pounding sensation. Test terminated owing to severe hypertensive response to exercise. RPP = 248.
	95			
	113	. . . . 220/136	<2	

ENDPOINT HR: 113 bpm　　　　　　　ENDPOINT BP: 220/136

CONCLUSION: Severe hypertensive response to exercise; severely deconditioned. No dysrhythmias or chest pain noted. Negative test for ischemia to level tested.

CASE STUDY 6

The patient is a 73-year-old man with a history of hypertension, chronic obstructive pulmonary disease (COPD), arthritis, and cancer of the colon. His body fat estimation is 30 percent; his medications are procainamide, Ativan, Antivert, Ecotrin, and Tylenol; and he is a smoker. The results of his GXTT are shown in Table 9–21.

TABLE 9–21 Raw Data—Case Study 6

AGE: 73	SEX: M	AAMHR: 147 bpm	80% AAMHR: 118 bpm

BRIEF HISTORY: Hypertension, COPD, Arthritis (generalized), CA (colon), Colostomy, Rectal Sensitivity, Hyperlipidemia

MEDICATIONS: Procainamide, Antivert, Ativan, Ecotrin, Tylenol

RESTING EKG: Normal

RESTING HR: 76 bpm   RESTING BP: 148/92

PROTOCOL: Adapted Bruce

STAGE:	HR (bpm)	BP (3-min)	METs	COMMENTS AND REASON FOR TEST TERMINATION:
1	98			
	98			
	98	194/98	2	
2	102			
	106			
	112	206/104	3	Slight Dyspnea
3	114			
	116			Moderate Hypertensive Response,
	122	220/106	5	Dyspnea, Fatigue, Achieved >83% AAMHR. RPP = 268.

ENDPOINT HR: 122 bpm   ENDPOINT BP: 220/106

CONCLUSION: No dysrhythmias noted during test but PACs were observed during recovery. ST-T depression of 1 mm in leads II, III and aVF indicate a mildly positive treadmill test suggesting possible right coronary artery disease. A moderate hypertensive response to exercise was noted.

CASE STUDY 7

The patient is a 51-year-old man with a history of CAD, post-MI, and hypertension. His body fat is estimated to be 25 percent, and his medications are Corgard and procainamide. Because the patient had been involved in a cardiac rehabilitation program, the Bruce protocol seemed appropriate for his GXTT. The results of his treadmill test are shown in Table 9–22.

TABLE 9–22 Raw Data—Case Study 7

AGE: 51	SEX: M	AAMHR: 169 bpm	80% AAMHR: 135 bpm

BRIEF HISTORY: CAD, Post-MI, Hypertension

MEDICATIONS: Corgard, Procainamide

RESTING EKG: Normal

RESTING HR: 56 bpm   RESTING BP: 126/86

PROTOCOL: Bruce

STAGE:	HR (bpm)	BP (3-min)	METs	COMMENTS AND REASON FOR TEST TERMINATION:
1	76			
	76			
	80	148/90	5	
2	92			Frequent PVCs, bigeminy,
	110			and 1 episode of coupling.
	110	168/94	7	Test terminated. RPP = 184.

ENDPOINT HR: 110 bpm   ENDPOINT BP: 168/94

CONCLUSION: At peak exercise, PVCs became more frequent with bigeminy and 1 episode of coupling, when test was terminated. No ST-T changes were noted, but the treadmill test is considered positive for ischemia due to dysrhythmias.

CASE STUDY 8

The patient is a 50-year old man with a history of an MI, CAD, CABG ($\times$ 3), peripheral vascular disease (PVD), and hyperlipidemia. His body fat is estimated to be 20 percent, and his medications are Cardizem, Isordil, and Transderm-Nitro 5. Table 9–23 shows the results of his GXTT.

TABLE 9–23 Raw Data—Case Study 8

AGE: 50	SEX: M	AAMHR: 170 bpm	80% AAMHR: 136 bpm

BRIEF HISTORY: CAD, Post-MI, CABG, PVD, Hyperlipidemia

MEDICATIONS: Cardizem, Isordil, Transderm-Nitro 5

RESTING EKG: Baseline ST abnormalities noted with ST-T flattening in II, III, and aVF

RESTING HR: 48 bpm   RESTING BP: 138/84

PROTOCOL: Adapted Bruce

STAGE:	HR (bpm)	BP (3-min)	METs	COMMENTS AND REASON FOR TEST TERMINATION:
1	68			
	78			
	82	138/84	2	
2	84			Patient complained of
	82			bilateral leg tightness,
	84	146/90	3	pain level 1.
3	94			Patient complained of
	94			bilateral leg pain. Some ST-T
	94	150/94	5	depression in V_5 noted.
4	98	156/98		Bilateral leg pain intense (pain level 2) and test was terminated after 1 min into Stage 4. ST-T depression apparent (−3 mm). RPP = 152.

ENDPOINT HR: 98 bpm   ENDPOINT BP: 156/98

CONCLUSION: Mild hypertensive response to exercise. Positive treadmill test for ischemia with 3 mm of depression noted in V_5 at maximal exercise. No angina occurred, but the test was positive for claudication. PVCs and occasional episodes of bigeminy were noted during cool-down and recovery.

CASE STUDY 9

The patient is a 55-year-old woman with a history of mitral valve prolapse (MVP), atypical angina, possible coronary artery spasms, hypertension, and hyperlipidemia. Her body fat is estimated to be 18 percent, and her medications are Inderal and HydroDIURIL. The results of her GXTT are shown in Table 9–24.

TABLE 9–24 Raw Data—Case Study 9

AGE: 55	SEX: F	AAMHR: 165 bpm	80% AAMHR: 132 bpm

BRIEF HISTORY: MVP, Atypical angina, Possible coronary artery spasms, Hypertension, Hyperlipidemia

MEDICATIONS: Inderal, HydroDIURIL

RESTING EKG: Resting ST flattening, T-wave inversion in V_4 during hyperventilation

RESTING HR: 62 bpm   RESTING BP: 150/86

PROTOCOL: Adapted Bruce

STAGE:	HR (bpm)	BP (3-min)	METs	COMMENTS AND REASON FOR TEST TERMINATION:
1	110			
	110			Some ST depression
	110	140/88	2	apparent.
2	112			ST depression continuing,
	114			patient complained of
	114	142/90	3	slight chest pain.
3	114			
	116			
	116	158/92	5	Same as for Stage 2.
4	130			Chest pain severe, radiating
	136			into neck and both arms.
	142	164/94	7	Test terminated. RPP = 232.

ENDPOINT HR: 142 bpm   ENDPOINT BP: 164/94

CONCLUSION: Positive treadmill test for angina and for ischemia, although it may be a false-positive for CAD due to MVP. Recommend thallium stress test for further evaluation.

The case histories provide examples of responses to graded exercise tolerance testing. In each case, the reason for test termination should be clear to the reader. Test termination guidelines have been provided in Table 9–10 and Chapters 7 and 8.

SUMMARY

The procedures commonly followed to evaluate patients with cardiovascular disease have been reviewed. The prudent clinician should be initially concerned with evaluating the medical status of a prospective patient through the comprehensive medical history. The information should include personal, medical, and family health histories, lifestyle health habits, and results from the most recent physical examination by the patient's physician.

Results from laboratory evaluations give valuable information about the medical status of a patient. Those of particular significance include blood test results, pulmonary function testing, and electrocardiograms. Information gathered through assessments, such as body weight and percent body fat, is also valuable to the understanding of the medical status of a patient.

Prior to the administration of the exercise evaluation or stress test, several forms must be read, completed, and in some cases signed by the patient. A primary concern for the clinician is the informed consent form, which should be devised with the aid of legal counsel and signed by each patient before any stress test or exercise program is undertaken.

The evaluation of cardiorespiratory capacity through stress testing has value not only for diagnosis of ischemic heart disease and similar disorders but also for formulating exercise prescriptions. Although the clinician may administer a stress test utilizing a treadmill, a bicycle ergometer, or a bench step, the mode of choice in most cases is the treadmill. Rather than the single level test, a graded test such as the adapted Bruce or the Bruce protocol is preferred.

The clinician administering the stress test should be alert for such patient symptoms as angina, dyspnea, and ECG changes that indicate the test should be terminated. Equipment and medications to be used in case of an emergency situation must be available during all testing and exercise sessions. Case studies illustrating criteria for test termination have been included.

REFERENCES

1. American College of Sports Medicine: Guidelines for Graded Exercise Testing and Prescription, ed 3. Lea & Febiger, Philadelphia, 1986.
2. Fardy, PS, Yanowitz, FG and Wilson, PK: Cardiac Rehabilitation, Adult Fitness and Exercise Testing, ed 2. Lea & Febiger, Philadelphia, 1988, pp 41–65.
3. Hellerstein, HK and Wenger, NK: Rehabilitation of the Coronary Patient, ed 2. John Wiley & Sons, New York, 1984.
4. Meizlish, JL, et al: Exercise nuclear imaging for the evaluation of coronary artery disease. In Wenger, NK (ed.): Exercise and the Heart, ed 2. FA Davis, Philadelphia, 1985, pp 105–123.
5. Fardy, PS, et al: Cardiac Rehabilitation: Implications for the Nurse and Other Health Professionals. CV Mosby, St. Louis, 1980.
6. Wilson, PK, et al: Policies and Procedures of a Cardiac Rehabilitation Program: Immediate to Long-Term Care. Lea & Febiger, Philadelphia, 1978.
7. Rogers, C: Client Centered Therapy. Houghton Mifflin, Boston, 1951.
8. Riffenburgh, RS: Active Listening in the Medical Interview. Postgrad Med J 55:91, 1974.
9. Rose, GA, et al: Cardiovascular Survey Methods, ed 2. World Health Organization, Geneva, 1982.

10. Diethrich, EB: The Heart Test. Simon & Schuster, New York, 1981.
11. Friedman, M and Ulmer, D: Treating Type A Behavior and Your Heart. Knopf, New York, 1984.
12. Gunderson, EK, Rahe, E and Rahe, RH: Life Stress and Illness. Charles C Thomas, Springfield, IL, 1974.
13. Guss, SB: Heart attack risk score. Cardiac Alert (newsletter) November, 1982.
14. Ruppel, G: Manual of Pulmonary Function Testing, ed 4. CV Mosby, St. Louis, 1986.
15. Chusid, LE: The Selective and Comprehensive Testing of Adult Pulmonary Function, Futura, Mount Kisco, NY, 1983.
16. Humberstone, N: Respiratory therapy and treatment. In Irwin, S and Tecklin, JS (eds.): Cardiopulmonary Physical Therapy, ed 2. CV Mosby, St. Louis, 1990, p 283.
17. Metropolitan Life Insurance Co: Four Steps to Weight Control, New York, 1969.
18. Wilmore, JH and Behnke, AR. Anthropometric estimation of body density and lean body weight in young men. J of Appl Physiol 27:25, 1969.
19. Wilmore, JH and Behnke, AR. Anthropometric estimation of body density and lean body weight in young women. Am J Clin Nutr 23:267, 1970.
20. McArdle, WD, Katch, FI and Katch VL. Exercise Physiology: Energy, Nutrition and Human Performance, ed 3. Lea & Febiger, Philadelphia, 1991.
21. Brooks, GA and Fahey, TD: Exercise Physiology: Human Bioenergetics and Its Applications. John Wiley & Sons, New York, 1984.
22. Brozek, J, et al: Densitometric analysis of body composition: Revision of some quantitative assumptions. Ann NY Acad Sci 110:113–140, 1963.
23. Siri, WE: The gross composition of the body. Biol Med Physics 4:239–280, 1956.
24. Jackson, JS and Pollock, ML: Practical assessment of body composition. Phys Sportsmed 13(5):76–90, 1985.
25. Naughton, J: Cardiac rehabilitation: Current status and future possibilities. In NK Wenger (ed): Exercise and the Heart, ed. 2. FA Davis, Philadelphia, 1985, pp 185–192.
26. Bruce, RA, Kusumi, F and Hosmer, D: Maximal oxygen intake and nomographic assessment of functional aerobic impairment in cardiovascular disease. Am Heart J 85:546–562, 1973.
27. Shephard, RJ: Physical Activity and Aging, ed 2. Aspen Publishers, Rockville, MD, 1987, pp 85–90.
28. Astrand, PO and Rodahl, K: Textbook of Work Physiology, ed 3. McGraw-Hill, New York, 1986, p 376.
29. Koppes, G et al: Treadmill testing: Part I. In Harvey, WP, (ed): Curr Prob Cardiol 7:8, 1977.
30. Wells, SJ, et al (eds): New York Heart Association: Manual of Cardiovascular Assessment. Reston Publishing, Reston, VA, 1983, pp 101–105.
31. Jorgenson, CR, et al: Effect of propranolol on myocardial oxygen consumption and its hemodynamic correlates during upright exercise. Circulation 50:1173, 1973.
32. Nelson, RR, et al: Hemodynamic predictors of myocardial oxygen consumption during static and dynamic exercise. Circulation 50:1179, 1974.
33. Redwood, DR, et al: Importance of design in an exercise protocol in evaluation of patients with angina pectoris. Circulation 43:618, 1971.
34. Barnard, RJ, et al: Ischemic responses to sudden strenuous exercise in healthy men. Circulation 48:936–942, 1973.
35. Brannon, FJ and Geyer, MJ: A study of electrocardiographic responses to various multi-stage treadmill tests in an adult cardiac population. Bio-Energetiks Rehabilitation, Prospect, PA, 1984. Unpublished study.
36. Golding, L, Myers, C and Sinning, W. The Y's Way to Physical Fitness, ed. 3. Human Kinetics Publishers, Champaign, IL, 1989.
37. Bruce, RA, et al: Cardiovascular function tests. Heart Bull 14:9, 1965.
38. Smith, EL and Gilligan, C: Physical activity prescription for the older adult. Phys Sportsmed 11:91–101, 1983.
39. Hamm, LF, et al: Short- and long-term prognostic value of graded exercise testing soon after myocardial infarction. J Am Phys Therapy Assoc 66(3):334–338, 1986.
40. American Heart Association Committee on Exercise: Exercise Testing and Training of Individuals with Heart Disease or at High Risk. American Heart Association, Dallas, 1975.
41. Ellestad, MH. Stress Testing: Principles and Practice, ed 3. FA Davis, Philadelphia, 1986, pp 343–344.
42. Priest, ML: Trauma Cardiorespiratory Arrest. In Campbell, JE (ed): Basic Trauma Life Support: Advanced Prehospital Care. Prentice-Hall, Englewood Cliffs, NJ, 1988, pp 226–237.
43. Ellis, DP and Billings, DM: Cardiopulmonary Resuscitation: Procedures for Basic and Advanced Life Support. CV Mosby, St. Louis, 1980, pp 183–200.
44. American Heart Association: Textbook of Advanced Cardiac Life Support. American Heart Association, Dallas, TX, 1987.
45. Weber, KT and Janicki, JS: Cardiopulmonary exercise testing for evaluation of chronic failure. Am J Cardiol 55:22A–31A, 1985.

CHAPTER 10

Pulmonary Assessment

The assessment of a patient's pulmonary status has several purposes applicable to pulmonary rehabilitation: (1) to evaluate the appropriateness of the patient's participation in a pulmonary rehabilitation program, (2) to determine the therapeutic measures most appropriate to the participant's treatment program, (3) to monitor the participant's physiologic response to exercise, and (4) to appropriately progress the participant's treatment program over a period of time.

Achieving those stated purposes necessitates an ongoing assessment throughout the entire rehabilitative process. The initial assessments of patients with pulmonary disease allow for a careful and appropriate selection of pulmonary rehabilitation candidates. Patients must be evaluated to verify the need for pulmonary rehabilitation and to predict those who will benefit within the given structure of the program.

An appropriate individualized rehabilitation treatment program can be formulated only after a comprehensive pulmonary evaluation has been performed. A pulmonary rehabilitation treatment program must be tailored to the individual's dysfunctions and his or her perceived needs. Mutually acceptable and realistic goals must be agreed on by the patient and the pulmonary rehabilitation staff.

Once the treatment program has been devised, the patient must be frequently assessed during the course of therapy. An evaluation of the participant's performance during each session makes it possible for the treatment program to reflect alterations in medical strategies, daily fluctuations in ability, and improvement in function. The success and safety of each rehabilitation session can be assured if the participant is continually assessed.

Exercise progression can be appropriately determined on the basis of an assessment of the participant's abilities to perform his or her exercise sessions. When heart rates plateau at lower levels and/or perceived exertion rates fall below the prescribed level during similar exercise intensity, exercise may be progressed. (This principle of exercise progression assumes all other parameters are within safe and acceptable ranges.)

Optimal care is continually formulated, and the overall success of the treatment program can be assured only by an ongoing assessment of the patient.

Assessment takes many forms. Information is obtained from the patient via patient interview and physical examination, which includes observation, inspection, palpation, and auscultation, and information is also received from the referring physician and

253

chart reviews regarding test results and interpretations including laboratory values, chest roentgenograms, pulmonary function tests, arterial blood gas analyses, and electrocardiograms (ECGs). Graded exercise tests are not always performed in a diagnostic work-up for chronic lung disease, but they are necessary prior to admission to a pulmonary rehabilitation program.

PATIENT INTERVIEW

A patient interview should begin with the "chief complaint," the patient's *perception* of why pulmonary rehabilitation is being sought. Commonly, the chief complaint will center around a loss of function. Participants differ in the type and degree of activity loss that motivates them to seek pulmonary rehabilitation. Identifying the chief complaint is the beginning of goal setting in the rehabilitation process.[1] Loss of activity should be translated into a measurable, achievable goal.

A medical history contains pertinent pulmonary symptoms specific to that patient: cough, sputum production, wheezing, and shortness of breath. By requesting the patient to relate his or her medical history, knowledge of the patient's disease processes can be evaluated. A medical history also addresses occupational, social, medication, and family histories.

Cough history is an important assessment when interviewing a patient with pulmonary disease. Participants often minimize the extent of cough and sputum production. That may not be a conscious deception of minimizing symptoms but instead may be due to the insidious onset of coughing that has become so incorporated in the patient's life that he or she is not aware of its frequency. It can be helpful to ask for such specific information as: Do you cough? Do you cough more in the morning upon arising from bed? Are you productive of sputum? If so, what is the amount?[2]

Participants are asked to relate episodes of shortness of breath and wheezing by answering such questions as these: How often do these episodes occur? When was the onset of these symptoms? Is there anything that either precipitates the occurrence or helps to alleviate the intensity of these symptoms? This information is necessary in order to devise the most appropriate individualized pulmonary rehabilitation program.

An occupational history for pulmonary patients provides information regarding exposures to toxins and irritants.[3] Inquiring about their *present* occupations will provide information on exposures that may put them at risk for hypersensitive occupational asthma. A *past* occupational history will contain information on exposure to hazardous materials that may cause a more chronic type of occupational lung disease. Asbestosis, silicosis, beryliosis, and many other occupational lung diseases have long latency periods between exposure to the toxin and the beginning of symptomatology.[4]

Social habits, such as smoking, alcohol consumption, and recreational or habitual drug use, should be documented. Each of the aforementioned has its own pulmonary issues that must be addressed.

Smoking history is usually calculated in pack-years. Total pack-years is equal to the number of packs smoked per day times the number of years smoked. A patient who smoked three packs per day for 10 years has a 30-pack-year history, and one who smoked one pack per day for 30 years also has a 30-pack-year history. The greater the pack-year history (especially over 60 pack-years), the more likely it is that that patient will have a smoking-related illness.[2]

An admission of excessive alcohol consumption may be difficult to obtain. Inquiring about extreme behaviors may make it easier for patients to be honest about the amount of alcohol they consume. For example, the interviewer might ask, "Do you ever drink between two to three cases of beer a day?"[5] Excessive alcohol consumption allows patients to harbor opportunistic pulmonary infections, and special precautions may need to be considered with this population.

Drug use of any sort involves health risks. Drugs that are smoked, such as marijuana and crack, deliver toxins directly to the lungs. The most common acute complication of these toxins is pulmonary edema.[2]

Knowing that cigarette smoking, excessive alcohol consumption, and drug usage are objectional health behaviors, patients may tend to minimize and understate the extent of consumption and use. By creating a nonjudgmental atmosphere, accurate information can often be gathered.[6] If there is a question of accuracy, the family may have to be consulted.

A medication history is necessary to alert the clinician to the need for special considerations when prescribing exercise. For example, a patient who has been maintained on long-term steroids for pulmonary bronchospasm is at risk for osteoporosis.[7] The resulting potential for fractures may necessitate a low-impact mode of exercise.

A patient's family history also is important. An environment of passive smoke may add to a pulmonary dysfunction,[8] and there may be a familial propensity for bronchospasm.[9] There are also pulmonary diseases that are genetic in origin, such as immotile cilia or alpha-antitrypsin deficiency.[10]

Finally, a patient's family/home environment should be assessed. What are the psychosocial issues surrounding the patient and his or her family? What is the housing situation? What are the patient's responsibilities within the family? What types of support systems are presently in place for this patient?

PHYSICAL EXAMINATION

Vital Signs

Vital signs are taken prior to the onset of exercise at each pulmonary rehabilitation session. Some of the vital signs and their significance are addressed in the following discussion.

Temperature elevation above normal (98.6°F or 37°C) commonly indicates an infection. Although the pulmonary system is a probable site for infection in patients with pulmonary disease, nonpulmonary infections can also be devastating to the pulmonary patient.

Resting heart rate values may be elevated in the patient with pulmonary disease as a result of bronchodilator drug therapy.[11] Heart rates may also be elevated in the presence of infection. If arrhythmias are suspected, heart rate should be determined by ECG tracings.

Respiratory rate and the character of ventilation should be closely evaluated. The normal resting respiration rate is 12 to 18 breaths per minute. Alterations in rate and character of ventilation can occur in the normal population for a variety of reasons including exercise and altitude changes and by simply drawing attention to a person's own respiratory pattern. The evaluator, therefore, must conceal the evaluation of respiratory rate from the client. One way to ensure an accurate measurement is to count the respirations while the patient assumes that the heart rate is being assessed. Respiratory rates may be elevated in patients with pulmonary dysfunction in an attempt to maintain as near normal $Paco_2$ value as possible. Respiratory breathing patterns can be described by the rhythm and amplitude of the respiratory cycle. Alterations in breathing patterns are not a common finding among patients enrolled in pulmonary rehabilitation programs.

An individual's height should be measured, since there is a direct relation between height and lung volumes. A stadiometer is recommended for this measurement. (See Chapter 9 for the procedure.)

Weight should be measured on a standard balance scale, and each evaluation of weight should be performed on the same scale. (See Chapter 9 for the procedure.) Weight gains should be interpreted as a possible decrease in activity and/or a decrease in cardiac function. An unexplained weight loss may be a sign of carcinoma.

Resting blood pressure measurements average from 90/60 to 120/90 mm Hg. Resting arterial blood pressures exceeding 160/95 mm Hg are considered to be hypertensive.[12] Blood pressures vary with age, drug therapy, stress, level of fitness, and pathological conditions. Blood pressure may be elevated in a patient with pulmonary disease during an infection. Pulsus paradoxus, an exaggerated decrease of 10 mm Hg or greater in the systolic blood pressure during inspiration, may be present in patients with severe airways obstruction.

Observation, Inspection, and Palpation

By observing the neck and shoulders of a patient with pulmonary disease, the use of the accessory muscles of ventilation can be observed. The severity of respiratory distress might well be judged by accessory muscle use at rest and the presence of paradoxical breathing.[13] Jugular venous distention (JVD) can also be discerned by observing the neck. It is a sign consistent with right ventricular failure from pulmonary disease (cor pulmonale).[14] Another external sign of right ventricular failure is peripheral edema.

A normal configuration of the thorax is necessary for proper ventilation. By observing and measuring the thorax, the anteroposterior (AP) and lateral dimensions of the thorax can be assessed. Any change in the normal configuration (AP to lateral ratio of 2:1) indicates structural abnormalities within the rib cage. Emphysema causes destruction of the lung parenchyma that results in an increase in the AP diameter and a narrowing of the ratio (1:1). Because of hyperinflation of the lungs, the chest appears rounder and is therefore referred to as a "barrel chest." The subcostal angle (the angle formed anteriorly by the borders of the costocartilage) is normally approximately 90°. Alterations in this angle often reflect a change in the underlying lung parenchyma.

The chest should appear symmetrical at rest. During inhalation and exhalation, both sides of the thorax should have equal lateral movement. By placing the clinician's hands over the anterior base of the lungs and aligning the thumbs over the costochrondral borders, symmetry can be grossly assessed during ventilatory maneuvers. Placement of the clinician's hands over the posterior bases of the lungs, with the thumbs parallel to the vertebral column, further enhances assessment of chest symmetry (Fig. 10–1).

By observing the skin and the nail beds, two characteristics of pulmonary disease can be seen. The first, cyanosis, is a bluish discoloration of the skin that indicates hypoxemia.[14] Common sites for observing cyanosis are the perioral and periorbital sites

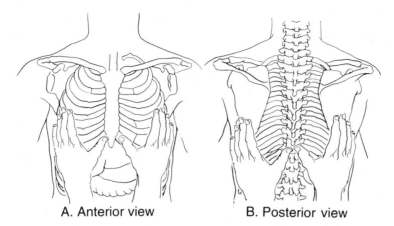

A. Anterior view   B. Posterior view

FIGURE 10–1. Placement of the clinician's hands to assess the symmetrical movement of the patient's thorax. (From Rothstein, JM, Roy, SH, and Wolf, SL: The Rehabilitation Specialist's Handbook. FA Davis, Philadelphia, 1991, p. 593, with permission.)

and the finger and toenail beds. The second observation, digital clubbing of the fingers and toes, is an increase in the angle created by the distal phalynx and the point at which the nail exits from the digit. The tip of the digit becomes bulbous. The condition is often associated with chronic hypoxia[14] (Fig. 10–2).

To assist their breathing, patients with chronic pulmonary disease will assume postures that structurally elevate and/or stabilize the shoulder girdle (Fig. 10–3). The

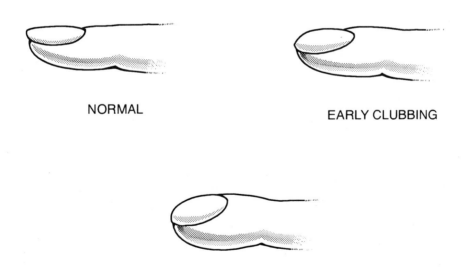

NORMAL   EARLY CLUBBING

ADVANCED CLUBBING

FIGURE 10–2. The progression of digital clubbing of the finger. (From Bell, C, et al: Home Care and Rehabilitation in Respiratory Medicine. JB Lippincott, Philadelphia, 1984, with permission.)

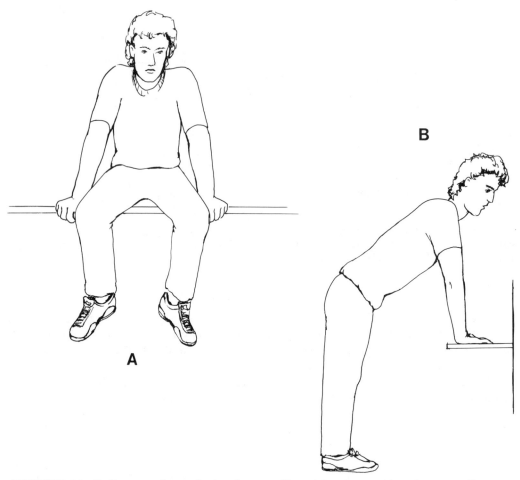

FIGURE 10–3. Postures that assist inspiratory efforts of patients with pulmonary disease.

thoracic attachments of the pectoralis major and minor and the serratus anterior can be used to expand the thorax and become muscles of inspiration.[15] By elevating and stabilizing the shoulder girdle, the thorax is already in the position to assist with inspiration. Some of the postures that assist in breathing are (1) sitting with hands clasping the edge of the chair or bed, elbows locked, and the shoulder girdle elevated, (2) standing while bending slightly forward and leaning on locked elbows on a window sill, (3) standing while leaning backwards against a wall with hands on knees, locked elbows, and so on. Observing the posture a patient assumes at rest and during exercise will help in an assessment of the severity of lung dysfunction.

Auscultation of the Lungs

Auscultation involves listening to air as it enters and exits the lungs. To perform it, a stethoscope is placed firmly on the patient's thorax over the lung tissue. The patient is

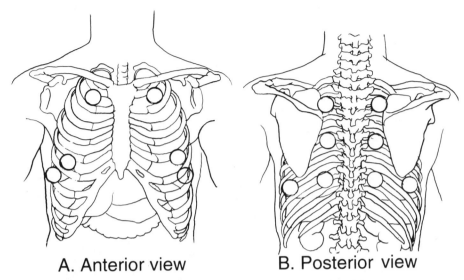

A. Anterior view   B. Posterior view

FIGURE 10–4. Anterior, lateral, and posterior auscultation sites. (From Rothstein, JM, Roy, SH, and Wolf, SL: The Rehabilitation Specialist's Handbook. FA Davis, Philadelphia, 1991, p. 593, with permission.)

asked to inspire fully through an open mouth and then to exhale quietly.[16] The clinician should listen for breath sounds over the anterior, lateral, and posterior chest wall. Breath sounds occurring on the right thorax should be compared with those on the left at comparable levels. A general auscultatory examination (Fig. 10–4) provides an overall assessment of the patient's breath sounds without risk of the patient tiring or hyperventilating. After the patient takes a brief rest, a more specific auscultatory examination in an area where abnormalities were heard can commence.

Inhalation and the beginning of exhalation normally emit a soft rustling sound. The end of exhalation is silent. This characteristic of a normal breath sound is termed "vesicular." It should be noted that, when listening over various portions of the thorax, different intensities will normally be heard. The bases of the lungs are quieter than the apices. A loud breath sound can be found over the right anterior upper thorax. When a louder, more hollow, and echoing sound occupies a larger portion of the ventilatory cycle, the breath sounds are referred to as "bronchial." Bronchial breath sounds can normally be heard over the trachea during quiet breathing. When the breath sounds are very quiet and barely audible, they are termed "diminished." With those three terms — vesicular, bronchial, and diminished — the listener can describe the intensity of the breath sound[17] (Fig. 10–5).

In addition to the normal and abnormal quality of the breath sound, there may be other sounds and vibrations — adventitious sounds — that can be heard during auscultation. They are superimposed on the already-described intensity of the breath sound. According to the American College of Chest Physicians and the American Thoracic Society, there are two types of adventitious sounds: crackles and wheezes.[18] Crackles, formerly termed "rales," are thought to occur when previously closed small airways and alveoli are rapidly reopened.[19] Patients with such problems as atelectasis, which is the collapse of alveoli, will present with crackles over the collapsed area.[20] As the patient inhales deeply, some of the airways open and the characteristic crackling is heard. In

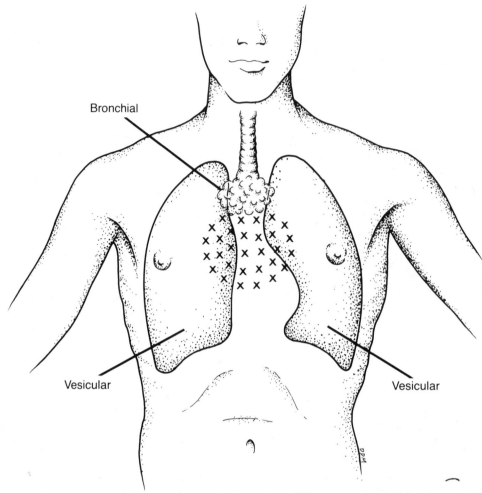

Bronchial

Vesicular

Vesicular

FIGURE 10–5. Normal auscultatory findings over different aspects of the thorax. (From Rothstein, JM, Roy, SH, and Wolf, SL: The Rehabilitation Specialist's Handbook. FA Davis, Philadelphia. 1991, p. 593, with permission.)

pulmonary edema, the fluid in the lung parenchyma may cause the small airways to close. Crackles can be heard on inhalation in a patient with pulmonary edema. The same is true of pneumonia, bronchiectasis, and other secretion-producing pulmonary pathologies.[21] Crackles are also heard in such restrictive pulmonary diseases as pulmonary fibrosis.[22]

Wheezes, on the other hand, are more musical in nature. They can be likened to blowing up a balloon and then pulling on its neck to produce a whistling sound as the balloon deflates. It is the decreased size of the neck of the balloon that produces the wheeze, and that is true within the lung also. Anything that can decrease the size of the lumen of the airway will create a wheezing sound. Asthma, with its bronchoconstriction, bronchial mucosal edema, and increased secretion production, typically produces a wheeze. Tumor growth into the lumen of an airway, an aspirated foreign body lodged in an airway, or excessive secretions also can produce a wheezing sound.[23] Under normal conditions, the size of the airway lumen increases during inspiration and decreases during expiration. Mild wheezing occurs at the end of expiration when the airway is the most narrow and the obstruction would further reduce the diameter of the airway. As wheezing worsens, it takes up more and more of the expiratory phase of breathing, and severe wheezing will affect both inspiration and expiration.

LABORATORY TESTS

Various laboratory studies should be performed to help in an evaluation of the appropriateness of a participant for pulmonary rehabilitation. They include chest roentgenograms (CXR), pulmonary function tests (PFT), graded exercise tests (GXT), arterial blood gas analysis (ABG), oxygen saturation measurements (Sao_2), and ECGs. The following discussion will focus on the use of ABG, Sao_2, and the ECG as they relate to an exercise-testing situation.

Chest Roentgenograms

A chest roentgenogram provides information pertaining to the bony thorax, the lungs, the heart, the structures of the hilum, the diaphragm, the interpleural space, and the soft tissues of the thorax.[24] As a diagnostic tool by itself, a CXR has limited capacities. Viewed in sequence, however, CXRs can show disease progression or resolution, and they are helpful for monitoring disease processes. Correlating clinical data with radiographic findings can make a CXR very useful in diagnosing disorders of the pulmonary system.

Pulmonary Function Tests

A PFT can assist in (1) establishing the diagnosis of lung disease, (2) documenting the extent of the abnormality, (3) determining the reversibility of the abnormality, (4) predicting the prognosis of a patient with pulmonary disease, and (5) deciding on appropriate exercise-testing protocols.

Five important pulmonary function measurements to be discussed are (1) the forced vital capacity (FVC), (2) the forced expiratory volume in 1 second (FEV_1), (3) maximum minute ventilation (VEmax), (4) the forced expiratory flow rate over 25 to 75 percent of the FVC ($FEF_{25\%-75\%}$), and (5) the diffusion capacity of the lung for carbon monoxide ($DLCO$). The measurements should be obtained with the patient in either the sitting or the standing position.[25] Maximal patient effort is needed to obtain reproducible values.[25] Each measurement of volume or flow can be compared to normative values based on a patient's height, age, and gender. A comparison of a subject's PFT values over a period of time can demonstrate stability or progression of the disease.

VITAL CAPACITY

Vital capacity (VC) is the amount of air that can be exhaled following a maximal inspiratory effort. When the VC is forcibly and quickly exhaled, the maneuver is called an FVC. VC is recorded in liters, and it may vary as much as 20 percent from the predicted normal values in healthy individuals. It may also vary somewhat from time to time in the same individual, depending on such factors as medical status, body position, bronchodilator therapy, and patient effort. It varies directly with height and indirectly with age. An equation that is useful to predict VC in males is

$$VC = 0.0481 \times H - 0.020 \times A - 2.81$$

For females, the equation[25] is

$$VC = 0.0404 \times H - 0.022 \times A - 2.35$$

where

$$H = \text{height, in centimeters}$$
$$A = \text{age, in years}$$

A VC less than 50 percent of predicted indicates severe respiratory impairment.[26]

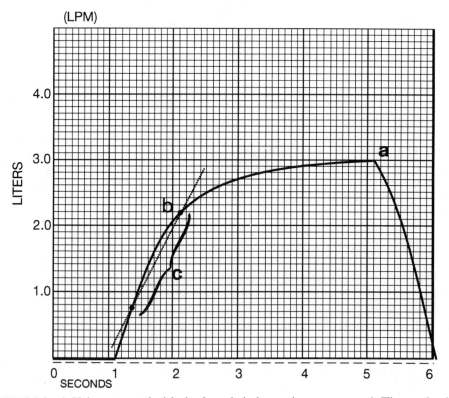

FIGURE 10-6. Values assessed with the forced vital capacity maneuver. *A*, The total volume of gas exhaled (FVC) is 3 liters. *B*, The volume of gas exhaled in the first second (FEV$_1$) is 2.2 liters. The volume of gas exhaled in the first second expressed as a percentage of the total volume exhaled (FEV$_1$/FVC) is 73%. *C*, The forced expiratory flow (FEF$_{25\%-75\%}$) is 1.66 liters per second.

MALES

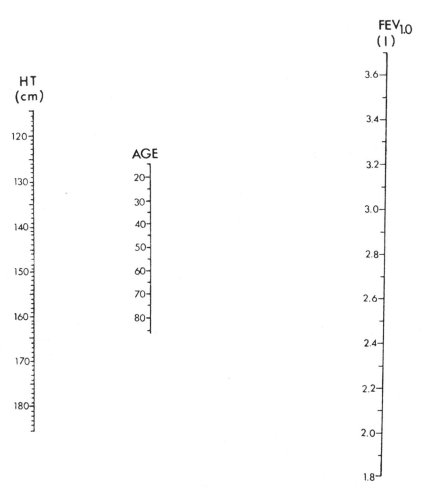

FIGURE 10−7. Nomogram for calculating FEV_1 in healthy nonsmoking males. (From Cherniack,[25] p. 245, with permission.)

FORCED EXPIRATORY VOLUME IN 1 SECOND

FEV_1 is the volume of gas expired during the first second of an FVC maneuver (Fig. 10−6). The FEV_1 is reported in liters per second, and it varies directly with height and indirectly with age. Because FEV_1 measures the volume of gas expired over time, it is a measurement of flow. Airway obstruction lengthens the exhalation time of a VC maneuver. By evaluating flow rates, the severity of airway obstruction can be determined. An individual whose FEV_1 is less than 40 percent of predicted is considered to have severe respiratory impairment.[26] Normative values for flow rates are shown in Figures 10−7 and 10−8.

Expressing FEV_1 as a percent of FVC (calculated by $FEV_1/FVC \times 100$, but commonly written FEV_1/FVC) corrects for variations in height, age, sex, and alterations in VCs.[27] FEV_1 as it relates to FVC then becomes a more reliable predictor of airway

FEMALES

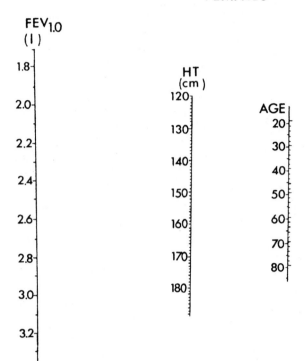

FIGURE 10–8. Nomogram for calculating FEV_1 in healthy nonsmoking females. (From Cherniack,[25] p. 246, with permission.)

obstruction. For example, compare the results of pulmonary function tests in a healthy 50-year-old man whose height is 180 cm (6 ft). His FVC is predicted to be 4.8 liters, and his FEV_1 is 4.1 liters per second. Normative values for a 160-cm (5 ft, 4 in), 60-year-old woman are predicted to be FVC of 2.79 liters and FEV_1 of 2.40 liters per second. Although the two individuals have very different FVC values (4.8 and 2.79 liters) and FEV_1 values (4.1 and 2.4 liters per second, respectively), they are quite similar in the FEV_1/FVC percents (84 and 86 percent). FEV_1/FVC is normally found to be greater than 75 percent.[22] An FEV_1/FVC of less than 40 percent indicates a severe respiratory impairment.[28]

MAXIMUM VOLUNTARY VENTILATION AND MAXIMUM MINUTE EXPIRED VOLUME

The maximum voluntary ventilation (MVV) is the maximum amount of air that can be moved in 1 minute. It is measured as follows: The patient is asked to breathe as hard and as fast as possible for 15 seconds. The volume is recorded and multiplied by 4 to convert the findings to liters per minute. The maximum voluntary ventilation can also be predicted by multiplying the FEV_1 by 35.[27] Since the former method is so dependent on effort for an extended period of time, the latter method may be preferred. The MVV is a definition of the ventilatory limit of the pulmonary system and is useful in conjunction with exercise testing.

The minute expired volume ($\dot{V}E$) is the amount of air expired per minute. $\dot{V}Emax$ is the amount of air expired per minute at peak exercise. During an exercise test, healthy subjects will not achieve their ventilatory limits, even when exercising at or near their maximum heart rate. The MVV in a healthy person may be 25 percent or more higher than $\dot{V}E$ at maximal exercise.[29] In contrast, a patient whose pulmonary system is the limiting factor to exercise will usually achieve nearly 100 percent of his or her ventilatory maximum before ever reaching the predicted maximum heart rate.[29] The pulmonary system then becomes the limiting factor in exercise.

FORCED EXPIRATORY FLOW

The $FEF_{25\%-75\%}$ reflects the amount of time required to exhale the middle half of a forced VC maneuver. The volume attained during a forced VC maneuver is divided into quarters. The first and last quarter are ignored, and the middle two quarters (half) of the volume is determined. That volume is then divided by the time it took to exhale it.[25] $FEF_{25\%-75\%}$ is recorded in liters per second. The test is sometimes called the maximum midexpiratory flow rate (MMEFR). Obstructive lung disease may be discovered in its early stages by the use of this test.[30] $FEF_{25\%-75\%}$ normally decreases with age.

DIFFUSION CAPACITY OF THE LUNGS FOR CARBON MONOXIDE

The DLCO is an analysis of the ability to transfer an inhaled gas from the pulmonary alveoli to the pulmonary capillary, and it is measured during a single held breath.[31] The subject is first asked to empty the lungs of all possible air, inhale as deeply as possible a combination of carbon monoxide and helium, and hold that breath for 10 seconds. Finally, the gas is fully exhaled and analyzed for carbon monoxide content. The amount of carbon monoxide that crossed the alveolar capillary membrane is then determined. The normal diffusing capacity is approximately 25 milliliters per minute per mm Hg.[22]

Although the DLCO test cannot be performed by simple spirometry, it is useful as a predictor of a subject's ability to oxygenate blood during exercise. Patients whose DLCO is greater than 55 percent of the normative value can be predicted to maintain their oxygenation during exercise.[32] Patients with chronic obstructive pulmonary disease (COPD) who are most likely to become hypoxic during exercise have DLCO values less than 55 percent of predicted.[32] A patient with other problems may have a different DLCO limit than one with COPD. Studying younger patients with cystic fibrosis, Lebecque et al.[33] showed that DLCO greater than 80 percent was predictive that a patient could maintain his or her oxygenation during exercise, whereas a patient with a DLCO less than 65 percent of predicted was likely to desaturate. The criterion for severe impairment is a DLCO less than 40 percent of predicted.[26,34]

EXERCISE TESTING IN PATIENTS WITH PULMONARY DISEASE

The evaluation of functional capacity is part of the assessment of a patient with pulmonary disease. A graded exercise test (GXT) can provide the objective information to document a patient's symptomatology and physical impairment. It can also provide the information necessary to prescribe safe exercise for the successful management of patients in a pulmonary rehabilitation program. Other uses of an exercise test are to document oxygen desaturation during exercise and to evaluate the need for supplemental oxygen.

Physiologic Testing Parameters

PULMONARY FUNCTION TESTS

Prior to the exercise testing session, pulmonary function tests previously mentioned in this chapter should be performed. The results of FEV_1 will help decide the appropriate protocol to use for the GXT. Maximum voluntary ventilation should be determined prior to the exercise test, because it is one of the criteria for test termination ($\dot{V}Emax = MVV$). The D_{LCO} can help predict patients who may not oxygenate their blood adequately during exercise. After exercise, especially in suspected asthmatic patients, the PFTs are again administered to assess the effects of exercise on lung function. A reduction of 10 percent in either FEV_1 or $FEF_{25\%-75\%}$ is an indication of need for bronchodilator therapy.[35]

ARTERIAL BLOOD GAS ANALYSIS AND OXYGEN SATURATION

An ABG analysis, performed either at rest or during exercise, provides the best method for determining arterial oxygenation and the adequacy of alveolar ventilation. Table 10–1 shows normal values obtained by an arterial blood gas sample. The recording of the partial pressure of oxygen (Pao_2) can detect hypoxemia, a decrease of PAO_2 in the blood. Hypercapnia, an increase in the partial pressure of carbon dioxide ($Paco_2$), indicates an abnormality in alveolar ventilation.

At rest, variations in arterial blood gas values can occur acutely, as during an acute pulmonary illness, or chronically, when they reflect ventilatory impairment. When analyzed during exercise, the ABG measurement provides information regarding the need for supplemental oxygen as well as information regarding anaerobic threshold and the ventilatory reserve.[36]

During exercise, arterial blood gas samples are drawn and analyzed from a catheter (which has been previously placed in the radial artery) every 1 to 1½ minutes. Although this is an invasive testing procedure, actual blood gas measurements are superior to measurements made by using noninvasive procedures, which provide estimates of the partial pressures of gases in the blood.

An estimate of Pao_2 can be made by using pulse oximetry, which measures the degree of saturation of hemoglobin with oxygen (Sao_2). Although there is not a perfect

TABLE 10–1 Normal Values for Arterial Blood Gas Sampling with the Subject Breathing Room Air

FIO_2	0.21
Pao_2	95–100 mm Hg
$Paco_2$	35–45 mm Hg
pH	7.35–7.45
HCO_3^-	24 mEq/m

FIO_2 = fraction of inspired oxygen, Pao_2 = partial pressure of oxygen, $Paco_2$ = partial pressure of carbon dioxide, HCO_3^- = bicarbonate ion.

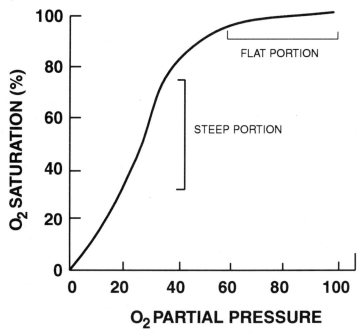

FIGURE 10–9. Oxyhemoglobin dissociation curve.

correlation between Sao_2 and Pao_2, according to the oxyhemoglobin dissociation curve, some correlation between the two values does exist. Changes in Sao_2 correlate closely with the changes in Pao_2 on the flat portions of the oxyhemoglobin desaturation curve, but when the Sao_2 falls to the steep slope of the curve, a small decrease in Sao_2 will produce a significant drop in Pao_2[37] (Fig. 10–9).

Anyone evaluating arterial oxygen saturation to predict Pao_2 must appreciate the limits in accuracy of oximeters. Confidence limits for measurement of arterial oxygen saturation by cutaneous oximetry is ± 4 to 5 percent.[35] Oximetry, unlike ABG testing, does not provide information about alveolar ventilation ($Paco_2$). On the other hand, oximetry is noninvasive and does provide a continuous stream of data. Those features may be valuable in some clinical situations.

Measuring exhaled volumes of gas for carbon dioxide (CO_2) content can predict $Paco_2$. However, the CO_2 levels of the expired air do not necessarily correspond accurately to the alveolar concentration of CO_2 or to the partial pressure of CO_2 in the blood. For those reasons, the risks involved with an invasive arterial line are thought to be worth the valuable information it provides.

THE EXERCISE ELECTROCARDIOGRAM

The ECG gives a recording of the electrical activity of the cardiac conduction system. Electrocardiography is used to detect cardiac arrhythmias, conduction abnormalities, and cardiac ischemia. Prior to exercise, patients are prepared for 12-lead exercise ECG tracings. Electrode sites, methods for checking poor tracings, and suggestions for recordings and interpretations are given in Chapters 8 and 9.

BLOOD PRESSURE

During the GXT, blood pressure measurements must be recorded frequently. Measurements should be recorded in supine, sitting, and standing positions at rest, at 2-minute intervals during exercise, and during recovery from the test. During the exercise test, systolic blood pressure should rise with increasing work loads, and the diastolic pressure should remain about the same. The highest systolic blood pressure should be achieved at the maximal work load, but the test should be terminated if and when the systolic pressure is 250 mm Hg and/or the diastolic pressure is 110 mm Hg or greater. The test should also be terminated if the systolic blood pressure falls more than 10 mm Hg with increasing exercise loads.

$\dot{V}o_2$max MEASUREMENT

Measurements of $\dot{V}o_2$max (Chapter 4) are used to identify vocational and leisure activities that lie within or outside the bounds of a participant's ability. According to some estimates, a person can perform a job for up to 8 hours if the maximal work load of that job requires no more than 40 percent of the worker's $\dot{V}o_2$max.[38] Justification for return to work or for disability can be objectively judged by the use of $\dot{V}o_2$max. If $\dot{V}o_2$max is below 15 milliliters per kilogram per minute or fewer than 5 METs (Chapter 9), the participant is considered to have a moderately impaired respiratory system[39] and to be physically impaired for practically all types of employment.[26]

Formulas are available to predict a participant's $\dot{V}o_2$max by using the amount of work accomplished on a specific exercise protocol (Chapter 9). Actual $\dot{V}o_2$max determinations necessitate the use of headgear with a mouthpiece and a nose clip to collect the gas samples necessary to make the actual $\dot{V}o_2$max determination. Although the actual $\dot{V}o_2$max is a valuable measurement, the anxiety produced by the equipment may be so objectionable to some pulmonary patients that a less than maximal test will result and therefore an inaccurate $\dot{V}o_2$max will be obtained. Decisions about the need for actual $\dot{V}o_2$max values versus predicted values should be made on an individual basis.

Exercise-Testing Protocols

Exercise testing of the pulmonary patient is not usually diagnostic; it is used to document the amount of impairment that is due to an existing diagnosis. The purposes of an exercise test are to establish a pulmonary patient's functional capacity, evaluate the need for oxygen therapy during exercise, and prescribe appropriate exercise intensity.

A graded (gradually increasing intensity) exercise test should stress the pulmonary patient to the point of limitation while vital signs are monitored to ensure safety. A number of testing procedures are available to assess the functional abilities of patients with pulmonary disease. Protocols and equipment requirements for measuring functional ability range from the very simple 12-minute walk test (which requires only the ability to measure heart rate, blood pressure, time, and distance) to more sophisticated treadmill and cycle protocols. The treadmill and cycle protocols may include any of the following measurements: $\dot{V}o_2$max, heart rate, electrocardiogram, blood pressure, respiratory rate, Pao_2, $Paco_2$, pH, Sao_2, A-ao_2 difference, A-Vo_2 difference, respiratory quotient (R), dead space volume (V_{DS}), and dead space to tidal volume ratio (V_{DS}/V_T).[40]

TABLE 10–2 Protocols Used for Exercise-Testing the Patient
with Pulmonary Disease

Mode	Author	Protocol
Walk test	Cooper[41]	Ambulate as far as possible in 12 min
	Guyatt et al.[43]	Ambulate as far as possible in 6 min
Cycle test	Jones[46]	Begin with 100 kpm (17 W), increase 100 kpm every min
	Jones and Campbell[47]	Begin with 25 W, 15-W increase every min
	Berman and Sutton[48]	Begin with 100 kpm/min, increase 100 kpm/min every min or 50 kpm/min every min when FEV_1 less than 1 liter/s
	Mass. Respiratory Hospital[49]	Begin at 25 W, increase 10 W every 20 sec or 5 W every 20 sec when FEV_1 less than 1 liter/s
Treadmill tests	Naughton et al.[51]	2 mph constant 0 grade 3.5% grade every 3 min
	Balke and Ware[52]	3.3 mph constant 0 grade 3.5% grade every 2 min
	Mass. Respiratory Hosptial[49]	1.5 mph constant 0 grade 4% grade every 2 min 2% grade every 2 min if FEV_1 is less than 1 liter/s

Testing protocols vary with the preference and training of the examiners, availability of equipment, and the abilities of the patient population. See Table 10–2 for examples of protocols used in exercise-testing patients with pulmonary disease.

THE 12-MINUTE WALK

The 12-minute walk is a simple way to assess functional ability: The subject is asked to cover as much distance as possible in 12 minutes.[41] Since functional ability increases with training, the distance walked in 12 minutes also should increase. Performance of a 12-minute walk has been shown to be positively correlated with FVC and $\dot{V}o_2max$ as determined by cycle ergometry and treadmill tests.[41,42] When used for pre-testing and post-testing, the 12-minute walk becomes an easy, inexpensive, and objective measurement of changes in ability. For pulmonary patients, the 12-minute walk may be modified to 6 minutes or sometimes 2 minutes.[43,44]

CYCLE ERGOMETER

Cycle ergometer protocols have advantages for patients who lack agility, coordination, and/or balance. Since the person is seated, the test performed can be safer. Blood pressure measurements, arterial blood gas samples, and ECG tracings are easier to obtain during a cycle ergometer test because of the stability of the upper body during exercise. One major disadvantage of using a cycle ergometer protocol is that leg fatigue often causes a test termination prior to the patient achieving maximal capability.[45]

There are a variety of testing protocols for cycle ergometers. Jones[46] uses a progression of 17 W every minute (speed is constant at 50 rpm). Another protocol suggested by Jones and Campbell begins with a workload of 25 W and increases by increments of 15 W every minute.[47]

According to the ability of each patient, an individualized protocol can be chosen for the exercise test session. Berman and Sutton[48] use increments of 100 kpm every minute with their patients whose FEV_1 was greater than 1 liter per second. If the FEV_1 is found to be less than 1 liter per second, the increments are lowered to 50 kpm per minute.

Some cycle protocols do not achieve steady states; instead, they use a more "ramped" increase in work load. With pedal speed kept constant, the work load is increased every 20 seconds. Again, these decisions should be based on the ability of each patient. For example, if a patient has an FEV_1 of less than 1 liter per second, he or she might be placed on a protocol that increases the work load 5 W every 20 seconds. If the FEV_1 is greater than 1 liter per second, then the work load can be increased 10 W every 20 seconds.[49] (See Chapter 9 for additional ergometry tests.)

TREADMILL TESTING

Treadmill tests provide a more accurate functional assessment of the patient with pulmonary disease than does a cycle ergometer test. The number of protocols available for treadmill testing allow accommodation to a number of individual abilities. For example, a patient who may have difficulty walking faster than 2 mph will perform best when following the Naughton protocol.[50,51] A patient who may be able to walk faster than 2 mph may be evaluated by the Balke test protocol.[50,52] A Bruce protocol is rarely indicated in exercise testing of pulmonary patients because the test is best suited for healthier patients capable of higher work loads.[53,54] Some patients cannot maintain speeds of 2 mph and require adaptations in protocols; treadmill speeds can be designed to run at 1.5 mph or less to accommodate that population.[49,54] One difficulty with a lower test speed is that not all treadmills can run below speeds of 2 mph. (Additional treadmill protocols can be found in Chapter 9.)

Test and Exercise Termination

The symptom-limited end point of an exercise test for pulmonary patients may be quite different from that already described for cardiac patients (Chapter 9). Criteria for stopping a pulmonary exercise test may include but not be limited to the following:[26,29,40]

1. Maximal shortness of breath
2. A fall in Pa_{O_2} of more than 20 mm Hg or a Pa_{O_2} less than 55 mm Hg
3. A rise in Pa_{CO_2} of more than 10 mm Hg or a Pa_{CO_2} greater than 65 mm Hg
4. Cardiac ischemia or arrhythmias
5. Symptoms of fatigue
6. Increase in diastolic blood pressure readings of 20 mm Hg, systolic hypertension greater than 250 mm Hg, decrease in blood pressure with increasing work loads
7. Leg pain
8. Total fatigue
9. Signs of insufficient cardiac output
10. Reaching a ventilatory maximum

Interpretation of Graded Exercise Test Results

By assessing functional abilities, an appropriate vocational assessment can be completed and documentation necessary for addressing disability is provided.[38]

The need for supplemental oxygen is identified if a patient becomes hypoxic during the exercise test session. A decrease in Pao_2 of more than 20 mm Hg or a Pao_2 less than 55 mm Hg are indications for oxygen supplementation.[55] Guidelines for supplemental oxygen prescription include a high flow rate with an Fio_2 of 24 to 27 percent.

For prescribing an exercise program based on the GXT, see Chapter 11. For emergency procedures, see Chapter 9.

PULMONARY TESTING CASE STUDIES

CASE STUDY 1

The patient is a 61-year-old woman with a diagnosis of COPD, asthma, and orthostatic hypotension. She is status postmastectomy. Medications are Tamoxatrin, imipramine, Ventolin MDI, Atrovent MDI, Ativan, and Slo-phyllin. Table 10-3 summarizes her exercise test.

CASE STUDY 2

The patient is a 77-year-old man with a diagnosis of COPD, asthma, chronic bronchitis, hypertension, and peptic ulcer disease. Medications are Beclovent MDI, Atrovent MDI, Robitussin, and Maxair MDI. Table 10-4 summarizes his exercise test.

CASE STUDY 3

The patient is a 69-year-old man with a diagnosis of COPD, pneumoconiosis (formerly a foundry worker—possible silicosis), HTN, CAD, MI (LVEF 43 percent), ulcers, L CVA, PVD, and gout. Medications are Lasix, ASA, diltiazem, Alipurinol, digoxin, Lanoxin, and NTG. Table 10-5 summarizes his exercise test.

CASE STUDY 4

The patient is a 73-year-old man with a diagnosis of COPD and glaucoma. Medications are Max Air MDI, Beclovent MDI, Atrovent MDI, prednisone, Dilantin, aminophylline, and Pilocar drops. Table 10-6 summarizes his exercise test.

TABLE 10–3 Raw Data—Case Study 1

Age: 61   Sex: F   AAMHR: 159   Ht: 162.6 cm   Wt: 56.4 kg
Smoking: 45 pack-years; quit 8 years ago
Occupation: Clerk, part-time
Resting ECG, Normal; Resting HR, 108; Resting BP, 130/70; Resting RR, 16
Resting PFTs: FVC, 1.77 liter (57%); FEV_1 0.68 liter/s (28%); FEV_1/FVC, 38%
Protocol: Modified cycle

Time	Work Load (W)	HR (bpm)	BP (mm Hg)	RR (br/min)	V_E (liter/min)	Vo_2 (liter/min)	METs	ABG Pao_2/$Paco_2$/pH
Rest	00.0	108	130/70	16	12.3	0.37	1.0	55/38/7.44
1:01	25.0	118		18.8	16.1	0.51	1.9	
2:01	40.0	120	136/82	19.1	16.8	0.55	2.6	41/44/7.36
2:14	45.0	123		23.4			2.8	

Reason for test termination: Leg fatigue

Exercise ECG: Normal

Max Values	Actual	Predicted	Percent of Predicted
HR	123	159	78
V_E	17.8	23.1	75
Vo_2	0.6	1.3	44

Postexercise PFTs: FVC, 1.55 L (50%); FEV_1, 0.60, liter/s (25%); FEV_1/FVC, 39%

Comments: There was a significant bronchospastic response after exercise. Also there was decrease in oxygenation with exercise.
Interpretation: Submaximal exercise test. Moderately severe ventilatory (pre- and post-PFTs) and diffusion (ABGs) limitations.

TABLE 10–4 Raw Data — Case Study 2

Age: 77   Sex: M   AAMHR: 143   Ht: 169 cm   Wt: 82.3 kg
Smoking: 75 pack-years, quit 2 years ago
Occupation: Retired
Resting ECG, Normal; Resting HR, 61; Resting BP, 128/82; Resting RR, 18.6
Resting PFTs: FVC, 2.76 liter (72%); FEV_1, 1.55 liter/s (53%); FEV_1/FVC, 56%
Protocol: Modified cycle

Time	Work Load (Ws)	HR (bpm)	BP (mm Hg)	RR (br/min)	V_E (liter/min)	Vo_2 (liter/min)	METs	ABG Pao_2/$Paco_2$/pH	Sao_2 %
Rest	00.0	61	128/82	18.6	8.9		1.0	71/34/7.40	94
1:00	25.0	74		19.0	13.8	0.49	1.7		92
2:03	55.0	84	170/86	21.3	20.4	0.83	2.9		90
3:01	85.0	94		21.7	25.4	0.98	3.4		90
4:00	115	111		25.5	32.3	1.20	4.2		87
4:30		123		29.7	39.3	1.31	4.5	57/45/7.33	87

Reason for test termination: Dyspnea

Exercise ECG: Normal

	Max Values		
	Actual	Predicted	Percent of Predicted
HR	123	146	87
V_E	44.2	54.3	81
Vo_2	1.3	1.6	80

Postexercise PFTs: FVC, 2.69 liter (70%); FEV_1, 1.70 liter/s (58%); FEV_1/FVC, 63%

Comments: There was a 10% improvement in FEV_1 postexercise. Oxygenation decreased during exercise, Sao_2 dropped to 87%.
Interpretation: Maximal test with moderately severe obstructive lung disease. Results indicate moderate ventilatory mechanical limitation with diffusion abnormality. No significant changes in ECG with exercise. Patient stopped exercise test because of pulmonary limitations.

TABLE 10–5 Raw Data — Case Study 3

Age: 69   Sex: M   AAMHR: 151   Ht: 181 cm   Wt: 66.8 kg
Smoking: 70 pack-years, quit 11 years ago
Occupation: Retired; former foundry worker
Resting ECG: 2–3mm ST depression; RHR, 84; RBP, 140/76; RRR, 13.1 br/min
Resting PFTs: FVC, 3.88 liter (82%); FEV$_1$, 1.61 liter/s; (44%); FEV$_1$/FVC, 41%
Protocol: Treadmill

Time	Work Load	HR (bpm)	BP (mm Hg)	RR (br/min)	V$_E$ (liter/min)	Vo$_2$ (liter/min)	METs	ABG Pao$_2$/Paco$_2$/pH	Sao$_2$ %
Rest		84	140/76	13.1	12.8		1.0	72/29/7.39	96
1:01	1.5 mph 0% grade	90		16.7	21.0	0.52	2.2		92
2:02		90		20.0	25.4	0.63	2.7		90
2:45		96		23.4	30.8	0.73	3.1		87
3:17	1.5 mph 0% grade	89	190/84	22.8	31.0	0.70	3.0	57/45/7.33	87

Reasons for test termination: Dyspnea and fatigue

Exercise ECG: No significant changes with exercise

	Max Values Actual	Predicted	Percent of Predicted
HR	96.0	152	63
V$_E$	36.9	56.4	66
Vo$_2$	0.8	1.9	40

Postexercise PFTs: FVC, 3.99 liter (84%); FEV$_1$, 1.59 liter/s (44%); FEV$_1$/FVC, 40%

Comments: Spirometry at rest showed moderately severe obstructive lung disease. There was no significant change postexercise.
Interpretation: Submaximal exercise test without reaching anaerobic threshold. Moderately severe gas exchange abnormality with diffusion-type limitations. Decrease in exercise heart rate at highest work load, indicating cardiac limitation or deconditioning. Suggest pulse oximetry on activity.

TABLE 10–6 Raw Data—Case Study 4

Age: 75   Sex: M   AAMHR: 145   Ht: 178 cm   Wt: 69.0 kg
Smoking: 50 pack-years, quit 3 years ago
Occupation: Retired, former truck driver
Resting ECG: PVCs, couplets twice; RHR, 93; RBP, 138/80; RRR, 22.5 br/min
Resting PFTs: FVC, 3.13 liter (71%); FEV_1, 1.41 liter/s (34%); FEV_1/FVC, 36%
Protocol: Treadmill

Time	Work Load	HR (bpm)	BP (mm Hg)	RR (br/min)	V_E (liter/min)	Vo_2 (liter/min)	METs	ABG $Pao_2/Paco_2/pH$
Rest		93	138/80	22.5	19.5		1.0	63/43/7.40
1:03	1.5 mph 0% grade	96		22.1	20.3	0.47	2.0	
2:01	1.5 mph 0% grade	98		19.7	22.0	0.61	2.5	52/45/7.40
3:01	1.5 mph 4% grade	114		23.2	24.6	0.68	2.8	44/47/7.38
4:01	1.5 mph 4% grade	113	190/84	26.4	28.5	0.78	3.2	42/50/7.36

Reason for test termination: Mouth and nose discomfort from mouthpiece and nose clip, some shortness of breath

Exercise ECG: Few PVCs seen; nonspecific ST-T-segment changes

	Max Values		
	Actual	Predicted	Percent of Predicted
HR	114.0	148	72
V_E	29.2	39.9	73
Vo_2	0.8	1.7	47

Postexercise PFTs: FVC, 3.35 liter (76%); FEV_1, 1.21 liter/s (36%); FEV_1/FVC, 36%

Comments: Spirometry at rest showed severe degree of airflow obstruction. Significant drop in Pao_2 during exercise, $Paco_2$ rose 7 mm Hg.
Interpretation: Submaximal exercise test because of pulmonary limitations and discomfort. Anaerobic threshold not reached. Heart rate reserve normal. Breathing reserve poor. Need for oxygen with exercise.

SUMMARY

Assessment of the pulmonary patient is a continuous process. A thorough assessment allows for the appropriate treatment program to be conceived, administered in a safe and effective manner, and altered, either progressed or regressed, according to the patient's needs. The value of the ongoing nature of pulmonary assessment is discussed.

Pulmonary assessment includes the interview, the physical examination, and the laboratory tests. Each area of assessment provides information that the clinician can use to tailor the treatment program to best suit the patient. It is of little benefit to develop a treatment program to which the patient either cannot or will not adhere.

The pulmonary assessment interview includes the chief complaint, that is, the patient's reason for seeking medical intervention, as well as medical, occupational, social, and family histories.

Physical examination includes observation of the patient's posture, breathing pattern (rate, rhythm, and use of accessory musculature), skin color and appearance of the distal extremities, and thoracic configuration. Palpation gives insight into symmetry and excursion of the thorax during the respiratory cycle. Auscultation allows the clinician to listen to the air movement within the thorax. Abnormal breath sounds (diminished or bronchial breath sounds) and adventitious sounds (crackles and wheezes) will, if heard, alert the clinician to the site of the abnormality.

Laboratory tests, including pulmonary function tests, chest roentgenograms, and arterial blood gas analyses, are used to diagnose pulmonary disease and to monitor the progress of the disease process. An exercise tolerance test, although not usually performed as a diagnostic test, is used to determine exercise prescription, document symptoms and functional capacity, assess the need for supplemental oxygen, and justify job-related abilities or disabilities. Case studies illustrating exercise testing and termination criteria have been included.

REFERENCES

1. Payton, O, Nelson, C and Ozer, M: Patient Participation in Program Planning. FA Davis, Philadelphia, 1990.
2. Hobson, L and Hammon, W: Chest assessment. In Frownfelter, D. (ed) Chest Physical Therapy and Pulmonary Rehabilitation, ed 2. Year Book Medical Publishers, Chicago, 1987, pp 150–151.
3. Surveillance for respiratory hazards in the occupational setting: The official ATS statement. Am Rev Respir Dis 126:952–956, 1982.
4. Luce, J: Lung Diseases of Adults. American Lung Association. 1986.
5. Cohen-Cole, S: The Medical Interview: The Three Function Approach. Year Book Medical Publishers, Chicago, 1991.
6. Purtilo, R: Health Professional/Patient Interaction, ed 3. WB Saunders, Philadelphia, 1984.
7. Ciccone, C: Pharmacology in Rehabilitation. FA Davis, Philadelphia, 1990.
8. Fielding, J: Smoking effects and control, part I. N Engl J Med 313(8):491–498, 1985.
9. Burki, N: Pulmonary Diseases. Medical Examination Publishing, New York, 1982.
10. Farzan, S: A Concise Handbook of Respiratory Diseases, ed 2. Reston Publishing, Reston, VA, 1985.
11. Zadai, C: Pulmonary pharmacology. In T Malone (ed): Physical and Occupational Therapy: Drug Implications for Practice. JB Lippincott, Philadelphia, 1989, pp 97–119.
12. Price, S and Wilson L: Pathophysiology: Clinical Concepts of Disease Processes, ed 2. McGraw-Hill, New York, 1982.
13. Gaskell, D and Webber, B: The Brompton Hospital Guide to Chest Physiotherapy, ed 2. Blackwell Scientific Publications, Oxford, 1973.
14. Bell, C., et al: Home Care and Rehabilitation in Respiratory Medicine. JB Lippincott, Philadelphia, 1984.
15. Goss, C (ed): Gray's Anatomy, ed 29. Lea & Febiger, Philadelphia, 1973.
16. Traver, G: Assessment of the Thorax and Lungs. Am J Nurs 73(3):466–471, 1973.
17. Murphy, R: Auscultation of the lung: Past lessons, future possibilities. Thorax 36:99–107, 1981.

18. Pulmonary terms and symbols: A report of the ACCP-ATS Joint Committee on Pulmonary Nomenclature. Chest 67:583–593, 1975.
19. Forgacs, P: Crackles and wheezes. Lancet 2:203–205, 1967.
20. Ploysongsang, Y and Schonfeld, S: Mechanism of the production of crackles after atelectasis during low volume breathing. Am Rev Respir Dis 126:413–415, 1982.
21. Loudon, R: The lung speaks out. Am Rev Respir Dis 126:411–412, 1982.
22. Harper, R: A Guide to Respiratory Care: Physiology and Clinical Applications. JB Lippincott, Philadelphia, 1981.
23. Hodgkin, J and Petty, T: Chronic Obstructive Pulmonary Disease: Current Concepts. WB Saunders, Philadelphia, 1987.
24. Downie, P (ed): Cash's Textbook of Chest, Heart and Vascular Disorders for Physiotherapists, ed 4. JB Lippincott, Philadelphia, 1987.
25. Cherniack, R: Pulmonary Function Testing. WB Saunders, Philadelphia, 1977.
26. American Thoracic Society: Evaluation of impairment secondary to respiratory disease. Am Rev Respir Dis 126:945–951, 1982.
27. Ruppel, G: Manual of Pulmonary Function Testing, ed 2. CV Mosby, St Louis, 1979.
28. Report of Snowbird Workshop on standardization of spirometry. Am Rev Respir Dis 119:831–838, 1979.
29. Weber, K and Janicki, J: Cardiopulmonary Exercise Testing. WB Saunders, Philadelphia, 1986.
30. Guenter, C and Welch, M: Pulmonary Medicine, ed 2. JP Lippincott, Philadelphia, 1982.
31. Jones, R and Mead, F: A theoretical and experimental analysis of anomalies in the estimation of pulmonary diffusing capacity by single breath holding method. Q J Exp Physiol 46:131–143, 1961.
32. Owens, G, et al: The diffusing capacity as a predictor of arterial oxygen desaturation during exercise in patients with chronic obstructive pulmonary disease. N Engl J Med 310:1218–1221, 1984.
33. Lebecque, P, et al: Diffusion capacity and oxygen desaturation effects on exercise in patients with cystic fibrosis. Chest 91:693–697, 1987.
34. Epler, G, Saber, F and Guensler, E: Determination of severe impairment (disability) in interstitial lung disease. Am Rev Respir Dis 121:647–659, 1980.
35. O'Ryan, J and Burns, D: Pulmonary Rehabilitation from Hospital to Home. Year Book Medical Publishers, Chicago, 1984.
36. Reis, A: Position paper of the American Association of Cardiovascular and Pulmonary Rehabilitation. Scientific basis for pulmonary rehabilitation. J Cardiopulmonary Rehabil 10:418–441, 1990.
37. Guyton, A: Textbook of Medical Physiology, ed 7. WB Saunders, Philadelphia, 1986.
38. Hodgkins, J, Zorn, E and Connors, G: Pulmonary Rehabilitation. Guidelines to Success. Butterworth Publishers, Boston, 1984.
39. Ostiguy, G: Summary of task force report on occupational respiratory diseases. Can Med Assoc J 121:414–421, 1979.
40. Zadai, C: Rehabilitation of the patient with chronic obstructive pulmonary disease. In Irwin, S and Tecklin, J (eds): Cardiopulmonary Physical Therapy. CV Mosby, St. Louis, 1985.
41. Cooper, K: A means of assessing maximal oxygen intake: Correlation between field and treadmill walking. JAMA 203:201–204, 1968.
42. McGavin, C, Gupta, S and McHardy, G: Twelve minute walking test for assessing disability in chronic bronchitis. BMJ 1:822, 1976.
43. Guyatt, G, Berman, L and Townsend, M: Long-term outcome after respiratory rehabilitation. Can Med Assoc J 137:1089–1095, 1987.
44. Butland, R, et al: Two, six and twelve minute walking tests in respiratory disease. Br Med J 284:1007–1008, 1982.
45. American College of Sports Medicine: Guidelines for Exercise Testing and Prescription, ed 4. Lea & Febiger, Philadelphia, 1991.
46. Jones, N: Exercise testing in pulmonary evaluation: Rationale, methods and the normal respiratory response to exercise. N Engl J Med 293:541–544, 1975.
47. Carter, R, et al: Exercise gas exchange in patients with moderate severe to severe chronic obstructive pulmonary disease. Journal of Cardiopulmonary Rehabilitation 9(6):243–248, 1989.
48. Berman, L and Sutton, J: Exercise for the pulmonary patient. Journal of Cardiopulmonary Rehabilitation 6(2):55–59, 1986.
49. Massachusetts Respiratory Hospital, Exercise Testing Protocol, Braintree, MA.
50. Bell, C: Exercise Stress Testing and Physical Conditioning Program in Pulmonary Rehabilitation Medical Manual, University of Nebraska Medical Center, pp 50–91, 1977.
51. Naughton, J, Balke, B and Poarch, R: Modified work capacity studies in individuals with and without coronary artery disease. J Sports Med 4:208–212, 1964.
52. Balke, B and Ware, R: An experimental study of physical fitness of Air Force personnel. US Armed Forces Med J 10:675–688, 1959.
53. Bruce, R: Methods of exercise testing: Step test, bicycle, treadmill, and isometrics. Am J Cardiol 33:715–720, 1974.
54. Ellestad, M: Stress Testing: Principles and Practice, ed 3. FA Davis, Philadelphia, 1986.
55. Wilson, P, Bell, C and Norton, A: Rehabilitation of the Heart and Lungs. Beckman Instruments, Fullerton, CA, 1980.

CHAPTER 11

The Exercise Prescription

In recent years, exercise training has become widely recognized as an important component in developing rehabilitation strategies for patients with coronary artery disease (CAD).[1,2] Recently, programs have expanded to include patients with other types of coronary heart disease (CHD) such as those recovering from coronary artery bypass graft surgery (CABG), myocardial infarction (MI), valve replacement, pacemaker implantation, percutaneous transluminal coronary angioplasty (PTCA), cardiac transplantation, and individuals with evidence of cardiovascular disease such as angina pectoris or a positive exercise test with evidence of disease from results of coronary angiography.[3-5]

The primary goal of cardiac rehabilitation programs is to restore patients with various cardiac disorders to active and productive lifestyles within the limitations imposed by their diseases.[6] Additional goals include preventing the progression and/or promoting reversal of the underlying atherosclerotic process in patients with CHD or at high risk for CHD, reducing the risk of sudden death and reinfarction, and alleviating angina.[3,7]

Largely because of the success of cardiac rehabilitation in returning cardiac patients to a better quality of life, patients with chronic obstructive pulmonary disease (COPD) are being referred to rehabilitation programs in increasing numbers. Rehabilitation programs for patients with COPD provide a valuable adjunct to medical therapy in helping to control the symptoms of lung disease and to improve functional capacity so that patients may achieve the highest possible level of independent function. A primary goal of pulmonary rehabilitation is to attempt to reverse a patient's disability from the disease rather than reverse a progressive disease process.[8]

The major goals of cardiac and pulmonary (cardiopulmonary) rehabilitation programs are therefore quite similar in that their objectives are to restore patients with cardiopulmonary diseases to their optimal physiological, psychological, social, and vocational status.[7,8] Although there are some differences in exercise prescription for cardiac and pulmonary patients, the basic guidelines for each group remain so similar that the two will be presented in a broad, general manner directed toward "cardiopulmonary" rehabilitation with more specific discussions included as needed. The case studies presented in this chapter are, of course, specific to cardiac and pulmonary patients.

278

To write a comprehensive exercise prescription for a cardiopulmonary patient, the clinician must (1) demonstrate an understanding of the physiologic factors that are essential to the attainment of normal cardiopulmonary function and physical fitness, (2) identify through evaluative procedures the status of an individual with regard to those factors, and (3) recognize and skillfully apply the training principles associated with physiologic adaptation to improve the functional status of impaired patients and assist patients in maintaining normalized function once it has been attained. The clinician who prescribes exercise for cardiopulmonary patients must consider the patient's age, sex, clinical status, related medical problems, habitual physical activity, and musculoskeletal integrity. The information obtained from multistage symptom-limited exercise tolerance tests (Chapters 9 and 10) will be the most useful tool to establish guidelines for exercise training for patients with known or suspected cardiopulmonary disease. Identification and definition of the physiologic and clinical basis for the prescription of exercise in cardiopulmonary patients will be presented. The exercise prescription will vary with the individual's development or recurrence of disease, and, as conditions warrant, it will ensure safety during exercise participation.[4] Examples of exercise prescriptions using case histories from the preceding chapters have been included in this section. In that way, knowledge of training principles can be integrated with the information attained from the evaluation procedures (Chapters 9 and 10) and applied to the formulation of initial exercise prescriptions that establish scientifically based, personalized goals for some of the patients whose case histories have been presented. This method of presentation will illustrate the process of writing an exercise prescription in a clear, practical manner. The cardiopulmonary rehabilitation staff should view the development of exercise prescriptions as a science as well as an art. Exercise program personnel should be prepared to modify exercise prescriptions in accordance with the responses and adaptations displayed by individual patients.

The major factors essential to the attainment and maintenance of physical fitness have been identified. Through regular exercise (training), they have been found to improve cardiorespiratory endurance, body composition, muscular strength and endurance, and flexibility (range of joint motion). The development of each factor requires a different training technique. To be effective, training methods designed to improve muscular strength must differ from those employed to improve flexibility. This requirement of variance in training methods illustrates the principle of "specificity of training."[9-11] Although training is specific and training programs differ, inherent in each well-designed program are principles relating to the type, intensity, duration, and frequency of exercise performed. All those factors are essential to the exercise prescription. The highest priority, however, must be placed on the development of cardiorespiratory endurance, which appears to be most beneficial in the prevention and progression of CHD,[11-13] and in improvement in exercise tolerance and endurance time.[8] The discussion of principles of exercise prescription that follows is included to illustrate the role each factor plays in cardiopulmonary exercise therapy. A comprehensive exercise prescription includes recommendations for the enhancement of all fitness factors, with emphasis on cardiorespiratory endurance training.

RISK STRATIFICATION

A recent addition to the rehabilitative process for the CHD patient initiated either during phase I or within a few weeks following hospital discharge is risk

TABLE 11-1 Guidelines for Risk Stratification of Cardiac Patients

Risk Level	Characteristics
Low-risk patients	Uncomplicated clinical course in hospital[18]
	No evidence of myocardial ischemia[14,15,18-20]
	Functional capacity ≥7 METs on 3-week exercise test[18]
	Normal left ventricular function (EF >50%)[14,15,18]
	Absence of significant ventricular ectopy[21]
Intermediate-risk patients (moderate)	ST-segment depression ≥2 mm flat or downsloping[14,15,18,19,22]
	Reversible thallium defects[15,23]
	Moderate to good left ventricular function (EF 35%-49%)[14]
	Changing pattern or new development of angina pectoris[17]
	Inability to self-monitor heart rate[16]
	Failure to comply with exercise prescription[16]
High-risk patients	Prior myocardial infarction or infarct involving ≥35% of left ventricle[14,15,20,22-24]
	EF <35% at rest[18]
	Fall in exercise systolic blood pressure or failure of systolic blood pressure to rise more than 10 mm Hg on exercise tolerance test[18,22,25]
	Persistent or recurrent ischemic pain 24 hours or more after hospital admission[18,22]
	Functional capacity <5 METs[19,23] with hypotensive blood pressure response or ≥1 mm ST-segment depression[20]
	Congestive heart failure syndrome in hospital[14,15,18]
	≥2-mm ST-segment depression at peak heart rate ≤135 bpm[14,18]
	Resting complex ventricular dysrhythmias (Low-grade IV or V)[16,21]

Note: From *Guidelines for Cardiac Rehabilitation Programs* (p. 5) by American Association of Cardiovascular and Pulmonary Rehabilitation, 1991, Champaign, IL: Human Kinetics, Copyright 1991 by American Association of Cardiovascular and Pulmonary Rehabilitation. Reprinted by permission.

stratification.[3,4,14-17] The levels of risk are outlined in Table 11-1. An assessment of the clinical course, the extent of myocardial damage, left ventricular function, and presence or absence of residual myocardia ischemia, ventricular arrhythmias, and other test results are used as guidelines for risk stratification.[3,25] A careful evaluation of those factors is needed to appropriately assess the patient's prognosis for reinfarction, cardiac arrest, or heart failure and determine his or her functional capacity.[4] The type, intensity, duration of medical supervision, and frequency of continuous electrocardiographic (ECG) monitoring should be guided by the level of risk, be it low, moderate, or high, in which the patient has been stratified.

After 3 weeks postdischarge, approximately one third to one half of the individuals having an acute MI and about three quarters of the patients who had CABG will be in the low-risk group and have less than a 2 percent annual mortality rate.[14,26] It is estimated that moderate-risk patients (severe resting or exercise-induced ischemia) will have a first-year mortality rate of approximately 10 to 25 percent and high-risk stratified patients (severe left ventricular dysfunction or heart failure) will have a mortality rate greater than 25 percent within the first year.[14] Risk assessment can be used to determine if more extensive cardiac evaluations are necessary, if cardiac rehabilitation, surgical, or other medical treatments are indicated, and the nature of the medical supervision to be provided for exercise training. In addition to assessing the patient's functional status and overall prognosis for a cardiac event, the objective of risk stratification when exercise-based rehabilitation is being considered is to evaluate the individual's risk of having a cardiac event during exercise.[4] Additional information on risk stratification will be discussed in Chapter 12 as it pertains to the exercise session, the degree of medical supervision, and the frequency of continuous ECG monitoring. CHD patients who exhibit significant left ventricular dysfunction or ischemia at rest are considered to be at high risk and usually are not ideal candidates for exercise training.[4] The risk stratification of a patient should be used as a guide in the medical management of the patient, including the nature and timing of the rehabilitation program.

Determination of Pulmonary Impairment

The status of a pulmonary patient can be classified by impairment of the pulmonary system. Although the results of a physical examination can be classified by degree of dyspnea, frequency of cough, amount of sputum, number of pack-years, findings upon auscultation, results of chest roentgenograms, and extent of occupational exposure, the results of pulmonary function testing are the most important criteria for documenting the degree of pulmonary impairment. Table 11–2 presents the criteria developed in 1986 by the Social Security Administration, the American Thoracic Society, and the American Medical Society.

The degree of pulmonary impairment is used to alert the rehabilitation staff to the individual needs of a pulmonary patient. For example, participants with mild pulmonary impairment may maintain their levels of oxygenation during exercise, whereas patients with a moderate or severe degree of impairment have been shown to decrease, increase, or maintain their oxygenation during exercise.[28] (See the section on exercise and oxygen therapy in this chapter.) The amount of pulmonary impairment also is considered when prescribing exercise intensity.[29,30] (See the section on intensity of exercise in this chapter.)

TABLE 11–2 Pulmonary Function Test Criteria for the Determination of Pulmonary Degree of Impairment*

Test	Normal (%)	Mildly Impaired (%)	Moderately Impaired (%)	Severely Impaired (%)
VC	80	60–79	51–59	50 or less
FEV_1	80	60–79	41–59	40 or less
FEV_1/FVC	75	60–74	41–59	40 or less
D_{LCO}	80	60–79	41–59	40 or less

*Values reported are given in units of percent of predicted.
Source: Adapted from the American Thoracic Society,[27] with permission.

Survival curves show the most predictive outcome measurements to be postbronchodilator forced expiration volume in 1 second (FEV_1) and age.[31] The Chicago study followed 200 subjects with COPD for 15 years. Patients with mild impairment—an FEV_1 of greater than 60 percent of predicted or greater—had survival rates equal to those of the general population.[34] For patients with severe pulmonary impairment, a mean FEV_1 of 33.5 percent of predicted, and a mean age of 59.1 years, the 3-year survival rate was found to be 67 percent. Also, 5-, 10-, and 15-year survival rates were found to be 52, 23, and 12 percent, respectively.[32]

CARDIORESPIRATORY ENDURANCE

No single exercise can promote improvement in all factors identified as major contributors to physical fitness. A complete exercise prescription for the cardiopulmonary patient, therefore, includes exercises to effect changes in all parameters. However, throughout this discussion the importance of one factor, cardiorespiratory endurance, is emphasized for the maintenance of health and the rehabilitation of individuals with cardiorespiratory disease. In writing an exercise prescription, no other component demands more specialized knowledge than cardiorespiratory endurance. The key purpose of the exercise prescription is to increase or maintain functional capacity.

Although health care providers are among those who strongly advocate exercise for health maintenance as well as to augment their patients' rehabilitation or treatment, not all of them receive formal training in exercise physiology. Many are unfamiliar with cardiorespiratory training principles and methodologies. Therefore, exercise prescription tends to be rather vague. "Walk as far as you feel you can each day"; "Do what you feel comfortable doing." As in all types of training, to be most effective, the cardiovascular exercise prescription must be specific about the intensity, duration, frequency, and type (mode) of exercise performed.

Intensity of Exercise

There is an intensity or level of aerobic exercise that is necessary to improve cardiorespiratory endurance. Although intensity and duration are separate entities and will be discussed separately, it is difficult to discuss intensity without mentioning duration because of the interaction between the two. Prescribing exercise intensity for all adults—cardiac, pulmonary, or apparently healthy—is the most difficult task in designing the exercise program because individualization and appropriate monitoring are required to ensure that the maximum prescribed intensity is not exceeded. The intensity of exercise is usually expressed in relative terms as a percent of functional capacity.[4] By using the data derived from the laboratory and clinical assessment (Chapters 9 and 10), the clinician can begin to formulate the exercise intensity portion of the rehabilitative exercise program. Table 11–3 outlines the data often used in developing the exercise prescription.

Three techniques are commonly used to prescribe and monitor exercise intensity: heart rate, metabolic energy expenditure ($\dot{V}o_2$ or metabolic equivalents [METs]) and rating of perceived exertion (RPE).[4,5,35–40]

TABLE 11–3 Data Obtained from the Exercise Test to Be Used in the Development of an Exercise Prescription

Subjective

  Angina pectoris
  Dyspnea
  Fatigue — weakness
  Leg discomfort
  Dizziness

Objective

  Physical examination
    Breath sounds
    Peripheral pulses
    Precordial examination for dyskinetic areas, murmurs, and gallops (before and after exercise)
    Blood pressure response
    Pulmonary function test results (before and after exercise)
    Heart rate response
    General appearance
    Oximetry/arterial blood gas results
  Physical performance
    Time on treadmill/cycle
    Maximum work load (watts, kg-m per minute, kp-m per minute)
    Rate of perceived exertion
    Rate pressure product (max HR × max systolic BP)
  Electrocardiogram
    Repolarization changes — ST segment and J point
    Rate response
    Dysrhythmias
    Conduction abnormalities — atrioventricular and ventricular
  Cardiorespiratory/metabolic measurements (limited availability)
    Anaerobic threshold (AT)
    Carbon dioxide output (Vco_2)
    Gas exchange ratio (R)
    Minute ventilation (VE)
    Oxygen uptake (Vo_2)
    Respiratory quotient (RQ)

Source: Adapted from Mikolich, JR and Fletcher, GF: The exercise prescription. In Fletcher, GF (ed): Exercise and the Practice of Medicine, ed 2. Futura Publishing Company, Mount Kisco, NY, 1988, p. 82, with permission.

HEART RATE

During dynamic exercise involving large muscle groups, a relatively linear relation exists between heart rate and oxygen uptake. There are several widely used methods for establishing target heart rate (THR) and target heart rate range (THRR) for apparently healthy adults, as well as patients with cardiac and pulmonary disease.

The method most commonly used to determine the THRR and the THR is the heart rate reserve method or Karvonen formula.[36] The heart rate reserve, or HRmax reserve, is the difference between the resting heart rate in the seated position and the maximal achieved heart rate on a graded exercise test (GXT). The heart rate reserve method of determining exercise intensity has been shown to have a positive correlation to functional capacity in young healthy men during a GXT.

TARGET HEART RATE RANGE

GIVEN:	LOWER LIMIT	UPPER LIMIT
Maximum HR	140	140
Resting HR	-70	-70
Heart rate reserve	70	70
Desired intensity	x.40	x.85
(40-85% HR range)	——	——
	28	59.5
Add resting HR	+70	+70.0
Target HR range	98	129 beat/min

FIGURE 11–1. The heart rate reserve or Karvonen[36] method for determining target heart rate range.

The THRR is determined to define safety guidelines for exercise intensity during the exercise session. To calculate the THRR for a patient, percents of the heart rate reserve are added to the resting heart rate. The heart rate reserve method, however, may give a slight overestimation of the training intensity appropriate for recently discharged (postevent) patients with cardiac disease[42,43] or patients with low levels of exercise tolerance. For that reason, the therapist should set the lower limit of the initial exercise prescription at 40 percent of HRmax reserve, and the high intensity limit should not exceed 85 percent of HRmax reserve. Therefore, the equation for determining the THRR for a cardiac or a pulmonary patient is:

$$(Maximal\ HR - resting\ HR)(40\%\ to\ 85\%) + resting\ HR = THRR$$

See Fig. 11–1 for an example of calculating the THRR at 40 to 85 percent of HRmax reserve.

The THR for a specific patient defines the most appropriate HR within the prescribed THRR to ensure cardiorespiratory endurance training. Determining the appropriate THR requires careful consideration of the patient's abilities and disabilities. For most individuals, the training intensity threshold for improvement in $\dot{V}o_2$max would require the use of approximately 50 percent of the HRmax reserve in the calculation of THR.[35] Subjects with a high functional capacity may require a higher percentage, for example, 80 percent of heart rate reserve. Recently discharged cardiac patients with low fitness levels who begin their exercise programs at the lower limit of the THRR (40 percent of HRmax reserve) have demonstrated significant training effects.[35,41] For pulmonary patients with mild to moderate impairment, the recommended THR should be calculated by using a minimum of 50 to 60 percent and up to 70 percent of the maximum functional capacity.[31] Patients with moderate to severe pulmonary impairment will reach their maximum voluntary ventilations (MVVs), equal to VEmax, before the cardiovascular maximums are approached. For those patients, exercise intensities that approach their maximum ventilatory limits or the upper end of the THRR can be used.[29,30] The formula for THR is then as follows:

$$\text{(Maximum HR} - \text{resting HR)(appropriate percent)} + \text{resting HR} = \text{THR}$$

Fluctuations of about 10 percent normally occur in a participant's exercise HR during a single exercise session.

A second way to calculate THR is to estimate or express THR as a percent of $\dot{V}o_2$max (percent of maximal METs). Assuming a relative linear relation between HR and oxygen uptake (expressed in either $\dot{V}o_2$ or METs), one can plot steady-state HR and estimated or observed oxygen uptake during at least two and preferably more submaximal work loads. The maximal HR is considered the peak HR measured at the highest exercise intensity attained during a symptom-limited maximal exercise test. The THRR can be determined by finding the HRs corresponding to the desired target range of functional capacity (i.e., 40 to 85 percent of $\dot{V}o_2$max). As with the first method, this method of determining exercise intensity may slightly overestimate the desired aerobic training intensity in the initial phases of cardiac rehabilitation.[43,44]

The third and least desirable way to determine the THRR is to take 55 to 85 percent of the maximal HR reported on the GXTT. Although this method is easier to calculate than the percent of HRmax reserve method, it is not recommended because it yields significantly lower HR values. In many cases, patients with high resting HR can have THRs lower than their resting HRs when calculated by using the method. Despite a number of limitations in the percent of HRmax method, a number of clinicians prefer its use. The therapist who uses the method should adjust the THR by adding 10 to 15 percent.[11,38,42,45]

PRESCRIPTION BY METABOLIC ENERGY EXPENDITURE

Some clinicians prefer to prescribe exercise intensity by using activities that require a percent of functional capacity, or maximal METs, achieved during the evaluation process (Chapters 9 and 10). Usually the activities chosen for prescription by this method correspond to 40 to 85 percent of maximal METs achieved during evaluation.[4] Table 11–4 provides a list of activities and their average exercise intensities in METs.

As with any method of exercise prescription, in the beginning phases of rehabilitation, the exercise intensity should be prescribed at the lower end of the target range, in this case, near 40 percent of maximal METs. It is a prudent practice, when prescribing exercise by METs, to also monitor HRs either by telemetry (in early rehabilitation) and/or by palpation (in later stages) of rehabilitation. Adding HR monitoring to prescription by METs ensures that maximal safe exercise will not be exceeded, especially in situations that naturally cause increases in HRs (e.g., hot, humid environment) and in the rate-pressure product (RPP) (Chapter 5).

The prescription of exercise intensity in METs should be adjusted as cardiorespiratory endurance increases, but the THRR should remain relatively the same. As training adaptation occurs, increases in work load will be necessary to maintain the work load at the prescribed MET level, even though the THRR will not change appreciably.

TABLE 11–4 Cardiorespiratory-Endurance-Promoting Potential
of Various Activities

Intensity (70-kg Person)	Endurance-Promoting	Occupational	Recreational
1½–2 METs 4–7 mL/kg/min 2–2½ kcal/min	Too low in energy level	Desk work, driving auto, electric calculating machine operation, light housework, polishing furniture, washing clothes	Standing, strolling (1 mph), flying, motorcycling, playing cards, sewing, knitting
2–3 METs 7–11 mL/kg/min 2½–4 kcal/min	Too low in energy level unless capacity is very low	Auto repair, radio and television repair, janitorial work, bartending, riding lawn mower, light woodworking	Level walking (2 mph), level bicycling (5 mph), billiards, bowling, skeet shooting, shuffleboard, powerboat driving, golfing with power cart, canoeing, horseback riding at a walk
3–4 METs 11–14 mL/kg/min 4–5 kcal/min	Yes, if continuous and if target heart rate is reached	Brick laying, plastering, pushing wheelbarrow (100-lb load), machine assembly, welding (moderate load), cleaning windows, mopping floors, vacuuming, pushing light power mower	Walking (3 mph), bicycling (6 mph), horseshoe pitching, volleyball (6-person, noncompetitive), golfing (pulling bag cart), archery, sailing (handling) small boat, fly fishing (standing in waders), horseback riding (trotting), badminton (social doubles)
4–5 METs 14–18 mL/kg/min	Recreational activities promote endurance. Occupational activities must be continuous, lasting longer than 2 min	Painting, masonry, paperhanging, light carpentry, scrubbing floors, raking leaves, hoeing	Walking (3½ mph), bicycling (8 mph), table tennis, golfing (carrying clubs), dancing (foxtrot), badminton (singles), tennis (doubles), many calisthenics, ballet
5–6 METs 18–21 mL/kg/min	Yes	Digging garden, shoveling light earth	Walking (4 mph), bicycling (10 mph), canoeing (4 mph), horseback riding (posting to trotting), stream fishing (walking in light current in waders), ice or roller skating (9 mph)

TABLE 11–4 Cardiorespiratory-Endurance-Promoting Potential
of Various Activities (*Continued*)

Intensity (70-kg Person)	Endurance-Promoting	Occupational	Recreational
6–7 METs 21–25 mL/kg/min 7–8 kcal/min	Yes	Shoveling 10 times/min (4½ kg or 10 lb), splitting wood, snow shoveling, hand lawn mowing	Walking (5 mph), bicycling (11 mph), competitive badminton, tennis (singles), folk and square dancing, light downhill skiing, ski touring (2½ mph), water skiing, swimming (20 yards/min)
7–8 METs 25–28 mL/kg/min 8–10 kcal/min	Yes	Digging ditches, carrying 36 kg or 80 lb, sawing hardwood	Jogging (5 mph), bicycling (12 mph), horseback riding (gallop), vigorous downhill skiing, basketball, mountain climbing, ice hockey, canoeing (5 mph), touch football, paddleball
8–9 METs 28–32 mL/kg/min 10–11 kcal/min	Yes	Shoveling 10 times/min (5½ kg or 14 lb)	Running (5½ mph), bicycling (13 mph), ski touring (4 mph), squash (social), handball (social), fencing, basketball (vigorous), swimming (30 yards/min), rope skipping
10+ METs 32+ mL/kg/min 11+ kcal/min	Yes	Shoveling 10 times/min (7½ kg or 16 lb)	Running (6 mph = 10 METs, 7 mph = 11½ METs, 8 mph = 13½ METs, 9 mph = 15 METs, 10 mph = 17 METs), ski touring (5 mph), handball (competitive), squash (competitive), swimming (greater than 40 yards/min)

Source: From Fox, Naughton, and Gorman,[46] pp. 26–27, by permission of the American Heart Association, Inc.

TABLE 11–5 Borg's Rate of Perceived Exertion Scale
and the Revised 10-Grade Scale

RPE	10-Grade Rating Scale	
6	0	Nothing at all
7 Very, very light	0.5	Very, very weak (just noticeable)
8	1	Very weak
9 Very light	2	Weak (light)
10	3	Moderate
11 Fairly light	4	Somewhat strong
12	5	Strong (heavy)
13 Somewhat hard	6	
14	7	Very strong
15 Hard	8	
16	9	
17 Very hard	10	Very, very strong (almost maximum)
18		Maximal
19 Very, very hard		

Source: Adapted from Borg, GV: Psychophysical bases of perceived exertion. Med Sci Sports Exerc 14:377–387, 1982, © by The American College of Sports Medicine.

RATE OF PERCEIVED EXERTION

As patients become familiar with the "feeling" associated with exercising at the appropriate target level, the need for an objective measurement (e.g., monitoring HR) declines. At that point, the "perceived exertion" provides a subjective means of monitoring exercise intensity.[47] Borg's Rate of Perceived Exertion (RPE) Scale[48,49] (Table 11–5) is used by the patient with cardiac disease to rate the intensity of an exercise activity. A rating of 12 to 13 (somewhat hard) on the 20-point scale corresponds to approximately 60 percent of the HR range, whereas a rating of 16 (hard) corresponds to approximately 85 percent. If the 10-point scale were used, these ratings would be between 4 and 6.[4] Borg's RPE scale may be particularly useful when evaluating patients on beta-blocking or calcium channel blocking medications and when supervising patients in atrial fibrillation. However, patients with aggressive, competitive personality traits may deny that they perceive the exertion to be "hard," even though their exercise HRs are at levels exceeding 85 percent of their maximum measured values. Denial of perceived exertion may limit the practical application of Borg's scale in some cases.

Pulmonary patients can use a similar scale by rating their perceived shortness of breath (Table 11–6). Since such patients often have poor ventilatory reserves but adequate HR reserves, the use of a scale of perceived shortness of breath becomes helpful for monitoring exercise intensity by subjective means. Ratings of between 4 and 6—mildly short of breath to moderately short of breath—define the range in which patients generally work. Pulmonary patients do not tend to deny their shortness of breath as cardiac patients may deny perceived exertion. Pulmonary patients, being aware of their inabilities to rapidly recover from shortness of breath, may tend to exaggerate their perception of shortness of breath so as not to exceed their abilities. With training, a patient's perception of shortness of breath may change because of an increase in physiologic training, an increase in motivation to exercise, and/or a desensitization to dyspnea. As those changes in training occur, exercise progression requires higher work loads to achieve the same RPE rating.

For the pulmonary patient, exercise targets and exercise progression during training

TABLE 11-6 Subjective Definitions for a 10-Point Perceived
Shortness of Breath Scale

Rate of Perceived Exertion/Shortness of Breath	
1 Rest	Not short of breath
2 Minimal activity	Minimally short of breath
3 Very light activity	Slightly short of breath
4 Light activity	Mildly short of breath
5 Somewhat hard activity	Mildly to moderately short of breath
6 Hard activity	Moderately short of breath
7	Moderately to severely short of breath
8 Very hard activity	Severely short of breath
9	Breathing is not in control
10 Very, very hard activity	Maximally short of breath

Source: Adapted from Pulmonary Rehabilitation Program, Massachusetts Respiratory Hospital, Braintree, MA.

should be based on symptoms of shortness of breath and fatigue more than on HRs or fixed work levels.[28,33] Clinicians usually prefer to prescribe exercise for both cardiac and pulmonary patients by utilizing a combination of prescription by HR and the RPE or shortness of breath. When prescribing exercise, the therapist should express the desired intensity as a range, because during exercise the patient usually shows fluctuations from prescribed THRs or METs of about 10 percent. It should also be emphasized that maximum aerobic capacity can be increased by either increasing the intensity of the activity or extending the duration of the exercise session. For persons with low functional capacities, extending the duration of the exercise session at a low intensity over a period of weeks is safer than increasing the intensity of the activity.[4]

OTHER CONSIDERATIONS

Additional considerations in prescribing the intensity of exercise should include such factors as age, gender, blood pressure response, and orthopedic limitations. Those factors are discussed in Chapters 4 and 12. Table 11-7 summarizes the relation among the various methods used to prescribe intensity.

TABLE 11-7 Classification of Intensity of Exercise Based
on 20 to 60 Minutes of Endurance Training

Relative Intensity			
HRmax (%)	$\dot{V}$omax or HRmax reserve (%)	RPE (20-point scale)	Intensity
<35	<30	<10	Very light
35-39	30-49	10-11	Light
60-79	50-74	12-13	Moderate
80-89	75-84	14-16	Heavy
>90	>85	>16	Very heavy

HRmax, maximum heart rate, bpm; $\dot{V}o_2$max, maximum oxygen uptake; RPE, rate of perceived exertion.
Source: From Pollock and Wilmore,[50] p. 105, with permission.

Duration of Exercise

Each cardiorespiratory (CR) session should consist of a 5- to 10-minute warm-up period, a CR training period of 15 to 60 minutes, and a 5- to 10-minute cool-down period. During the 15 to 60 minutes of CR exercise, the HR should be maintained, as nearly as possible, at the target level and within the THRR (see page 284).[4,51]

Most commonly, the CR exercise session lasts from 20 to 30 minutes at a functional capacity of 40 to 60 percent (moderate activity level). Since there is a relation between the intensity and the duration of activity, and since CR improvement is dependent on the total energy expended during any single bout of activity, current policy is to prescribe CR exercise at moderate levels (lower intensities – longer duration) rather than at more intense levels (higher intensities – shorter duration). This moderate approach to exercise prescription reduces musculoskeletal injury and decreases cardiac risk.[4,51] A reduction in cardiovascular mortality of 9 to 15 percent has been reported in persons who engage in moderate exercise activity such as 30 to 60 minutes of daily walking.[52] In patients with cardiac or pulmonary disease whose functional capacities are low, several short bouts of CR activity may be prescribed rather than activity of longer duration.[4] As functional capacity increases and physiological adaptation to CR activity improves, the exercise prescription should be adjusted accordingly. The reduction is accomplished by increasing the intensity and/or duration of CR exercise.

Frequency of Exercise

"Frequency of exercise" refers to the number of exercise sessions scheduled per day and/or per week. Depending on individual functional capacities, frequency of CR exercise may vary from several short exercise sessions per day to three to five bouts per week. In patients whose functional capacities are less than 3 METs, short sessions of 5 minutes (more or less) that are performed several times a day may be prescribed. Generally, patients with functional capacities greater than 5 METs should exercise three to five times per week.[4]

Exercise Prescription Progression

The rate of progressing patients from light CR activities (lower functional capacities) to more difficult CR activities (requiring higher functional capacities) usually involves three stages: (1) the initial conditioning stage, (2) the improvement stage, and (3) the maintenance stage. Of course, rate of exercise progression is dependent on such factors as age, functional capacity, health status, compliance, and various individual needs.[4]

INITIAL CONDITIONING STAGE

One goal that is especially important in the early stages of initial conditioning is to ensure that each exercise session is undertaken at low levels of intensity and duration. Taking that approach will help to avoid muscle soreness, musculoskeletal, or other injury that is likely to result if the exercise sessions are undertaken at higher levels of intensity and/or duration. During the first few weeks of the initial conditioning stage,

HRs should be monitored frequently so that patients exercise fairly close to their THRs (which should be prescribed at the lower end of their HR ranges). Whether patients need to exercise by interspersing activity of short duration with periods of rest will depend on individual needs and abilities, but the duration of the total activity performed usually does not exceed 10 to 15 minutes. The role of the clinician in prescribing activity for patients at the appropriate intensity and duration is extremely important, because the clinician must be able to adjust the exercise prescription to meet individual needs. Although there is considerable variation among patients, usually the initial conditioning stage lasts from 4 to 6 weeks.[4]

IMPROVEMENT STAGE

The improvement stage usually lasts for 4 to 5 months. It is during this stage that the intensity and duration of the exercise sessions are gradually increased so that the patient is exercising within the THRR and within his or her functional capacities (40 to 85 percent of $\dot{V}O_2$max. Durations of aerobic activity also are gradually increased (every 2 to 3 weeks) so that patients are exercising for at least 20 to 30 minutes per exercise session as the end of the improvement stage approaches. It is especially important for older patients and/or those with disease to begin this stage with intermittent activity (if necessary) and progress gradually to activity that is continuous. The duration of the exercise should be increased before the intensity is increased.[4]

MAINTENANCE STAGE

Most patients require about 6 months of exercise training to reach the maintenance stage of conditioning. Usually this stage involves continuing the exercise routine that was acquired at the end of the improvement stage. To maintain fitness levels, the workouts must be continued on a regular basis, because levels of CR fitness have been found to decrease significantly after 2 weeks of training. Missing an occasional exercise session or decreasing the duration of the bout apparently does not decrease functional capacity provided the training intensity remains at the maintenance level.[53-56]

Type of Aerobic Exercise

The rules of specificity of training apply to CR endurance, and the clinician must prescribe the activities that are most useful in improving functional capacity. Generally, any physical activity that is rhythmical, that can be sustained for prolonged periods of time, and that uses large muscle groups can be classified as an aerobic activity. High-impact activities (e.g., running and jumping) are not generally recommended for promoting CR endurance because of the increased risk of injury inherent in their use. Low-impact and/or non-weight-bearing activities have a lower incidence of injury and are generally recommended for cardiopulmonary patients.

Since it is necessary to maintain an appropriate intensity of exercise, activities that are particularly useful for improving functional capacity include walking, perhaps jogging, and riding stationary bicycles.[4,10,57,58] A recent meta-analysis of several studies investigated the roles that intensity, duration, frequency, and mode of activity play in improving functional capacity through central and peripheral physiologic changes. The data indicated that the intensity of the exercise prescription was more important than duration, frequency, or mode in eliciting positive central adaptations, provided the exercise was performed at an intensity of at least 80 percent of Vo_2max.

Peripheral adaptations to aerobic training appeared to be a more significant factor in improving functional capacity when the exercise was performed at an intensity below 80 percent of Vo_2max.[59] For some cardiopulmonary patients, exercising at a functional capacity of 80 percent of Vo_2max is unrealistic and unsafe and should be prescribed with caution. No doubt the future will bring more study into the relations of intensity, frequency, duration, and mode of aerobic activity as they apply to improving functional capacity.

Percent Body Fat

Various factors have important roles in the development of obesity and/or overfatness. Genetic, hormonal, metabolic, and behavioral variables contribute to the development of obesity, but the main reason for increased body fat in individuals is believed to be an imbalance between energy input (caloric intake) and energy output (energy expenditure). Recent evidence, however, indicates that obesity and overfatness may not be a result of overeating but instead may result from eating a diet with a high fat-to-carbohydrate ratio.[60,61] Recent research also indicates that fat deposited primarily in the trunk and abdominal area (central obesity) seems to be associated with a higher risk for the development of hypertension, diabetes, and CAD.[4]

Although considerable variations exist among individuals in their responses to weight loss regimens and body composition changes, generally programs developed for managing body weight should include some type of CR endurance training. The benefits of CR endurance training in helping to control body weight include increased caloric expenditure, a decrease in body fat, and a possible increase in lean body weight. To be effective in helping to control excess body fat, the CR activity should use approximately 300 kcal per exercise session and be performed for at least 20 minutes for a minimum of 3 days per week. Aerobic exercise for longer durations and at lower intensities and performed for 4 or 5 days per week might be prescribed for persons needing to maximize the weight-controlling effects of regular, aerobic activity.[4,50,63] Additional guidelines that have been reported to be effective and should be considered in providing diet therapy for overfat patient include:[4,60,61,63]

1. Generally, do not restrict caloric intake to less than 1200 kcal per day.
2. Allow for a gradual weight loss of approximately 2 lb per week.
3. Gradually reduce the amount of fat and increase the amount of complex carbohydrates and fiber consumed.
4. Include behavioral techniques to help manage eating and exercise behaviors.
5. Include participation in peer social support groups.
6. Include regular counseling from therapists for approximately 6 months as well as regular follow-up contacts.

Muscular Strength and Endurance

Two components of total physical fitness—muscular strength and muscular endurance—are usually discussed together because the acquisition of one (strength) usually causes improvement in the other (endurance), and vice versa. Both are acquired through adhering to the overload principle, which simply stated means that, to improve, an individual must increase the intensity, duration, and perhaps the frequency of the activity. If the goal is to maximize strength gains, an individual must increase the resistance (intensity) and decrease the number of repetitions (frequency) per exercise bout. Maximal gains in muscular endurance are acquired through an increase in repetitions and a decrease in resistance.[63]

A second principle that is important in the acquisition of strength and/or endurance is that of specificity of training: strength and/or endurance improvement is gained only in the muscle groups actively involved in the resistance training. Effects of training (improvement) are also specific to the range of motion through which the resistance is moved or lifted. For best results, the resistance activity should be performed through the full range of motion.[63]

Controversy exists as to the feasibility of including resistance training in cardiopulmonary rehabilitation (Chapter 4). However, recent research indicates that static (isometric), dynamic (isotonic or isokinetic), and isodynamic (the combination of isometric with dynamic) can be safe for selected patients, particularly when the activity is of low intensity, is progressed fairly slowly, and is properly supervised.[64,65]

Most patients should not begin a resistance training program until they have participated in a CR exercise program for at least 3 months.[66] Additional criteria to be utilized for patient entrance into a resistance training program include functional capacity of at least 7 METs, ejection fraction of approximately 45 percent, no evidence of ischemic ECG changes, fairly normal blood pressure responses to activity, and absence of uncontrolled arrhythmias.[64,66]

Patients who generally are not candidates for resistance training include those with unstable angina, uncontrolled hypertension, uncontrolled arrhythmias, congestive heart failure (CHF), and a functional capacity of less than 6 to 7 METs.[64,66]

The clinician must supervise patients involved in the resistance training program. HRs and blood pressures must be taken, and evidence of patient activity evoking the Valsalva manuever (straining to lift a weight) should not be tolerated.[64]

Guidelines to follow in prescribing the resistance program include the following:

1. Use low resistance (30 percent of one maximum lift when beginning the program).
2. Increase the repetitions (12 to 15).
3. Perform one to three sets.
4. Train for two to three times per week.
5. Exercise large muscle groups before smaller groups.
6. Perform the activity in an even, rhythmical manner.

Table 11–8 presents the resistance training guidelines recommended for cardiac patients who are candidates for a resistance training program.

Flexibility

Flexibility, or range of motion in a joint, is necessary for normal bodily movement. This component of total physical fitness is important to include in the rehabilitative process, especially for the older adult who may lack flexibility and, consequently, may

TABLE 11–8 Weight Training Guidelines for Low-Risk Cardiac Patients

- To prevent soreness and injury, initially choose a weight that will allow the performance of 12 to 15 repetitions comfortably, corresponding to approximately 30%–50% of the maximum weight load that can be lifted in one repetition. (Note: Selected stable, aerobically trained cardiac patients may eventually use loads corresponding to a more traditional program of weight training [i.e., 60%–80% of 1 RM])
- Perform one to three sets of each exercise.
- Avoid straining. Ratings of perceived exertion (6–20 scale) should not exceed fairly light to somewhat hard during lifting.
- Exhale (blow out) during the exertion phase of the lift. For example, exhale when pushing a weight stack overhead and inhale when lowering it.
- Increase weight loads by 5 to 10 lb when 12 to 15 repetitions can be comfortably accomplished.
- Raise weights with slow, controlled movements; emphasize complete extension of the limbs when lifting.
- Exercise large muscle groups before small muscle groups. Include devices (exercises) for the upper and lower extremities.
- Weight-train at least two to three times per week.
- Loosely hold hand grips when possible; sustained, tight gripping may evoke an excessive blood pressure response to lifting.
- Stop exercise in the event of warning signs or symptoms, especially dizziness, arrhythmias, unusual shortness of breath, and/or angina pectoris.
- Allow minimal rest periods between exercises (e.g., 30–60 sec) to maximize muscular endurance and aerobic training benefits.

Note: From *Guidelines for Cardiac Rehabilitation Programs* (p. 11) by American Association of Cardiovascular and Pulmonary Rehabilitation, 1991, Champaign, IL: Human Kinetics. Copyright 1991 by American Association of Cardiovascular and Pulmonary Rehabilitation. Reprinted by permission.

have difficulty in performing activities of daily living. In including flexibility exercises in the rehabilitation program, particular attention should be given to the range of motion in the lower back and posterior thigh, since "stiffness" in that region is often associated with chronic low back pain. Flexibility activities should also be prescribed for the upper and lower trunk, neck, hips, and muscles in the lower legs.[4] (Examples of flexibility activities are given in Appendix E.)

Stretching activities are usually performed as part of the warm-up preceding aerobic activity as well as during the cool-down following completion of the aerobic activity. Flexibility exercises should be performed slowly, and progression to greater ranges of motion should be gradual. Generally, the recommended procedure to follow in prescribing flexibility exercises is to perform a slow dynamic movement that is followed by a static stretch that is "held" for 10 to 30 seconds. Each flexibility activity should be repeated three to five times, and the flexibility regime should be performed at least three times per week. During the execution of the flexibility exercises, the range of motion should not be so great as to cause pain.[4]

EXERCISE AND OXYGEN THERAPY

Supplemental oxygen improves the mortality and morbidity in hypoxemic patients with COPD.[67] The physiologic goals of oxygen therapy are to reverse or prevent tissue hypoxia. The benefits of supplemental oxygen for patients who are hypoxemic only during exercise remains controversial, because there have not been any reports that hypoxemia only during exercise causes any long-term ill effects.[68] Therefore, the rationale for using supplemental oxygen during exercise sessions would be to prevent the immediate effects of hypoxemia, for example, cardiac ischemia or rhythm disturbances,[69] and to increase exercise tolerance. Nixon and co-workers[70] reported that supplemental oxygen minimized oxygen desaturation during the exercise session and enabled patients to exercise with a lower ventilatory and cardiovascular demand. Other authors also have reported an increase in exercise tolerance with the use of supplemental oxygen.[71-73]

Supplemental oxygen to decrease arterial hypoxemia during exercise becomes warranted when the Sao_2 dips below 85 percent saturation, Pao_2 dips below 55 mm Hg, or the Pao_2 drops more than 20 mm Hg during exercise.[74] Arterial blood gases should be monitored during the graded exercise test to document changes in Pao_2 during exercise (Chapter 10). Pulse oximetry can evaluate a patient's arterial oxygen saturation during an exercise test or during the session, since it is a noninvasive procedure.

Supplemental oxygen is prescribed by the attending physician. Oxygen therapy should be based on the patient's diagnosis, age, amount of hypoxemia during different living conditions, and lifestyle or mobility.[67] Common practice suggests the use of oxygen in patients who desaturate to a clinically significant degree during exercise. A usual prescription may include a variety of liter flow rates according to the patient's activity level. Oxygen flow rate during exercise, when minute ventilation is higher than at rest, may have to be increased to provide an Fio_2 of 24 to 27 percent and maintain Pao_2 above 55 mm Hg or Sao_2 above 85 percent.[67,75] Flow rates may have to be readjusted when the patient is at rest or during sleep.[67] The necessary liter flow may dictate the portability of the oxygen source.

Supplemental oxygen can be provided in a variety of ways. The most common device used during rehabilitation sessions is the nasal cannula using either liquid O_2 or compressed gas in a portable canister. More recent advances in oxygen delivery are transtracheal O_2 and inspiratory phased oxygen delivery (Oxymizer). Because none of the oxygen is "wasted" when those methods of oxygen delivery are used, lower liter flows and longer durations of the portable oxygen source are possible.[76]

By transtracheal administration, oxygen is delivered directly into the trachea through an opening in the neck. The method has been shown to use only 50 percent as much oxygen as the nasal cannula delivery system.[77] Other benefits from transtracheal oxygen are improved cosmesis, increased comfort, and improved compliance.[78] There are also disadvantages to the use of transtracheal oxygen that must be considered. Surgical emphysema, catheter fracture, local infection, catheter dislodgement, and mucus plugging have been reported.[77,79] Exercise studies using transtracheal oxygen demonstrate that exercise performance is enhanced with this method of oxygen delivery as compared with more traditional methods, although the mechanisms for the improvement are not readily apparent.[80]

Inspiratory phased delivery of oxygen, or demand oxygen delivery system (DODS), uses a reservoir attached to the apparatus of oxygen delivery. Inhalation removes oxygen from the reservoir during high inspiratory flow rates, as in early inspiration, but not during expiration. That method of oxygen delivery also is more efficient than the nasal cannula delivery system: less oxygen is wasted.[76] Tiep and co-workers[81] showed that DODS during exercise used only one seventh the amount of oxygen as compared with the more traditional oxygen delivery system.

FORMULATING THE EXERCISE PRESCRIPTION (CASE STUDIES)

The information presented in this chapter should provide guidelines for writing exercise prescriptions for cardiopulmonary patients. Tables 11–9 to 11–18 illustrate the use of intensity, duration, frequency, and mode of activity as they apply to the prescription of total fitness programs for rehabilitating cardiopulmonary patients. The examples presented integrate the information obtained from the assessment (Chapters 9 and 10), and case studies 1, 5, 7, and 8 from Chapter 9 have been included to show exercise prescriptions for four patients with cardiovascular disease. Case studies 1, 2, 3, and 4

TABLE 11–9 Sample Exercise Prescription Form for the Cardiac Patient

Exercise Rx

Name _____ F   M   Age _____ Date _____
                                        Ht. (in) _____ Wt. (lb) _____

Dx: _____

Meds: _____

Comments: _____
_____

GXT Data: Date Performed ____/____/_____   Where: _____

        Rest HR _____   Protocol: _____

        Max HR _____   Max METs: _____

        Re-evaluation scheduled ____/____/____

C-R Rx:

    Target Zone (METs) = 50 to 85% of Max METs
                = 0.50 to 0.85 × _____
                = _____ METs

    Target HR (bpm) = (Max HR − Rest HR) (65% to 90%) + (Rest HR)
              = (_____ − _____) (0.65 to 0.90) + (_____)
              = _____ bpm

    Type of Exercise: _____ bike   _____ row   _____ walk   _____ walk/jog

    Length of session: _____ Frequency: _____

    Comments: _____
    _____
    _____

Flexibility Rx: _____
_____
_____

Muscular S & End Rx: _____
_____
_____

% Body Fat Rx:
_____ %   Desirable M   15%
                                                   F   25%

Body Wt. _____ lb
        _____ kg   Desired Range _____ to _____ lb

from Chapter 10 have been included to illustrate prescriptions for the pulmonary patient. The exercise prescriptions presented in Tables 11–9 to 11–13 and 11–15 to 11–18 are the initial exercise prescriptions that were written following the assessment and prior to initiating exercise therapy. Progressions and exercise prescription adjustments will be presented in Chapter 12.

TABLE 11–10 Exercise Prescription for Case Study 1, Chapter 9

Exercise Rx

Name   Case Study 1   (F) M   Age 57   Date _____
                            Ht. (in) 59   Wt. (lb) 149.5

Dx: CAD, CABG, Angina

Meds: Persantine, Synthroid

Comments: ST-T sagging—2mm at Max HR GXT & Dyspnea, Fatigue

GXT Data: Date Performed 3/19/87   Where: X Hospital
          Rest HR   65   Protocol: Adapted Bruce
          Max HR   118   Max METs: 7
          Re-evaluation scheduled   6/20/87

C-R Rx:
    Target Zone (METs) = 50 to 85% of Max METs
                       = 0.50 to 0.85 × 7
                       = 3.5 to 6.0 METs
    THRR (bpm) = (Max HR − Rest HR) (65% to 90%) + (Rest HR)
               = (118 − 65) (0.65) + (65)
               = ~99 bpm
    Type of Exercise: X bike ____ row X walk ____ walk/jog

    Length of session: 20–30 min. Frequency: 2–3/wk
    Comments: Initial HR determined from Target Zone & THR = 99 bpm
    RPP = 198
Flexibility Rx: Begin with flex for calf, hamstring, quads, hip flexors.
Hold 10 sec, progress to 30 sec. Add shoulder, trunk, neck and back exercises
as needed. 3Xs/week prior to Ex. 1X/day at home.
Muscular S & End Rx: N/A Begin if needed p̄ re-evaluation 6/20/87

% Body Fat Rx:
    32   %   Desirable M 15%
                                          F 25%

Body Wt. 149.5 lb
           68   kg   Desired Range 115 to 125 lb
Referred also for nutrition education and weight reduction.

TABLE 11–11 Initial Exercise Prescription for Case Study 5, Chapter 9

Exercise Rx

Name __Case Study 5__   Ⓕ M Age _70_   Date _____
                               Ht. (in) _59_   Wt. (lb) _180_

Dx: __Hypertension, Obesity, Arthritis (knees, wrists, spine)__

Meds: __HydroDIURIL, Aldomet__

Comments: __Severe hypertensive response to exercise Max BP 220/186,__
__severely deconditioned, orthopedic limitations.__

GXT Data: Date Performed _2/7/87_   Where: __Clinic X__
          Rest HR __62__   Protocol: __Adapted Astrand-Rhyming__
          Max HR __113__   Max METs: __2__
          Re-evaluation scheduled __5/15/87__

C-R Rx:

    Target Zone (METs) = 50 to 85% of Max METs
                       = .50 to .85 × __2__
                       = __~1 to 2__ METs (↓40% due to age & BP = ~1 MET)
        THRR (bpm) = (Max HR − Rest HR) (65% to 90%) + (Rest HR)
                   = (__113__ − __62__) (.65) + (__62__)
                   = __~95__ bpm
    Type of Exercise: X bike ____ row ____ walk ____ walk/jog
                      (no arms on Schwinn Airdyne until adapt. occurs)
    Length of session: __20–30 min.__ Frequency: __3×s/week__
    Comments: __Initial HR based on Target Zone and THR = 95 bpm.__
    __Limited by BP response. Intermittent CR exercise initially 2–3 min of__
    __exercise with 1–2 min rest. Progress to continuous. RPP = 248__

Flexibility Rx: __General program with emphasis on affected joints performed__
__3×s/day.__

Muscular S & End Rx: __Mild strengthening program for quadriceps & hamstrings—__
__10 reps, 3×s/day—no weights.__

% Body Fat Rx:
    __44__ %   Desirable M __15%__
                                              F __25%__

Body Wt. __180__ lb
         __82__ kg   Desired Range __115__ to __125__ lb
Referred also for nutrition education and weight reduction.

TABLE 11–12 Exercise Prescription for Case Study 7, Chapter 9

Exercise Rx

Name __Case Study 7__   F Ⓜ Age __51__   Date _____
                               Ht. (in) __74__   Wt. (lb) __238__

Dx: __CAD, s/pMI, Hypertension, Rhythm Disturbance__

Meds: __Corgard, Procainamide__

Comments: Mild hypertensive response GXT, PVCs, Coupling (1), Bigeminy at Max HR on GXT.

GXT Data: Date Performed __1/24/87__   Where: __Hospital X__

        Rest HR __56__   Protocol: __Bruce__

        Max HR __110__   Max METs: __7__

        Re-evaluation scheduled __4/25/87__

C-R Rx:

    Target Zone (METs) = 50 to 85% of Max METs

$$= .50 \text{ to } .85 \times \underline{7}$$
$$= \underline{3.5 \text{ to } 6} \text{ METs}$$

    THRR (bpm) = (Max HR − Rest HR) (65% to 90%) + (Rest HR)

$$= (\underline{110} - \underline{56}) (.65) + (\underline{56})$$
$$= \underline{{\sim}91} \text{ bpm}$$

    Type of Exercise: __X__ bike ____ row __X__ walk ____ walk/jog

    Length of session: __20 – 30 min.__   Frequency: 3×s/week

    Comments: __Initial HR based on Target Zone, THR response = 91 bpm.__
__Patient referred to Physician for Med. change to stabilize Arrhythmia prior to beginning exercise therapy, RPP = 184__

Flexibility Rx: __Flex for calf, hamstrings, quads, hip flexors, 3×s/week prior__ to therapy, 1×/day home, progress from 10 sec to 30 sec. Add shoulders, trunk, neck as needed.

Muscular S & End Rx: __N/A at this time.__

% Body Fat Rx:
    __25__ %   Desirable M __15%__
                               F __25%__

Body Wt. __238__ lb
        __108__ kg   Desired Range __200__ to __210__ lb
Referred also for nutrition education and weight reduction.

TABLE 11–13 Initial Exercise Prescription for Case Study 8, Chapter 9

Exercise Rx

Name __Case Study 8, Chapter 9__ — F Ⓜ Age __50__ Date _____

Ht. (in)__69__Wt. (lb) __160__

Dx: CAD, Post-MI, Post CABG, Hyperlipidemia, PVD

Meds: Cardizem, Isordil, Transderm 5

Comments: Mild hypertensive response on GXTT, ST-T depression of 3 mm in V_5 at Max

HR on GXT, Leg claudication—bilateral at 3 METs on GXTT, PVCs, Bigeminy during

cool-down and recovery.

GXT Data: Date performed __2/4/91__   Where: Clinic X

Rest HR 48   Protocol: Bruce Treadmill

Max HR 98   Max METs: 5

Re-evaluation scheduled __5/7/91__

Risk Stratification: HIGH

C-R Rx:

Functional Capacity (METs) = 40% to 85% of Max METs
$$= .40 \text{ to } .85 \times \underline{5}$$
$$= \underline{2.0 - 4.25 \text{ METS}}$$

THRR (bpm)   = (Max HR − Rest HR)(.40% − .85%) + (Rest HR)
$$= (\underline{98} - \underline{48}) \, (.40 \text{ to } .85) + (48)$$
$$= \underline{68 \text{ to } 91} \text{ bpm}$$

Type of Exercise:__X__ bike ____ row __X__ walk ____ walk/jog

(Intermittent, progressing to continuous as able.)

Length of session: __20–60 min__ Frequency 3Xs/week

Comments: Initial HR: 68 bpm based on Target Heart Rate. Longer cool-down. Subjective

gradation of pain = 2 at Max HR on GXT. RPP = 152

Flexibility Rx: Stretching for calves, hamstrings, quads, hip flexors—3X/wk prior to exercise

and daily on alternate days

Muscular S & End Rx: N/A begin as needed as need

% Body Fat Rx:
__20%__

Desirable M __15%__
          F __25%__

Body Wt.__160__lbs   Desired Range __150__ to __160__ lbs
        __73__kg

Referred for lipid-lowering diet plan and nutrition education.

TABLE 11–14 Sample Pulmonary Exercise Prescription Form

Exercise Rx

Name_____ F M Age_____ Date_____

Pack-years_____ Ht. (in)_____ Wt. (lb)_____

Dx:_____

Meds:_____

Comments:_____

_____

GXT Data: Date performed / / _____   Where:_____

Rest HR _____   Protocol: _____

Max HR _____   Max METs: _____

Re-evaluation scheduled: / / _____

PFT Interpretation:_____

_____

C-R Rx:

Functional Capacity (METs) = 40% to 85% of Max METs

= .40 to .85 × _____

= _____ METs

THRR (bpm) = (Max HR − Rest HR) (.40% to .85%) + (Rest HR)

= _____ bpm

RPE (10-point scale)   = _____

Type of Exercise: _____ bike _____ row _____ walk

_____ walk/jog _____ stairs

_____ arm ergometry

_____

_____

Length of session: _____ Frequency _____

Comments: _____

_____

Flexibility Rx: _____

_____

Monitoring and Oxygen Needs:

Telemetry _____   Oximetry _____

Supplemental oxygen _____

Comments _____

_____

TABLE 11–15 Exercise Prescription for Case Study 1, Chapter 10

Exercise Rx

Name __Case Study 1, Chapter 10__   F M Age __61__   Date _____

Pack-years __45__   Ht. (in) __65__   Wt. (lb) __124__

Dx: COPD, Asthma, Orthostatic hypotension, S/P Mastectomy

Meds: Tamoxatrin, imipramine, Ventolin MDI, Atrovent MDI, Slo-phyllin, Ativan

Comments: ECG normal before and after exercise. Quit smoking 8 years ago. Termination: Leg fatigue

GXT Data: Date performed __4/5/91__   Where: Clinic X

Rest HR __108 bpm__   Protocol: Modified cycle

Max HR __123 bpm__   Max METs: 2.8

Re-evaluation scheduled: __7/12/91__

PFT Interpretation: Bronchospastic response to exercise moderately severe mechanical and diffusion limitations

C-R Rx:

Functional Capacity (METs) = 40% to 85% of Max METs

$$= .40 \text{ to } .85 \times \underline{2.8}$$
$$= \underline{1.1 \text{ to } 2.4} \text{ METs}$$

THRR (bpm) = (Max HR − Rest HR)(.40 to .85) + (Rest HR)

$$= \underline{114-121} \text{ bpm}$$

RPE (10 point scale) $= \underline{4 \text{ to } 5}$

Type of Exercise: __X__ bike ____ row __X__ walk

____ walk/jog ____ stairs

__X__ arm ergometry

Circuit program: 10-min walk, 5-min bike (20 watts), 5 minutes arm ergometer, RPE not to exceed 5

Length of session: __20 min of total__   Frequency: __4–5×/wk__

Comments: Suggest Ventolin and Atrovent MDIs prior to exercise rest periods as needed. 16 stairs to home, work on pacing, not ex program yet.

Flexibility Rx: General flexibility exercises with emphasis on head, neck, and shoulders.

Muscular strength and endurance Rx: Not applicable at this time. If METs increase, consider light weights later.

Monitoring and Oxygen Needs:

Telemetry _____   Oximetry __X__

Supplemental oxygen 3 liters

Comments: Dropped Pao_2 during exercise. Oximetry eval with 3 liters of oxygen with exercise. Keep sats above 85%.

TABLE 11-16 Exercise Prescription for Case Study 2, Chapter 10

Exercise Rx

Name Case Study 2, Chapter 10   F (M) Age 77   Date _____

Pack-years 75   Ht. (in) 67.6   Wt. (lb) 180

Dx: COPD, Asthma, Chronic bronchitis, HTN, Peptic ulcers

Meds: Atrovent MDI, Beclovent MDI, Max Air, Robitussin

Comments: No significant ECG changes, termination due to dyspnea. Quit smoking 2 years ago

GXT Data: Date performed 6/12/91   Where: Clinic X

Rest HR 61   Protocol: Modified cycle

Max HR 123   Max METs: 4.5

Re-evaluation scheduled 9/ /91

PFT Interpretation: Moderately severe obstruction.

Moderate ventilatory mechanical and diffusion limitations

C-R Rx:

Functional Capacity (METs) = 40% to 85% of Max METs

$$= .40 \text{ to } .85 \times \underline{4.5}$$
$$= \underline{1.8 \text{ to } 3.8} \text{ METs}$$

THRR (bpm) = (Max HR − Rest HR)(.40 to .85) + (Rest HR)

$$= \underline{85 \text{ to } 114 \text{ bpm}}$$

RPE (10-point scale)   = 4 to 5

Type of Exercise: __X__ bike ____ row __X__ walk

____ walk/jog ____ stairs

__X__ arm ergometry

Cycle 60 to 80 watts for 10 minutes, walking 10 minutes.

Arm ergometry for 5 minutes at 25 watts

Length of session: __25 minutes__ Frequency: __3×/wk__

Comments: Intersperse rest periods only if needed during each stage of circuit. Rest

between modes as needed.

Flexibility Rx: General flexibility program with attention to low back

Monitoring and Oxygen Needs:

Telemetry_____   Oximetry_____

Supplemental oxygen_____

Comments: Pao_2 57 with sats at 87% at 4.5 METs. Dyspnea correlated well with

decreased sats. No supplemental O_2 indicated since sats above 85%.

TABLE 11–17 Exercise Prescription for Case Study 3, Chapter 10

Exercise Rx

Name __Case Study 3, Chapter 10__   F (M) Age __69__ Date_____
                                          Pack-years __70__ Ht. (in) __72.4__ Wt. (lb) __147__

Dx: COPD, Pneumoconiosis, HTN, CAD, S/P MI, L CVA, PVD, Gout, Ulcers

Meds: Lasix, ASA, diltiazem, Alipurinol, digoxin, Lanoxin, NTG

Comments: ST seg depression pre- and post-exercise. HR is disproportionately increased indicating cardiac limitation. Smokefree 11 years. Termination: Dyspnea and fatique.

GXT Data: Date performed 5/11/91   Where:_____

    Rest HR 84   Protocol: Modified treadmill

    Max HR 96   Max METs: 3.1

    Re-evaluation scheduled 8/ /91

PFT Interpretation: Moderately severe obstructive disease, no change with exercise.

C-R Rx:

    Functional Capacity (METs) = 40% to 85% of Max METs

$$= .40 \text{ to } .85 \times \underline{3.1}$$
$$= 1.2 \text{ to } 2.6 \text{ METs}$$

    THRR (bpm) = (Max HR − Rest HR)(.40 to .85) + (Rest HR)

$$= \underline{88-94} \text{ bpm}$$

    RPE (10-point scale) $= \underline{\quad 4 \quad}$

    Type of Exercise: __X__ bike ____ row __X__ walk

    ____ walk/jog ____ stairs

    __X__ arm ergometry

    Cycle 50 rpm no resistance 2 sets of 3 min each with rests 1–2 minutes.

    Walking 3–5 minutes with 1–2 min rests

Length of session: 12–15 min ex, 4–8 min rest Frequency: 4–5X/wk

Comments: Intersperse rest periods as needed. No upper extremity work as yet.

Progression: 15 min continuous exercise

Flexibility Rx: General flexibility, special attention to L upper and lower extremity

Monitoring and Oxygen Needs:

Telemetry__X__   Oximetry__X__

Supplemental oxygen Only if indicated during ex session

Comments: Decreased O_2 sats to 87% and increased heart rate with low-level exercise.

Suggest telemetry and oximetry during exercise session.

TABLE 11–18 Exercise Prescription for Case Study 4, Chapter 10

Exercise Rx

Name Case Study 4, Chapter 10   F (M) Age 73 Date_____

Pack-years 50   Ht. (in) 71.5 Wt. (lb) 152

Dx: COPD, Glaucoma

Meds: Beclovent MDI, Max Air MDI, Atovent MDI, prednisone, Dilantin, aminophylline,

Pilocar drops

Comments: Few PVCs, nonspecific ST-T changes. Smokefree 3 years. Termination: Nose/

mouth discomfort, some dyspnea

GXT Data: Date performed 4/5/91   Where: Clinic X

Rest HR 93   Protocol: Treadmill

Max HR 114   Max METs: 3.2

Re-evaluation scheduled 7/ /91

PFT Interpretation: Severe airflow obstruction. No change pre- and post-exercise test

C-R Rx:

Functional Capacity (METs) = 40% to 85% of Max METs

$= .40$ to $.85 \times \underline{3.2}$

$= \underline{1.3 \text{ to } 2.7}$ METs

THRR (bpm) = (Max HR − Rest HR)(.40% to .85%) + (Rest HR)

$= \underline{101\text{–}111}$ bpm

RPE (10-point scale) $= \underline{\quad 4 \text{ to } 5 \quad}$

Type of Exercise: ____ bike ____ row X walk

____ walk/jog X stairs

X arm ergometry

Never been on a bike. Lives on 3rd floor walk-up walking 5 min,

1–2 min rest. Stairs 2–3 min within THRR

Length of session: 3 sets walk   Frequency: 4–5×/wk

Comments: Keep within THRR during 5-min walk, progress to 15 min continuous

walking. Consider arm erg as progression

Flexibility Rx: General flexibility, begin with LE and low back, add UEs as progression

occurs.

Monitoring and Oxygen Needs:

Telemetry_____   Oximetry____X____

Supplemental oxygen 3 liters

Comments: Heart rate reserve adequate, breathing reserve poor. Pao_2 drop to 42, $Paco_2$

up to 50. Keep sats above 85%.

SUMMARY

Guidelines for writing exercise prescriptions for cardiopulmonary patients have been presented. Training principles associated with the development of each of the components of physical fitness (cardiorespiratory endurance, percent body fat, muscular strength and endurance, and flexibility) have been included. The principles of intensity, duration, frequency, and mode of activity have been described and interpreted as they relate to the improvement in functional capacity and normalization of daily activities so that patients may be able to lead more productive lives. Examples of exercise prescriptions and four case histories of patients with cardiovascular disease and four case histories for patients with pulmonary disease have been included. These case studies should assist students and clinicians in the application of the guidelines presented for writing complete exercise prescriptions.

REFERENCES

1. Fletcher, GF: Survey of current cardiac exercise programs. In Fletcher, GF and Cantwell, JD (eds): Exercise and Coronary Heart Disease. Charles C Thomas, Springfield, IL, 1979, p 250.
2. Franklin, BA, et al: Exercise prescription for the myocardial infarction patient. J Cardiopulmonary Rehabil 6:62, 1986.
3. American Association of Cardiovascular and Pulmonary Rehabilitation, Position Paper: Scientific evidence of the value of cardiac rehabilitation services with emphasis on patients following myocardial infarction. Section I. Exercise conditioning component. J Cardiopulmonary Rehabil 10:79, 1990.
4. American College of Sports Medicine. Guidelines for Exercise Testing and Prescription, ed 4. Lea & Febiger, Philadelphia, 1991.
5. American Heart Association Medical/Scientific Statement: Special report. Exercise standards: A statement for health professionals. From the American Heart Association. Circulation 82:2286, 1990.
6. National Center for Health Services Research and Health Care Technology Assessment. Health Technology Assessment Reports. Cardiac Rehabilitation Services. US Department of Health and Human Services. DHHS Publication No. (PHS) 88- 3427, Rockville, MD, 1987.
7. Recommendations of the American College of Cardiology on cardiovascular rehabilitation. J Am Coll Cardiol 7:451, 1986.
8. Ries, AL: Position Paper of the American Association of Cardiovascular and Pulmonary Rehabilitation: Scientific basis of pulmonary rehabilitation. J Cardiopulmonary Rehabil 10:418–441, 1990.
9. Sharkey, BJ: Specificity of exercise. In Resource Manual for Guidelines for Exercise Testing and Prescription. American College of Sports Medicine. Lea & Febiger, Philadelphia, 1988, p 55.
10. DeVries, HA: Physiology of Exercise, ed 4. Wm C Brown Group, Dubuque, IA 1986.
11. Franklin, BA, et al: Cardiac patients. In Franklin, BA, Gordon, S, and Timmis, GC (eds): Exercise in Modern Medicine. Williams & Wilkins, Baltimore, 1989, p 69.
12. Oldridge, NB, et al: Cardiac rehabilitation after myocardial infarction: Combined experience of randomized clinical trials. JAMA 260:945, 1988.
13. O'Connor, GT, et al: An overview of randomized trials of rehabilitation with exercise after myocardial infarction. Circulation 80:234, 1989.
14. DeBusk, RF, et al: Identification and treatment of low risk patients after acute myocardial infarction and coronary artery bypass graft surgery. N Engl J Med 314:161, 1986.
15. Beller, GA and Gibson, RS: Risk stratification after myocardial infarction. Mod Concepts Cardiovasc Dis 55:5, 1986.
16. Greenland, P and Chv, J: Health and Public Policy Committee, American College of Physicians. Position paper: Cardiac rehabilitation services. Ann Intern Med 109:671, 1988.
17. American Association of Cardiovascular and Pulmonary Rehabilitation: Guidelines for Cardiac Rehabilitation Programs. Human Kinetics Publishers, Champaign, IL, 1991, p 5.
18. DeBusk, RF, Kraemer, HC and Nash, E: Stepwise risk stratification soon after acute myocardial infarction. Am J Cardiol 52:1161, 1983.
19. McNeer, JF, et al: Role of the exercise test in evaluating patients for ischemic heart disease. Circulation 57:64, 1978.
20. Weiner, DA, et al: Value of exercise test in determining the risk classification in the response to coronary artery bypass grafting in three vessel coronary artery disease: A report from the CASS registry. Am J Cardiol 60:262, 1987.

21. Bigger, JT, et al: The relationships among ventricular arrhythmia, left ventricular dysfunction and mortality in the first two years after myocardial infarction. Circulation 69:250, 1984.
22. Waters, DD, et al: Comparison of clinical variables and variables derived from a limited predischarge exercise test as predictors of early and late mortality after myocardial infarction. J Am Coll Cardiol 5:1, 1985.
23. Hung, J, et al: Comparative value of maximal treadmill testing, exercise thallium myocardial perfusion scintigraphy, and exercise radionuclide ventriculography for distinguishing high and low risk patients soon after myocardial infarction. Am J Cardiol 53:1221, 1984.
24. Madsen, EB, et al: Prediction of late mortality after myocardial infarction from variables measured at different times during hospitalization. Am J Cardiol 53:47, 1984.
25. Krone, RJ, et al: Low level exercise testing after myocardial infarction: Usefulness in enhancing clinical risk stratification. Circulation 71:80, 1985.
26. DeBusk, RF: American College of Physician Position Paper: Evaluation of patients after recent acute myocardial infarction. Ann Intern Med 110:485, 1989.
27. American Thoracic Society: Evaluation of impairment/disability secondary to respiratory disorders. Am Rev Respir Dis 133:1205–1209, 1986.
28. Ries, A: Position Paper of the American Association of Cardiovascular and Pulmonary Rehabilitation: Scientific basis of pulmonary rehabilitation. J Cardiopulmonary Rehabil 10:418–441, 1990.
29. Reis, A: Endurance exercise training at maximal targets in patients with chronic obstructive pulmonary disease. J Cardiopulmonary Rehabil 7:594–601, 1987.
30. Carter, R, et al: Exercise conditioning in the rehabilitation of patients with chronic obstructive pulmonary disease. Arch Phys Med Rehabil 69:118–121, 1988.
31. Hodgkins, J: Prognosis in chronic obstructive pulmonary disease. Clin Chest Med 11(3):555–569, 1990.
32. Traver, G, Cline, M and Burrows, B: Predictors of mortality in chronic obstructive pulmonary disease: A 15 year follow up study. Am Rev Respir Dis 119:895–902, 1979.
33. Belman, M: Exercise in chronic obstructive pulmonary disease. Clin Chest Med 7(4):585–596, 1986.
34. Burrows, B, et al: The course and prognosis of different forms of chronic airway obstruction in a sample from the general population. N Engl J Med 317:1304–1309, 1987.
35. American College of Sports Medicine 1990 Position Stand. The recommended quantity and quality of exercise for developing and maintaining cardiorespiratory and muscular fitness in healthy adults. Med Sci Sports Exerc 22(2):265, 1990.
36. Karvonen, M, Kentala, K and Mustala, O: The effects of training on heart rate: A longitudinal study. Ann Med Exp Biol Fenn 35:307, 1957.
37. Davis, JA and Convertino, VA: A comparison of heart rate methods for predicting endurance training intensity. Med Sci Sports Exerc 7:295, 1975.
38. Pollock, ML and Wilmore, JH (eds): Exercise in Health and Disease: Evaluation and Prescription for Prevention and Rehabilitation, ed 2. WB Saunders, Philadelphia, 1990.
39. Borg, GAV: Psychophysical bases of perceived exertion. Med Sci Sports Exerc 14:377, 1982.
40. Noble BJ: Clinical applications of perceived exertion. Med Sci Sports Exerc 14:406, 1982.
41. Wenger, NA and Bell, GJ: The interactions of intensity, frequency, and duration of exercise training in altering cardiorespiratory fitness. Sports Med 3:346, 1986.
42. Pollock, ML, et al: Exercise prescription for rehabilitation of the cardiac patient. In Pollock, ML and Schmidt, DH (eds): Heart Disease and Rehabilitation, ed 2. John Wiley & Sons, New York, 1986, p 417.
43. Dressendorfer, RH and Smith, JL: Predictive accuracy of the maximum heart rate reserve method for estimating aerobic training intensity in early cardiac rehabilitation. J Cardiac Rehabil 4:484, 1984.
44. Franklin, BA, et al: Exercise prescription for the myocardial infarction patient. J Cardiopulmonary Rehabil 6:62, 1986.
45. Metier, CP, Pollock, ML and Graves, JE: Exercise prescription for the coronary artery bypass graft surgery patient. J Cardiopulmonary Rehabil 6:236, 1986.
46. Fox, SM, Naughton, JP and Gorman, PA: Physical activity and cardiovascular health. Part 3. The exercise prescription: Frequency and type of activity. Mod Concepts Cardiovasc Dis 41:25–30, 1972.
47. Borg, GV and Linderholm, H: Perceived exertion and pulse rate during graded exercise in various groups. Acta Med Scand (Suppl)472:194–206, 1967.
48. Borg, GV: Perceived exertion: A note on history and methods. Med Sci Sports Exerc, 5:90–93, 1973.
49. Borg, GV: Psychophysical bases of perceived exertion. Med Sci Sports Exerc 14:377–387, 1982.
50. Pollock, ML and Wilmore, JH: Exercise in Health and Disease: Evaluation and Prescription for Prevention and Rehabilitation, ed 2. WB Saunders, Philadelphia, 1990.
51. Pollock, ML and Froelicher, VF: Position stand of the American College of Sports Medicine: The recommended quantity and quality of exercise for developing and maintaining cardiorespiratory and muscular fitness in healthy adults. J Cardiopulmonary Rehabil 10:235–245, 1990.
52. Blair, SN, et al: Physical fitness and all-cause mortality: A prospective study of healthy men and women. JAMA 262:2395–2401, 1989.
53. Coyle, EF, et al: Time course of loss of adaptation after stopping prolonged intense endurance training. J Appl Physiol 57:1857–1864, 1984.
54. Hickson, RC and Rosenkoelter, MA: Reduced training frequencies and maintenance of increased aerobic power. Med Sci Sports Exerc 13:13–16, 1981.

55. Hickson, RC, et al: Reduced training duration effects on aerobic power, endurance, and cardiac growth. J Appl Physiol 53:225–229, 1982.
56. Hickson, RC, et al: Reduced training intensities and loss of aerobic power, endurance, and cardiac growth. J Appl Physiol 58:492–499, 1985.
57. Blair, SN, Kohl, HW and Goodyear, NN: Rates and risks for running and exercise injuries: Studies in three populations. Rev Quart Exerc Sports 58:221–228, 1987.
58. Powell, KE, et al: An epidemiological perspective of the causes of running injuries. Phys Sportsmed 14:100–114, 1986.
59. LeMura, LM, von Duvillard, SP and Bacharach, DW: Central versus peripheral adaptations for the enhancement of functional capacity in cardiac patients: A meta-analytic review. J Cardiopulmonary Rehabil 10:217–223, 1990.
60. Miller, WC: Introduction: Obesity, diet composition, energy expenditure, and treatment of the obese patient. Med Sci Sports Exerc 23:273–274, 1991.
61. Miller, WC: Diet composition, energy intake, and nutritional status in relation to obesity in men and women. Med Sci Sports Exerc 23:280–284, 1991.
62. Foreyt, JP and Goodrick, GK: Factors common to successful therapy for the obese patient. Med Sci Sports Exerc 23:292–297, 1991.
63. Graves, JE, et al: Specificity of limited range of motion variable resistance training. Med Sci Sports Exerc 21:84–89, 1989.
64. Franklin, BA, et al: Resistance training in cardiac rehabilitation. J Cardiopulmonary Rehabil 11:99–107, 1991.
65. Stewart, KJ: Resistive training effects on strength and cardiovascular endurance in cardiac and coronary prone patients. Med Sci Sports Exerc 21:678–682, 1989.
66. Kelemen, MH: Resistive training safety and assessment guidelines for cardiac and coronary prone patients. Med Sci Sports Exerc 21:675–677, 1989.
67. Tiep, B: Long term home oxygen therapy. Clin Chest Med 11:505–521, 1990.
68. American Thoracic Society: Standards for the diagnosis and care of patients with chronic obstructive pulmonary disease (COPD) and asthma. Am Rev Respir Dis 136(1):225–244, 1987.
69. Cox N, et al: Exercise and training in patients with chronic obstructive lung disease. Sports Med 6:180–192, 1988.
70. Nixon P, et al: Oxygen supplementation during exercise in cystic fibrosis. Am Rev Respir Dis 142:807–811, 1990.
71. Zack, M and Palange, A: Oxygen supplemented exercise of ventilatory and non-ventilatory muscles in pulmonary rehabilitation. Chest 88:669–675, 1985.
72. Bradley, B, et al: Oxygen assisted exercise in chronic obstructive lung disease: The effect on exercise capacity and arterial blood gas tensions. Am Rev Respir Dis 118:239–243, 1978.
73. Davidson A, et al: Supplemental oxygen and exercise ability in chronic obstructive airway disease. Thorax 43:965–971, 1988.
74. Wilson P, Bell, C and Norton, A: Rehabilitation of the Heart and Lungs. Beckman Instruments, Inc. Fullerton, CA, 1980.
75. Hodgkin, J: Pulmonary rehabilitation: Structure, components and benefits. J Cardiopulmonary Rehabil 11:423–434, 1991.
76. Stewart, A and Howard, P: Devices for low flow O_2 administration. Eur Respir J 3:812–817, 1990.
77. Russi, E, et al: Experiences with long term transtracheal oxygen therapy (abstract). Schweiz Rundsch Med Prox 79:850–853, 1990.
78. Tiep, B, et al: Pulsed nasal and transtracheal oxygen delivery. Chest 97(2):364–368, 1990.
79. Walsh, D and Govan, J: Long term continuous domiciliary oxygen therapy by transtracheal catheter. Thorax 45(6):478–481, 1990.
80. Wesmiller, S, et al: Exercise tolerance during nasal cannula and transtracheal oxygen delivery. Am Rev Respir Dis 14:789–791, 1990.
81. Tiep, B, et al: Demand oxygen delivery during exercise. Chest 9:15–20, 1987.

CHAPTER 12

The Exercise Therapy Session

CANDIDATES FOR REHABILITATION

Patients may be referred for cardiopulmonary exercise therapy following interpretation of their clinical data previously obtained via invasive and noninvasive testing procedures. Important results of the clinical evaluations are to determine (1) whether a patient is likely to benefit from exercise training, (2) the patient's ability to return to employment, (3) the success of current medical management, and (4) the amount of supervision and/or monitoring needed during the exercise session by each patient.

Cardiac Patients

Following completion of the clinical evaluation, cardiac patients are "stratified" according to the degree of risk, that is, low, medium, or high (see Table 11–1). Some cardiac patients are considered to be too high-risk during exercise to gain benefit and are excluded from exercise therapy programs.[1,2] Table 12–1 summarizes the conditions that would preclude a patient from being referred for exercise training.

Major reasons for risk stratification include establishing the prognosis a patient is likely to have, predicting the risk of further major events, and determining the patient's chance for survival, especially during the first year following an acute myocardial infarction (AMI) or coronary artery bypass graft surgery (CABG). Patients found to be at low risk following AMI or CABG have a first-year mortality rate of 2 percent[3] compared to a 10 to 25 percent mortality in moderate-risk patients. High-risk individuals' first-year mortality rates exceed 25 percent.[4]

Risk stratification is also being currently employed in the decision-making process to determine which patients should be continuously monitored during the exercise session. Although this topic is still controversial and some clinicians feel that all patients in phase II should be monitored, guidelines have been established to indicate which patients should probably be continuously monitored. The guidelines are presented in Table 12–2.[5]

An additional benefit of risk stratification is to determine the amount of supervision (staff-to-patient ratio) recommended for individual patients during the exercise training

TABLE 12–1 Absolute Contraindications to Exercise Training

Unstable angina
Uncontrolled congestive heart failure
Dysrhythmias compromising hemodynamic status
Uncontrolled hypertension
Acute myocarditis
Severe valvular stenosis
Hypertrophic cardiomyopathy
Acute pulmonary embolism or deep venous thrombosis

Source: From Balady, GJ and Weiner, DA: Risk stratification in cardiac rehabilitation. J Cardiopulmonary Rehabil 11:39–45, 1991, with permission.

sessions. The recommended staff-to-patient ratio for phase II cardiac rehabilitation is one staff member to supervise each five patients. The minimum staff required for operation of any cardiac rehabilitation program includes a supervising physician, program director, and registered nurse (the latter may also be the program director).[5,6]

Pulmonary Patients

Pulmonary patients can be grouped according to their degree of impairment. Patients most likely to benefit from a pulmonary rehabilitation program are those who (1) have moderate to moderately severe pulmonary disease, (2) are stable on current medical management for their diseases, (3) have minimal disease in other organ systems, (4) are willing to learn about their disease, and (5) are motivated to participate in an exercise program. Motivation seems to be the most important of all of the factors.[8,9]

Grouping patients according to their degree of disease may allow predictions of benefit, untoward events, return to work, and so on. Patients with mild disease may not recognize their disease or may not be willing to be active participants in a pulmonary rehabilitation program, and, therefore, may not benefit from the program. Patients whose severe pulmonary impairment results in a lack of adequate reserve in lung function may be too limited to benefit significantly.[8]

Patients with moderate to severe impairment may experience exercise hypoxemia, which will necessitate oximetric monitoring during the exercise session. Patients with

TABLE 12–2 Characteristics of Patients Most Likely to Benefit from Continuous Electrocardiogram Monitoring during Cardiac Rehabilitation

Severely depressed left ventricular function (ejection fraction less than 30%)
Resting complex ventricular arrhythmia
Ventricular arrhythmias that appear or increase with exercise
Survival of sudden cardiac death
Survival of myocardial infarction complicated by congestive heart failure, cardiogenic shock, and/or serious ventricular arrhythmias
Severe coronary artery disease and marked exercise-induced ischemia (ST depression >2 mm)
Inability to self-monitor heart rate (physical or intellectual impairment)

Source: Reprinted with permission from The American College of Cardiology (Journal of the American College of Cardiology 7(2):453, 1986.)

moderate to severe pulmonary disease with signs of cor pulmonale, ischemic heart disease, ventricular arrhythmias, and/or who are unable to self-monitor appropriately should be initially monitored by electrocardiogram (ECG).

Patients with mild pulmonary impairment do not correlate with diminished ability to perform most jobs, whereas moderate impairment is correlated with diminishing ability to meet the physical demands of many jobs. Severe impairment precludes gainful employment and reflects total disability.[10]

There are patients who may benefit from pulmonary rehabilitation who are not classified as having obstructive pulmonary disease. Persons in that category include those with restrictive pulmonary disease and/or with mixed diseases. However, pulmonary rehabilitation is not appropriate for some patients, especially those with such diseases as terminal lung cancer or acute respiratory failure.

Once a patient has been referred for cardiopulmonary rehabilitation, the rehabilitation team must provide a comprehensive program involving weight control, nutrition counseling, smoking cessation, social and psychologic support, and, of course, the exercise program. The goal is to return the patient to a productive lifestyle and to prevent or reverse (when possible) the progression of the disease process.[11]

This chapter will present the principles discussed in Chapter 11, The Exercise Prescription, and give examples of exercise prescription and progressions as they apply to cardiopulmonary rehabilitation. Case studies will be presented to illustrate the events that transpire during the exercise session. A discussion of patients with special needs in exercise training also will be briefly discussed.

COMPONENTS OF THE EXERCISE SESSION

Each exercise session usually includes a 5- to 10-minute warm-up, a cardiorespiratory (CR) exercise period of 20 to 60 minutes, a 5- to 10-minute cool-down, and perhaps some resistance training activities. The warm-up period may include flexibility exercises, and it should always include low-intensity CR activities performed below target heart rate (THR) levels and below the exercising rate of perceived exertion (RPE). The goal is to gradually elevate the heart rate (HR) from the resting level to just below the THR within the 5- to 10-minute period. Activities selected for the CR warm-up phase may include the same as those used for the CR endurance training, but they are performed at a lower intensity and heart rate. Longer warm-up periods may be needed for older and/or deconditioned patients, but the 5-minute warm-up is considered to be the minimal amount of warm-up prior to CR endurance training.[12]

Cardiorespiratory Endurance Training

The CR endurance training period should follow the warm-up phase. To produce the desired CR adaptations (increased functional capacity and so on), the goal of the CR endurance training period is for patients to perform 20 to 60 minutes of continuous aerobic activity. However, as indicated in Chapter 11, this is the goal, and especially in the early stages of CR conditioning, patients may not be able to perform continuous activity. It is fairly common for patients to initiate their CR programs by using discontinuous activity with frequent rest periods. No one part of the exercise prescription is more challenging to the clinician than that of prescribing the appropriate CR activity. It should be emphasized that it is best to increase the duration of the activity before the intensity of the CR activity is increased.[12,13] As functional capacity increases and physiological adaptation improves, the exercise prescription should be adjusted accordingly (Chapter 11).

Cool-Down

The CR endurance training period should be followed by a 5- to 10-minute cool-down period. Abrupt cessation of exercise may cause pooling of blood in the extremities. As a result of peripheral pooling, the brain, heart, or intestines may have insufficient blood supplies and such symptoms as vertigo, syncope, palpitations, or nausea may occur. Cardiac arrhythmias are sometimes precipitated following CR exercise, and a cool-down seems to be beneficial in preventing the potentially lethal irregularities that may result from increased catecholamine levels in the blood that are due to exercise.[14] Exercises similar to those used for the warm-up and/or the CR endurance training period are appropriate, but they should be performed at lower intensities. The heart rate should return to near resting levels before the patient is considered to be cooled down.

Resistive Exercises

As stated in Chapter 11, resistive exercise may be appropriate for cardiopulmonary patients provided it is undertaken with caution. When it is so prescribed, it is usually performed after the cool-down period that follows the CR endurance training. Blood pressures should be monitored before, during, and after the resistive training period, since the rate-pressure product (RPP) will increase, largely because of increases in systolic blood pressure. The resistive part of the rehabilitation process is usually prescribed after a patient has been aerobically conditioned for at least 3 months. The intensity begins gradually (usually at 30 percent of maximal effort) and progresses gradually until the patient can perform one to three sets of 12 to 15 repetitions. The resistance may be gradually increased to 60 percent of one maximal effort, but the decision to do so is based on each individual's responses to resistive training.[12,15]

CASE STUDIES

To enhance the clinician's decision-making skills with regard to modification of the exercise prescription, this section includes case studies that describe a 12-week course of treatment for two patients with cardiovascular disease and two case studies that describe an 8- to 12-week course of treatment for two patients with pulmonary disease. Each case study includes the initial exercise prescription and rationale as well as a summary of the data obtained during the exercise training sessions that justify change in the exercise prescription. In that way, the developmental progression of the training sessions, as well as many of the factors that enter into the decision-making process for writing and adjusting an exercise prescription, can be more easily understood. Additional guidelines for outpatient cardiac exercise are included in Appendix F.

CASE STUDY 8, CHAPTER 9

This section describes the course of rehabilitative treatment for Case Study 8, Chapter 9. The initial exercise prescription written for this patient is given in Table 12–3. The prescription is based on the results of his graded exercise tolerance test (GXTT) (Chapter 9, Table 9–23) and the information gathered from his completed preliminary forms and interview.

Aspects of this 50-year-old male cardiac patient's history that have particular significance in relation to the patient's exercise prescription include hypertensive response to exercise, ST-T depression of 3 mm in V_5 with the absence of angina, bilateral leg claudication (pain level 1) at 3 metabolic equivalents (METs), and ventricular arrhythmias that occurred during the cool-down and recovery periods. His risk stratification is high, and he is therefore classified as a high-risk cardiac patient who should be monitored during the exercise sessions.

In formulating his training THR, both the functional capacity (METs) achieved on his GXTT and a formula for THR were considered. The MET level achieved on the GXTT was 5 METs, and his exercise prescription according to his functional capacity was calculated to be 2 to 4.25 METs (0.40 to 0.85 × 5; see Chapter 11). Using the Karvonen formula[17] (Fig. 11–1) for calculating his THR, his target heart rate range (THRR) was found to be 68 to 91 beats per minute (bpm). Considering that the maximal HR achieved on the GXTT was 98 bpm, that his blood pressure at that level was 156/98, and that he experienced claudication and ST-T depression (Table 9–23), the initial exercise prescription should be written for the lowest THR within his range, that is, 68 bpm.

As well as continuously monitoring the ECG of this patient, the blood pressure (BP) response to exercise should be monitored at regular intervals as needed. The bicycle ergometer and treadmill (or other means of walking) should be selected as the primary mode of exercise to be used in CR training because alternate bouts of walking and cycling will minimize his leg pain. If the Schwinn Airdyne or similar ergometer is used, the patient should be instructed, initially, to refrain from using his arms to maintain his work load on the bike, because to maintain it may increase his BP response to exercise (Chapter 4). As his functional capacity improves, the patient may be allowed to use his arms in CR activity. Work load performed on the bicycle and the walking distance covered per exercise bout should be carefully recorded to give the patient and staff objective feedback on the intensity of the exercise. Accurate recording of the data makes it easier to identify the point at which training adaptations occur. Educating the patient regarding training adaptations (Chapter 4) and linking the adaptations to changes in daily exercise data help to motivate the patient to proceed with training. That is also helpful in the self-education process the patient is given in a structured rehabilitation program, so that regular exercise becomes a lifelong commitment once the patient graduates from the formal program.[5,11,16]

Initially, this patient may require longer than average warm-up and cool-down periods to prevent ventricular irritability. Also, his pain tolerance may not permit continuous exercise, and his walking and cycling bouts might have to be limited to 2 to 3 minutes of exercise followed by 1 or 2 minutes of rest. Intermittent exercise should be extended to continuous exercise as soon as possible. That is done by gradually decreasing the rest period, increasing the exercise period, or both. The length of the total CR training period (excluding warm-up and cool-

TABLE 12–3 Initial Exercise Prescription for
Case Study 8, Chapter 9

Exercise Rx

Name __Case Study 8, Chapter 9__ F (M) Age __50__ Date _____

Ht. (in) __69__ Wt. (lb) __160__

Dx: __CAD, Post-MI, Post CABG, hyperlipidemia, PVD__

Meds: __Cardizem, Isordil, Transderm 5__

Comments: __Mild hypertensive response on GXTT, ST-T depression of 3 mm in V_5 at__
Max HR on GXT, Leg claudication-bilateral at 3 METs on GXTT, PVCs, bigeminy
during cool-down and recovery.

GXT Data: Date performed __2/4/91__   Where: __Clinic X__
           Rest HR __48__   Protocol: __Bruce Treadmill__
           Max HR __98__   Max METS: __5__
           Re-evaluation scheduled __5/7/91__

Risk Stratification: High

C-R Rx:

  (METs) = 40% to 85% of Max METs
         = .40 to .85 X __5__
         = __2.0–4.25 METs__

  THRR (bpm) = (Max HR − Rest HR) (.40 − .85) + (Rest HR)
             = (___98___ − ___48___)(.40 TO .85) + (48)
             = __68–91__ bpm

  Type of exercise: __X__ bike ____ row __X__ walk ____ walk/jog
                    (Intermittent progressing to continuous as able.)

  Length of session: __20–60 min__ Frequency: __3Xs/week__
  Comments: __Initial HR: 68 bpm based on Target Heart Rate. Longer cool-down__
  Subjective gradation of pain = 2 at Max HR on GXT. RPP = 152

Flexibility Rx: __Stretching for calves, hamstrings, quads, hip flexors — 3Xs/week prior to__
exercise and daily on alternate days

Muscular S & End Rx: __N/A begin as needed as need p re-eval. 5/7/91__

% Body Fat Rx:
    __20%__   Desirable M __15%__
                                                F __25%__

Body Wt. __160__ lbs Desired Range __150__ to __160__ lbs
         __73__ kg
Referred for lipid-lowering diet plan and nutrition education.

TABLE 12-4 Summary of 12-Week Cardiac Exercise Program for Case Study 8, Chapter 9

Date	Rest HR	Rest BP	TARGET HR	W-UP	C-R Work Type-Min.*	C-R HR	Laps Wkload.	Cool-Down HR	Cool-Down BP	Wt. lb.	Comments: BPs, Arrhythmias, Med. Changes, Symptoms, etc.
WEEK 1	50	140/84	78	72	B-3, R-2 / W-3, R-2	76–72 / 78–74 / 76–72 / 78–74	0.8 KP / 3 Laps / 0.8 KP / 3 Laps	48	128/80	160	BP 1stB—144/82; BP 2ndW—138/82; 20' Inter. CRE$_x$. Pt. tolerance good. No pain on bike, pain level 1 walking. 7 min. cool-down. No arrhythmias
WEEK 2	48	138/82	78	70	B-4, R-1 / W-4, R-1 / B-4, R-1	78 / 78 / 76	0.9 KP / 5 Laps / 0.9 KP	68	118/78	159	BP 1stW—138/80; BP 3rdB—126/80; 25' Continuous CRE$_x$. Pt. tolerance good. Pain level 1 walking. 7 min. cool-down
WEEK 3	60	138/74	78–80	72	B-5 / W-5 / B-5 / W-5 / B-5	76 / 80 / 78 / 80 / 78	0.8 KP / 6 Laps / 0.8 KP / 5 Laps / 0.8 KP	70	126/70	158	BP 2ndB—132/72; 25' Continuous CRE$_x$. Pt. tolerance good. Pain level 1 to 2 walking. 6 min. cool-down. No arrhythmias
WEEK 4	60	126/74	78–80	72	B-5 / W-5 / B-5 / W-5 / B-5	78 / 80 / 80 / 80 / 80	0.9 KP / 6 Laps / 1.0 KP / 6 Laps / 0.9 KP	60	126/70	158	BP only prn; 25' Continuous CRE$_x$. Pt. tolerance good. 6 min. cool-down. No arrhythmias

Continued

315

TABLE 12–4 continued

Date	Rest HR	Rest BP	HR TARGET W-UP	C-R Work Type-Min.*	C-R HR	Laps Wkload.	Cool-Down HR	Cool-Down BP	Wt. lb.	Comments — BPs, Arrhythmias, Med. Changes, Symptoms, etc.
	54	128/72	80 / 72	B-5	80	1.0 KP	60	124/70	158.5	Pt. tolerance good
				W-5	78	6 Laps				6 min. cool-down
				B-5	80	1.0 KP				No arrhythmias
				W-5	80	6 Laps				BP only prn
				B-5	80	0.9 KP				30′ Continuous CRE$_x$
WEEK 5				W-5	80	6 Laps				
	72	160/90	76 / 72	B-5	74	0.7 KP	70	128/80	158	↓Target Hr. Pt. tired, worked overtime all week
				W-5	76	4 Laps				BP p̄ 2nd Bike—132/84
				B-5	74	0.7 KP				BP p̄ 2nd Walk— 130/80
				W-5	76	5 Laps				30′ Continuous CRE$_x$
				B-5	74	0.7 KP				7 min. cool-down
WEEK 6				W-5	74	4 Laps				
	54	120/70	80 / 72	B-5	78	1.0 KP	62	118/70	157	Pt. tolerance good
				W-5	80	6 Laps				6 min. cool-down
				B-5	78	1.0 KP				No arrhythmias
				W-5	80	6 Laps				BP only prn
				B-5	78	1.0 KP				35′ Continuous CRE$_x$
WEEK 7				W-5	80	6 Laps				

WEEK				Activity*							Notes
WEEK 8	54	80	68	B-5	78	1.0 KP					Pt. tolerance good
			118/70	W-5	80	6 Laps					6 min. cool-down
				B-5	80	1.1 KP					No arrhythmias
				W-5	80	6 Laps	70	114/68	157	BP prn / 40' Continuous CRE$_x$	
WEEK 9	50	80	72	B-5	80	1.1 KP					Pt. tolerance good
			118/70	W-5	80	6 Laps					6 min. cool-down
				B-5	80	1.1 KP					No arrhythmias
				W-5	80	6 Laps					
				B-10	80	1.1 KP					
				W-5	80	6–7 Laps					
				B-10	80	1.1 KP					
				W-5	80	7 Laps					
				B-10	80	1.1 KP	68	112/68	156	BP prn / 40' Continuous CRE$_x$	
WEEK 10	48	80	74	B-10	80	1.2 KP					Pain Level 1 s/t cramping
			120/70	W-7	80	10 Laps					5 min. cool-down
				B-10	80	1.2 KP					No arrhythmias
				W-7	80	10 Laps					
				B-10	80	1.2 KP	64	114/68	156	BP prn / 44' Continuous CRE$_x$	
WEEK 11	48	80	68	B-10	78	1.2–1.3 KP					Pt. tolerance good
			118/68	W-10	80	13 Laps					Pain level 1
				B-10	80	1.3 KP					5 min. cool-down
				W-10	80	14 Laps	62	112/64	156	BP prn / 45' Continuous CRE$_x$	No arrhythmias
WEEK 12	46	80	72	B-10	80	1.3 KP					Pt. tolerance good
			118/70	W-10	80	14–15 Laps					Pain level 1
				B-10	80	1.3 KP					5 min. cool-down
				W-10	80	14–15 Laps	64	110/60	156	BP prn / 45' Continuous CRE$_x$	No arrhythmias
				B-5							

*B = Bike; W = Walk; R = Rest
Re-evaluation:

317

down) should be increased gradually from 20 to 45 minutes over a period of weeks. The patient should be encouraged to exercise at home in addition to the on-site therapy sessions, which should be scheduled a minimum of three times per week on alternate days.

The flexibility program for this patient should emphasize the muscles and joints of the legs and hips and exclude any exercises that may place excessive stress on a joint or change BP. Stretching may be performed prior to or after CR training, and the exercises should be clearly explained and demonstrated. This patient should be checked periodically to make sure that, while stretching, no straining or actual pain occurs and that he is breathing slowly and rhythmically and not holding his breath.

A muscular strength and endurance training program is not indicated for this patient at this time. The instability of his medical status rules out, initially, any type of training other than CR and mild flexibility exercises.

This patient should be referred for nutrition education regarding cardiovascular disease and a lipid-lowering diet regimen (Chapter 13). He is within his ideal weight range, and his percent body fat should decline as a result of the CR training.

A summary of this patient's course of treatment is recorded on a sample data sheet (Table 12–4). Note that although the THR remained relatively the same (78 to 80 bpm), the work load was increased to compensate for the improvements made in CR endurance.

As the patient's BP response to exercise improved, the need for BP measurement during exercise bouts declined and BP during exercise was not measured again except for week 6, when he worked overtime and his resting values were unusually high. Note also that his unusually high BP at rest that week required an adjustment in both the THR and the work load.

By keeping the THR low and increasing the length of the cool-down period during the 12 weeks, the patient was able to tolerate the CR exercise well and exhibited no dysrhythmias. Gradual increases in the length of time he walked enabled him to exercise with manageable pain (<2 subjective gradation of pain).

CASE STUDY 5, CHAPTER 9

The following is a description of the rehabilitative treatment for Case Study 5, Chapter 9. An initial exercise prescription written for this patient is given in Table 12–5. The prescription is based on the results of her GXTT (Table 9–20) and the information obtained from her completed preliminary forms and interview.

Although not a coronary artery diseased patient, certain features of the 70-year-old hypertensive female patient's medical history and response to the GXTT have special significance; namely, her age, arthritic condition (which limits her orthopedically), severe hypertensive response to exercise, and extremely deconditioned state (<2 METs on GXTT).

Her CR training heart rate should be determined after careful consideration of both the functional capacity and the Karvonen method[17] for calculating THR (see Fig. 11–1). Her functional capacity is approximately 2 METs. During the performance of her GXTT, the 2-MET level elicited an HR response of 113 bpm and a BP response of 220/136 (see Table 9–20). The THR calculations result in a THR range

TABLE 12–5 Initial Exercise Prescription for
Case Study 5, Chapter 9

Exercise Rx

Name _Case Study 5, Chapter 9_ (F) M   Age _70_ Date _____

Ht. (in) _59_ Wt. (lb) _180_

Dx: _Hypertension, Obesity, Arthritis (knees, wrists, spine)_

Meds: _HydroDIURIL, Aldomet_

Comments: _Severe hypertensive response to exercise Max BP 220/136 severely_
deconditioned, orthopedic limitations.

GXT Data: Date performed _6/7/91_   Where: _Clinic X_

Rest HR _62_   Protocol: _Adapted Astrand-Rhyming_
Bike

Max HR _113_   Max METS: _2_

Re-evaluation scheduled _9/15/91_

Risk Stratification: Intermediate

C-R Rx:

$$(\text{METs}) = 40\% \text{ to } 85\% \text{ of Max METs}$$
$$= .40 \text{ to } .85 \times \underline{2}$$
$$= \underline{1-2 \text{ METS}} \quad (\text{low end is due to age \& BP} = 1 \text{ MET})$$
$$\text{THRR (bpm)} = (\text{Max HR} - \text{Rest HR})(.40 - .85) + (\text{Rest HR})$$
$$= (\underline{113-62})(.40) + (\underline{62})$$
$$= \underline{82-105} \text{ bpm}$$

Type of exercise: _X_ bike ____ row ____ walk ____ walk/jog
(no arms on Schwinn Airdyne until adapt. occurs)

Length of session: _20–30 min_ Frequency: _3Xs/week_

Comments: _Initial HR based on Functional Capacity and THR = 82 bpm. Limited_
by BP response. Intermittent CR exercise initially 2–3 min of exercise with
1–2 min rest. Progress to continuous.

RPP = 248. Take more frequent BPs.

Flexibility Rx: _General program with emphasis on affected joints performed 3Xs/day_

Muscular S & End Rx: _Mild strengthening program for quadriceps and hamstrings—_
10 reps, 3Xs/day—no weights

% Body Fat Rx:
_44%_
                          Desirable M _15%_
                                   F _25%_

Body Wt. _180_ lbs Desired Range _115_ to _125_ lbs
_82_ kg

Referred also for nutrition education and weight reduction.

of 82 to 114 bpm. However, considering the rapid rise in both systolic and diastolic BP (to 220/136) in 3 minutes, it may be dangerous (see the section on rate-pressure product in Chapter 9) for her to exercise at an HR above the lower end of her THR (40 percent in the Karvonen formula). Therefore, her initial THR should be 82 bpm, and since she is extremely deconditioned, her CR training will have to be intermittent training, at least initially. The duration of the CR training should be adjusted by gradually increasing the rest periods between them. Once she is able to perform 20 to 30 minutes of continuous activity, the THR, and therefore the intensity, may be adjusted upward.

This patient's BP response to exercise should be monitored at regular intervals during the CR exercise session, because her BP response is another indicator of the intensity of her CR exercise and it, not her HR, may be her limiting factor. Remember that a diastolic BP of 120 mm Hg is considered to be a criterion for termination of exercise (Chapter 9).

The bicycle ergometer is the mode of choice for CR training of this patient. Because of her arthritic condition and her obesity, it is important to reduce the pressure on her weight-bearing joints. Also, with the bicycle ergometer, lower initial work loads and smaller work-load increments can be prescribed to avoid overtaxing her in her deconditioned state. The Schwinn Airdyne or other bicycle ergometer may be used, and the patient should be instructed not to use her arms to maintain her work load (Chapter 4). The work load performed on the bicycle ergometer during each exercise bout should be carefully recorded. If weight loss and orthopedic conditions permit, walking may be added to her CR training program after initial improvements in strength and CR endurance are noted.

Initially this patient may require shorter than average warm-up and cool-down periods because of her deconditioned state. Her muscular weakness will not permit continuous exercise, and her cycling should be limited to bouts of 2 or 3 minutes of exercise followed by 1 or 2 minutes of rest. Intermittent exercise should be extended to continuous exercise as soon as possible. This patient should not be encouraged to perform CR exercise at home until her BP response is under control.

The flexibility program for this patient should emphasize range-of-motion exercises for her affected joints. All stretching exercises should be performed in comfortable positions, most of which should be supported. A seated position should minimize the amount of strength required for stretching and permit the patient to concentrate on stretching technique. As muscular strength improves, the position in which the flexibility exercises are performed may be modified. The patient should be encouraged to perform the flexibility exercises daily.

Mild strengthening exercises should be prescribed for this patient because her quadriceps muscle weakness will limit her ability to perform CR training exercises. However, her BP response to even mild strengthening exercises must be evaluated when she performs the exercises for the first time (Chapter 11). If her BP response is too high, the exercises should be added only after her BP response to exercise improves or her medication is adjusted.

This patient's medical problems are compounded by her obesity, and she should be referred for nutritional counseling (Chapter 13). Fortunately, she is neither diabetic nor hyperlipidemic and should be able to tolerate a low-calorie general meal plan.

The following is a summary of this patient's course of treatment recorded on a sample data sheet (Table 12–6). Note that the patient was unable to tolerate CR

TABLE 12-6 Summary of a 12-Week Cardiovascular Exercise
Program for Case Study 5, Chapter 9

Date	Rest HR	Rest BP	HR TARGET / W-UP	C-R Work Type-Min.*	C-R HR	Laps Wkload.	Cool-Down HR	Cool-Down BP	Wt. Lb.	BPs, Arrhythmias, Med. Changes, Symptoms, etc. (Comments)
WEEK 1	66	162/92	88 / 76	B-3, R-2	80	0.5 KP	78	160/90	180	B1st BP—170/103 Exercise terminated p 3rd bike due to hypertensive response to ex.
				B-3, R-3	82	0.5 KP				B2nd BP—172/106
				B-3, R-3	86	0.5 KP				B3rd BP—180/112
				B-3, Terminate						9' CRE$_x$ Intermittent
										10 minute cool-down
WEEK 2	52	152/84	78 / 68	B-2, R-2	72	0.5 KP	60	148/82	178	B2nd BP—160/86 Medication change: Tenormin Lower Target HR Good tolerance
				B-2, R-2	76	0.5 KP				B4th BP—168/90
				B-2, R-2	78	0.5 KP				10' CRE$_x$ Intermittent
				B-2, R-2	75	0.5 KP				10' cool-down
				B-2, R-2	78	0.5 KP				
WEEK 3	52	140/78	78 / 66	B-3, R-1	70	0.5 KP	58	138/76	176	B2nd BP—156/82 Good tolerance, below THR
				B-3, R-1	70	0.5 KP				B4th BP—154/80
				B-3, R-1	70	0.5 KP				12' CRE$_x$ Intermittent
				B-3, R-1	70	0.5 KP				8' cool-down
WEEK 4	50	152/74	78 / 68	B-5, R-1	78	0.6 KP	56	142/74	173	B2nd BP—148/76 Good tolerance, on target
				B-5, R-1	72	0.6 KP				B4th BP—144/74
				B-5, R-1	78	0.6 KP				20' CRE$_x$ Intermittent
				B-5, R-1	78	0.6 KP				8' cool-down

TABLE 12–6 continued

Date	Rest HR	Rest BP	TARGET HR	W-UP HR	C-R Work Type-Min.*	C-R HR	Laps Wkload.	Cool-Down HR	Cool-Down BP	Wt. Lb.	BPs, Arrhythmias, Med. Changes, Symptoms, etc.
WEEK 5	48	130/82	78	60	B-5	78	0.6–.7 KP	60	132/78	172	B3rd BP-132/80 20'CR Continuous — Good tolerance 6' cool-down
					B-5	73	0.6–.7 KP				
					B-5	78	0.6–.7 KP				
					B-5	78	0.6–.7 KP				
WEEK 6	50	136/74	78	66	B-5	72	0.7 KP	54	132/72	170	3rdB BP— 130/76 25' CR Continuous — Good tolerance 6' cool-down
					B-5	72	0.7 KP				
					B-5	73	0.7 KP				
					B-5	72	0.7 KP				
					B-5	78	0.7 KP				
WEEK 7	50	130/74	78	66	B-5	78	0.8 KP	58	128/72	168	BPs prn 30' CR Continuous — Good tolerance 6' cool-down
					B-5	76	0.8 KP				
					B-5	78	0.8 KP				
					B-5	76	0.8 KP				
					B-5	78	0.8 KP				
					B-5	78	0.8 KP				
WEEK 8	48	130/68	78	66	B-5	78	0.8–.9 KP	54	128/74	165	BPs prn 30' CR Continuous — Good tolerance 5' cool-down
					B-5	78	0.8–.9 KP				
					B-5	78	0.8–.9 KP				
					B-5	76	0.8–.9 KP				
					B-5	78	0.8–.9 KP				
					B-5	78	0.8–.9 KP				

Week	Rest HR	Rest BP	Ex HR	Post HR	Activity	HR	Intensity	HR	BP	Peak HR		Comments
WEEK 9	48	128/70	78	66	B-5 B-5 B-5 B-5 B-5 B-5	76 76 78 76 76 76	1.0 KP 1.0 KP 1.0 KP 1.0 KP 1.0 KP 1.0 KP	50	110/70	163	BPs prn 30' CR Continuous	Good tolerance 5' cool-down
WEEK 10	48	128/72	78	64	B-5 W-5 B-5 B-5 W-5 B-5	76 78 76 78 78 76	1.0 KP 5 Laps 1.0 KP 5 Laps 1.0 KP 5 Laps	50	114/70	160	BPs prn 30' CR Continuous	Add walk to CR Ex. Good tolerance 5' cool-down
WEEK 11	50	118/74	78	66	B-5 W-5 B-5 W-5 B-5 W-5	76 76 76 78 76 78	1.1 KP 6 Laps 1.1 KP 6 Laps 1.1 KP 6 Laps	48	110/70	158	BPs prn 30' CR Continuous	Increase Walking to ½ of Cr Ex Good tolerance 5' cool-down
WEEK 12	50	114/72	78	68	W-5 B-10 W-5 B-10	76 76 76 76	7 Laps 1.2 KP 7 Laps 1.2 KP	48	110/68	156	BPs prn 30' CR Continuous	↑Length of CR bouts Good tolerance 5' cool-down

*B = Bike; W = Walk; R = Rest.
Re-evaluation:

exercise bouts of 3 minutes and had to be referred to her physician regarding her continuation in the program (see example re-referral form in Appendix B). Her physician added Tenormin to her HydroDIURIL and eliminated Aldomet. Tenormin, a beta-blocking drug, reduced her resting heart rate from 66 bpm to approximately 50 bpm. The medication change necessitated a change in her THR prescription. Although general guidelines regarding the effect of a beta-blocking agent on maximum heart rate are available, the true effect is difficult to predict because it is influenced by both dosage and individual patient response. A practical approach to changing the THR in this case is to exercise the patient at the same work load as prior to the medication change and establish a THR range based on the response. The patient's HR response to the same work load was approximately 8 to 10 bpm lower as a result of the beta-blocking medication. Thus, her new THR range became 72 to 95 bpm.

As the patient's BP response to exercise improved, the need for frequent BP measurement during exercise bouts declined. BP was not measured during exercise after the sixth week of CR training. Her flexibility and muscular strength training also were adjusted at this time. Her improved recovery from CR exercise resulted in a decrease in the time of her cool-down period.

The patient's compliance to her weight-reducing regimen was demonstrated by her weight loss of 24 lb over the 12-week period. Her weight loss enhanced her CR training response and enabled her to tolerate more walking exercise and longer bouts of continuous cycling.

CASE STUDY 1, CHAPTER 10

This section will describe the rehabilitative course for the patient in Case Study 1, Chapter 10. The initial exercise prescription is summarized in Table 12–7. The prescription is based on the results of a symptom-limited cycle ergometer test. (Table 10–3 gives the results of this exercise test.)

This patient's assessment was remarkable for her severe obstructive pulmonary disease, desaturation during exercise, and the recorded bronchospastic response to exercise. Reviewing Table 10–3, $\dot{V}Emax$ was predicted to be 23.1 liters per minute based on pre-exercise FEV_1 of 0.68 liters per minute ($FEV_1 \times 35 = \dot{V}Emax$). However, if the post-exercise FEV_1 of 0.6 liters per minute were used in the calculation, the predicted $\dot{V}Emax$ would be only 21.0 liters per minute. This patient achieved 17.8 maximum ventilation, which is 88 percent of the adjusted predicted $\dot{V}Emax$, certainly close to her predicted respiratory maximum. Her ECG was normal throughout her exercise session, and her termination was due to leg fatigue.

Using the Karvonen formula, her THRR is calculated as follows:

(Maximum HR − resting HR)(40% to 85%) + resting HR = THR
(123 − 108)(40% to 85%) + 108 = 114 to 121 bpm

Since this patient tested quite close to her respiratory maximum and has severe obstructive pulmonary disease with no compounding system disease, it was decided that she could exercise close to the maximum THRR. Using a THR of 80 percent of the HR reserve results in a THR of 120 bpm.

TABLE 12–7 Pulmonary Exercise Prescription for
Case 1, Chapter 10

Exercise Rx

Name __Case Study 1, Chap. 10__ (F) M   Age __61__ Date _____

Pack-years __45__ Ht. (in) __65__ Wt. (lbs) __124__

Dx: __COPD, Asthma, Orthostatic hypotension, S/P Mastectomy__

Meds: __Tamoxatrin, imipramine, Ventolin MDI, Atrovent MDI,__
Slo-phyllin, Ativan

Comments: __ECG normal before and after exercise. Quit smoking 8 years ago. Termination:__
Leg fatigue

GXT Data: Date performed __4/5/91__   Where: __Clinic X__

Rest HR __108__   Protocol: __Modified cycle__

Max HR __123__   Max METs: __2.8__

Re-evaluation scheduled __7/12/91__

PFT Interpretation: __Bronchospastic response to exercise moderately severe mechanical__
and diffusion limitations

C-R Rx:

$$\text{Functional Capacity (METs)} = 40\% \text{ to } 85\% \text{ of Max METs}$$
$$= .40 \text{ to } .85 \times \underline{2.8}$$
$$= \underline{1.1 \text{ to } 2.4} \text{ METs}$$

$$\text{THRR (bpm)} = (\text{Max HR} - \text{Rest HR})(.40 - .85) + (\text{Rest HR})$$
$$= \underline{114-121} \text{ bpm}$$

$$\text{RPE (10-point scale)} = \underline{4 \text{ to } 5}$$

Type of exercise: __X__ bike _____ row __X__ walk

_____ walk/jog _____ stairs
__X__ arm ergometry

Circuit program: __10-min walk, 5 min bike (20 watts), 5 min arm ergometer, RPE not to__
exceed 5

Length of session: __20 min__   Frequency: __3X/wk__

Comments: __Suggest Ventolin and Atrovent MDIs prior to ex. 16 stairs at home, work on__
pacing.

Flexibility Rx: __General flexibility exercises with emphasis on head, neck, and shoulders.__

Muscular strength and endurance Rx: __Not applicable at this time. If METs increase,__
consider light weights later

Monitoring and Oxygen Needs

Telemetry _____   Oximetry __X__

Supplemental oxygen __3 liters__

Comments: __Dropped Pao$_2$ during exercise. Oximetry evaluation with 3 liters of oxygen__
with exercise. Keep sats above 85%

It was suggested that the patient use her metered dose inhaler (MDI) bronchodilators prior to the exercise session to help avoid the bronchospasm induced by exercise. As she was always encouraged to use those drugs just prior to exercise, her resting heart rate was often elevated prior to the beginning of exercise. Therefore, the THR was not strictly utilized; instead, symptoms and RPE dictated the exercise session.

The patient was placed (by the attending physician) on 3 liters per minute of nasal cannula oxygen during exercise sessions, which resulted in oxygen saturation of no less than 92 percent. Because of oximetry monitoring, the patient initially was required to exercise on the following stationary equipment: treadmill, cycle, and arm ergometer. Midway through the second week of exercise, oximetry readings were stable and oxygen saturation was checked only periodically. She was then free to ambulate out-of-doors on the track. Since the ability to walk out-of-doors was one of the goals she had set for the rehabilitation process, outdoor walking was strongly encouraged. Compliance with the rehabilitation program and her own home program might increase if her goals were incorporated in the rehabilitation program.

This patient had a 15 minute warm-up session that included general flexibility with special attention to the shoulders and neck. Care was taken to perform the exercises properly so that stretching was done on exhalation only to discourage the Valsalva maneuver. No pain should be experienced with the flexibility exercises. This patient was able to do the exercises on a mat on the floor. The warm-up was done on a treadmill at a perceived slow pace (RPE of 3). A cycle ergometer pedaled at 10 to 15 mph with no resistance could have been chosen as a warm-up as well. The warm-up period for this patient was especially important because of her exercise-induced bronchospasm. Her warm-up was maintained at 15 minutes throughout the rehabilitative process because of her potential for bronchospasm.

The CR endurance training began with ambulation, cycle ergometry, and arm ergometry. A circuit program allows for a variety of exercise modes to increase the specificity of training as well as to maintain interest in the activities. The patient accomplished three exercise sessions the first week with no symptoms of muscle soreness, fatigue, or joint pain. The program included 5 minutes of activity interspersed with rest periods. Exercise progression would be accomplished by increasing the amount of continuous activity until 30 minutes could be completed. Table 12-8 provides a weekly summary of the exercise performed. Exercise progression can be inferred from reviewing the chart.

Cool-down was accomplished by ambulating again on the treadmill at an RPE of 3. Flexibility exercises were repeated, and the HR was taken. Occasionally, this patient had an elevated HR after her 10 minutes of cool-down. When that occurred, diaphragmatic breathing was practiced for 5 to 10 minutes with a continued decline in HR approaching resting. The patient was not dismissed from the rehabilitation session until her HR had returned to a reasonable resting level.

At week 3, pulsed portable home oxygen was supplied by a home care service company. A home exercise program was begun, and compliance was fair. The patient was hindered by the 16 stairs at home. Therefore, during week 4 of the rehabilitation program, stair climbing was substituted for biking.

During the final week of her pulmonary rehabilitation program, her physician asked her to perform exercise using a reduced amount of oxygen: 2 liters per minute. Oxygen saturation was found to decrease to 86 percent during exercise,

TABLE 12-8 Summary of 8-Week Pulmonary Exercise Program for Case Study 1, Chapter 10

Date	Rest		HR		C-R Training					Cool-Down		O₂	Comments
	HR	BP	THRR THR	W-UP	C-R Work Type-Min*	HR	RPE	RR %Sat	Distance Work Load	HR	BP	Liters/Min	BPs, Arrhythmias, Med. Changes, Symptoms, etc.
WEEK 1	114	144/92	114–121 / 120	114	W-5 / R-5 / W-5 / R-5 / B-5 / A-2 / R-2 / A-2	116 / 120 / 120	3-4 / 5	28 / 30 / 92	1400 ft / 20 W / 15 W	108	136/90	3L	Meds prior to exercise, 15-min warm-up % sats remain 90–93 range throughout program Spot check & paddles—NSR 10-min cool-down
WEEK 2	108	130/84	114–121 / 120	112	W-5 / R-2 / W-5 / B-5 / R-3 / A-3 / R-2 / A-3	120 / 120 / 120	4 / 4 / 5	30 / 92	1800 ft / 20 W / 15 W	114	134/88	3L	Meds prior to exercise, 15-min warm-up Ambulated out of doors Sats on 3L remain good Oximeter spot check only 10-min cool-down
WEEK 3	114	140/80	114–121 / 120	114	W-10 / R-2 / W-10 / A-3 / R-2 / A-3	120 / 120	4 / 5 / 5	24 / 30 / 30	1700 ft / 1700 ft / 15 W	108	144/86	3L	Meds prior to exercise, 15-min warm-up Walk out-of-doors—enjoying being outside. Oxygen at home delivered. Port pack filled. Walking 10–15 min/day 10-min cool-down

Continued

TABLE 12-8 continued

Date	Rest HR	Rest BP	HR THRR/THR	W-UP	C-R Work Type-Min*	HR	RPE	RR	%Sat	Distance Work Load	Cool-Down HR	Cool-Down BP	O₂ Liters/Min	Comments BP's, Arrhythmias, Med. Changes, Symptoms, etc.
WEEK 4	114	134/76	114–121 / 120		W-15 R-2 W-13 B-5	120 120	5	30		3200 ft 3000 ft 20 W	114	134/80	3L	Meds taken, 15-min warm-up Stairs & pacing taught 2 flight 2 stairs per exhalation 10-min cool-down
WEEK 5	112	128/74	114–121 / 120	116	W-23½ A-4 R-2 A-4	123	5	28		4500 ft	120	126/78	3L	Meds prior to exercise, 15-min warm-up, 10-min cool-down Diaphraquatic breathing after cool-down, HR down to 116 Stairs: 2/stairs breath pacing 1 floor Enjoys walking out-of-doors (hates arm ergometer!)
WEEK 6	108	126/80	114–121 / 120	108	W-25 A-3½ R-2 A-4	120 123	4½	30 28		5000 ft 20 W	114	124/80	3L	Meds taken, 15-min warm-up Stairs: 1 flight 2/stairs breath pacing Home program increased to 25 min, walking 5 times a week 10-min cool-down

									Notes
WEEK 7	106	114–121 / 120	134/80	W-30 / A-5 / 110	126 / 120 / 3 / 4	30 / 30	5000 ft / 20 W	110 / 140/84	3L	Meds taken, 15-min warm-up; Stairs: 2 flights up, 2:1 pacing; Continuous down whole flight; Home program—good compliance; 10-min cool-down
WEEK 8	108	114–121 / 120	134/90	W-30 / A-5 / 110	126 / 118 / 4	30	5000 ft / 20 W	112 / 136/88	2–3	Oximetry checked on 2 L during exercise SaO$_2$ down to 86%; Returned to 3L/min; Stairs done 2 flights; All goals met—D/C from rehab = 1 mo follow-up

and the patient showed changes in her exercise performance and RPE values. At that time, 3 liters per minute of oxygen delivered by nasal cannula was reinstituted.

By week 8 of pulmonary rehabilitation, all the patient's goals and the goals of the staff had been met. She was ambulating out of doors for 30 continuous minutes. She was able to climb two flights of stairs by using the pacing technique without becoming short of breath. She was able to descend two flights of stairs with no sensation of dyspnea. All formal lectures had been attended, and all informal teaching had been completed. The patient graduated from the program with a follow-up scheduled 1 month later.

CASE STUDY 3, CHAPTER 10

This section describes the course of rehabilitation for Case Study 3, Chapter 10. The initial exercise prescription written for this patient is given in Table 12–9. The prescription is based on the results of a physical assessment, including a symptom-limited graded exercise test. (Table 10–5 gives the results of the exercise test.)

Important considerations in the assessment of this patient are the moderately severe obstructive pulmonary disease, baseline ST-segment depression of 2 to 3 mm that does not change with exercise, an exercise test that did not reach anaerobic threshold, and a disproportionately increased HR to work load (a sign of cardiac limitation or deconditioning). The test was stopped because of fatigue and dyspnea, although V̇Emax was only 66 percent of predicted.

Using the Karvonen formula, the patient's THRR was calculated as follows:

(Maximum HR − resting HR)(40% to 85%) + resting HR = THRR
$$(96 - 84)(40\% \text{ to } 85\%) + 84 = 88 \text{ to } 94 \text{ bpm}$$

Since he had signs of deconditioning and/or cardiac involvement and he stopped his exercise test prior to reaching his ventilatory maximum, the THR was set at the lowest end of THRR, or 88 bpm. This patient was monitored during exercise by both telemetry and oximetry, which necessitated walking on a treadmill and using a stationary bicycle for the exercise modes. Distance walked and bicycle work loads should be recorded, as should be physiological parameters (subjective and objective) at those work levels. Both the patient and the rehabilitation staff were used to assess functional gains and to motivate the patient to continue with the exercise program. Upper extremity work was not begun until it was clear that the patient had developed some cardiopulmonary endurance. Education sessions, both group (formal) and individual (informal), began immediately.

At first, this patient required 15 minutes to get through the warm-up sessions. His warm-up included flexibility exercises modified so that he could do them in the sitting position. The therapist who demonstrated the exercises to the patient made it clear that the actual stretching motion of each exercise should be made during exhalation. That is important, because patients with cardiac and pulmonary problems must take care to avoid the Valsalva maneuver. At first, it was continually necessary to remind the patient to continue to breathe throughout each exercise.

**TABLE 12–9 Pulmonary Exercise Prescription for
Case Study 3, Chapter 10**

Exercise Rx

Name __Case Study 3, Chapter 10__ (F) M   Age __69__ Date _____

Pack-years __70__ Ht. (in) __72.4__ Wt. (lb) __147__

Dx: __COPD, Pneumoconiosis, HTN, CAD, S/P MI, L CVA, PVD, gout, ulcers__

Meds: __Lasix, ASA, Diltiazem, Alipurinol, digoxin, Lanoxin, NTG__

Comments: __ST-seg depression pre- and post-exercise. HR is disproportionately increased__
indicating cardiac limitation, smokefree 11 years. Termination: Dyspnea and fatigue.

GXT Data: Date performed __5/11/91__   Where: _____

Rest HR __84__   Protocol: __Modified treadmill__

Max HR __96__   Max Mets: __3.1__

Re-evaluation scheduled __8/ /91__

PFT Interpretation: __Moderately severe obstructive disease no change with exercise.__

C-R Rx:

Functional Capacity (METs) = 40% to 85% of Max METs

= .40 to .85 × __3.1__

= 1.2 to 2.6 METs

THRR (bpm) = (Max HR − Rest HR)(.40 − .85) + (Rest HR)

= __88–94 bpm__

RPE (10-point scale) = __4__

Type of exercise: __X__ bike ____ row __X__ walk

____ walk/jog ____ stairs

____ arm ergometry

Cycle 50 rpm no resistance 2 sets of 3 min each with rests 1–2 minutes. Walking
3–5 minutes with 1–2 min rests

Length of session: __12–15 min ex, 4–8 min rest__ Frequency: __5×/wk__

Comments: __Intersperse rest periods as needed. No upper extremity work as__
yet. Progression: 15 min continuous ex.

Flexibility Rx: __General flexibility, special attention to L upper and lower extremity__

Monitoring and Oxygen Needs

Telemetry __X__   Oximetry __X__

Supplemental oxygen __Only if indicated during ex session__

Comments: __Decreased O₂ sats to 87% and increased heart rate with low-level exercise.__
Suggest telemetry and oximetry during exercise session.

After stretching, the patient continued the warm-up session by performing, at a low effort level, the activity that he was to perform for the cardiopulmonary endurance exercise. In this case, the activity was treadmill walking, and the warm-up level was the perceived slow pace of 3 on the RPE scale. (An alternative warm-up and cardiopulmonary endurance exercise was pedaling on a stationary bicycle.)

The cardiorespiratory endurance training involved short bouts of aerobic activity interspersed with rest periods. The patient initially was able to perform 3 minutes of exercise with 2 minutes of rest. Oximetry showed a S_{NO_2} decrease from 96 to 86 percent. Telemetry revealed some HR irregularities, including occasional unifocal PVCs and three couplets. The ST segment did not change from baseline. A rhythm strip was recorded and sent to his physician for further evaluation. He did not achieve his THR of 88. However, since his resting HR was 12 bpm below his resting HR on the day of his test, and because he had increased his HR linearly with this work load while maintaining an appropriate RPE, the CR training session was felt to be adequate.

The CR endurance training activity was modified to promote cool-down and was completed in 10 minutes. This time, since the patient was already on the bicycle, cycling at 25 rpm, no resistance was added. Flexibility exercises followed the cool-down, again with emphasis on the need for a continuous breathing pattern during all phases of activity.

The patient returned to the program 2 days later with no symptoms of joint pain, muscle soreness, or fatigue. The program was then determined to be adequate for him. The physician ordered 1 liter of oxygen via nasal cannula during the exercise session. Exercise progression was undertaken, as tolerated, by increasing the amount of time within each activity until 15 to 30 minutes of continuous activity could be accomplished.

On the Sunday preceding the second week of pulmonary rehabilitation, the patient was seen in the emergency room (ER) for shortness of breath and headache. He was treated with bronchodilators and 3 liters of nasal cannula oxygen. His symptoms resolved, and he was released from the ER. There was no change in his medication schedule.

His second week of pulmonary rehabilitation showed an increase in his resting BP. Therefore, his BP was taken during the exercise session rather than only at rest and after cool-down. His BP rose to 182/94 with an oxygen saturation of 84 percent during his second set of walking. A rhythm strip was taken; it showed one couplet and multifocal PVCs. The patient began the normal cool-down phase of the rehabilitation program, and his physician was called. The patient was excluded from pulmonary rehabilitation until physician clearance to continue was obtained.

The patient returned for week 3 of rehabilitation with no medication changes. During exercise, 2 liters per minute of oxygen were administered, and nocturnal oxygen was used at home. The patient continued in the exercise program with no further incidents. Telemetry was discontinued during week 4, although spot checking with paddles was continued for the duration of the exercise sessions. Oximetry was discontinued on week 5, and the patient began ambulating on the outdoor track. Arm ergometry began on week 6. Progression of exercise is shown in Table 12–10 on the sample data sheets.

By the end of 12 weeks of pulmonary rehabilitation, this patient had achieved all the long-term goals established at the onset of his program. He had attended all of the formal lectures in the series and had completed all of the individual counseling sessions. He was independent in his exercise program, was able to accomplish 30 minutes of continuous exercise, and was successful in the use of the RPE scale. Since he made such significant gains in abilities, he was elected "valedictorian" of his graduating class. He was encouraged to continue his exercise

TABLE 12–10 Summary of 12-Week Pulmonary Exercise Program for Case Study 3, Chapter 10

Date	Rest HR	Rest BP	HR THRR/THR	HR W-UP	C-R Work Type-Min*	HR	RPE	RR	%Sat	Distance Work Load	Cool-Down HR	Cool-Down BP	O$_2$ Liters/Min	Comments
WEEK 1	72	162/74	88–96 / 88	82	W-3 R-3 W-3 R-3 B-3 R-3 B-3	78 78 86	5 4–6	24 30 30	86	800 ft 50 rpm No resistance	78	162/78	—	15-min warm-up HR irregular—send strip Good understanding of RPE scale Oxygen sats down from 96 to 86 MD orders 1 liter/min oxygen exercise 10-min cool-down
WEEK 2	72	148/100	88–96 / 88	82	W-4 R-3 W-2	84 90	5–6	30	84	1200 ft	80	182/94	1 L/min	15-min warm-up Patient to ER on Sunday for shortness of breath, headache; no change in med.; BP up today BP during 2nd set walking 182/94, HR 80 MD notified. MD increases O$_2$ to 2 L/min. Telemetry shows occasional PVCs at max ex. and recovery; no couplets 10-min cool-down
WEEK 3	78	148/80	88–96 / 88	80	W-9 R-3 W-9 B-5 R-3 B-5	84 84–90	5	24 30	90	2400 ft 20 W	82	160/80	2 L/min	15-min warm-up, patient able to tolerate much longer periods of exercise Telemetry shows occasional PVCs at max ex. & recovery No couplets 10-min cool-down

Continued

333

TABLE 12–10 *continued*

Date	Rest HR	Rest BP	HR THRR/THR	HR W-UP	C-R Work Type-Min*	C-R HR	RPE	RR	%Sat	Distance Work Load	Cool-Down HR	Cool-Down BP	O₂ Liters/Min	Comments (BPs, Arrhythmias, Med. Changes, Symptoms, etc.)
WEEK 4	72	164/80	88–96 / 88	80	W-12 / R-2 / W-10 / R-2 / B-5	78 / 84	5	30	90	2600 ft / 20 W	78	150/74	2 L/min	15-min warm-up / 2 unifocal PVCs at max ex. / Began stairs with pacing / Begin spot check HR/remove telemetry / 10-min cool-down / Began home program of walking 10 min/rest/10 min.
WEEK 5	66	150/74	88–96 / 88	72	W-15 / R-3 / B-5	84 / 78	5	24	90	2400 ft / 20 W	72	148/80	2	15-min warm-up / Discontinue oximetry / Normal sinus rhythm / Add arm ergometry / 10-min cool-down
WEEK 6	72	166/82	88–96 / 88	74	W-15 / A-3 / R-3 / A-3	84 / 84	5	24 / 26	90	2400 ft / 15 W	76	164/86	2	15-min warm-up / Normal sinus rhythm / Arm ergometry begin at 15 W / 10-min cool-down

WEEK 7										
72	88–96 / 88	76	162/82	W-15 / R-3 / W-15 / B-5 / A-3	78 / 88	5	30	5000 ft / 25 W / 20 W	74 / 156/84	2	15-min warm-up 13 stairs up & down, pacing 10-min cool-down

WEEK 8										
72	88–96 / 88	76	156/80	W-20 / B-10 / A-5	78 / 90	5	30	3800 ft / 25 W / 20 W	76 / 152/84	2	15-min warm-up Good control of respiration Pacing during ADLs reported Home program: 20 min continuous exercise 10-min cool-down

WEEK 9										
74	88–96 / 90	78	164/86	W-25 / B-10 / A-5	90 / 90 / 90	5 / 30	30	4000 ft / 25 W / 20 W	78 / 158/84	2	10-min warm-up Independent in warm-up & cool-down Increase THR to 90—with RPE at 5 Occasional PVC's at peak seen on scope 5-min cool-down

Continued

TABLE 12–10 *continued*

Date	Rest HR	Rest BP	THRR/THR	W-UP	C-R Work Type-Min*	HR	RPE	RR	%Sat	Distance Work Load	Cool-Down HR	Cool-Down BP	O₂ Liters/Min	Comments (BPs, Arrhythmias, Med. Changes, Symptoms, etc.)
WEEK 10	72	148/84	88–96 / 90	76	W-30	90		27		4800 ft	80	154/80	2	10-min warm-up
					B-10	90	5	30		25 W				Spot checks show occasional unifocal PVCs
					A-5	90		30		20 W				5-min cool-down
WEEK 11	72	150/82	88–96 / 90	74	W-30	90		30		4800 ft	76	154/82	2	10-min warm-up
					B-10	90	5			25 W				Continue with previous ex. program
					A-5	90				20 W				Home program 30 min continuous ex.
														5-min cool-down
WEEK 12	74	154/86	88–96 / 90	76	W-30	90		30		4800 ft	76	156/86	2	Exuberant graduation ceremony
					B-10	90	5			25 W				
					A-5	90				20 W				

regimen at home and was given the opportunity to join the open exercise program that meets every other week at the clinic. It was hoped that he would continue his compliance with the exercise program.

PATIENTS REQUIRING SPECIAL CONSIDERATION

Although some mention has been made of the problems arthritic or elderly cardiac patients may have in attempting an exercise program, a large number of patients seen in rehabilitation programs have multiple problems worthy of special consideration. This population includes the cardiopulmonary diseased patient with one or more of the following conditions: angina pectoris, diabetes mellitus, peripheral vascular disease, restrictive pulmonary disease, pulmonary hypertension, exercise-induced broncho-spasm, arthritis or other orthopedic limitations, and obesity. In such cases, the exercise prescription must be modified to enable the patient to adjust physiologically and psychologically to exercise therapy.

Angina Pectoris

Patients with stable angina are excellent candidates for exercise therapy. The object of the exercise therapy is to increase the functional capacity of the patient so that more physical exercise can be performed before the onset of limiting angina. In this case, special consideration must be given to the ongoing evaluation of the angina, the extent of warm-up and cool-down periods, and the intensity of the cardiovascular endurance training period. Evaluation of the angina involves carefully documenting each episode as the patient describes it according to the type of pain, the location of the pain, factors that may have precipitated the episode, the duration and frequency of the episodes, and the methods used to relieve the pain. Also, the therapist can usually observe and should record unique mannerisms or other subtle changes in coloring or demeanor exhibited by the patient during an episode. Ongoing evaluation of patients with stable angina is critical, because any change in either the frequency or the intensity of the episodes warrants immediate medical investigation. In addition, careful observation is required of patients for whom prophylactic use of nitroglycerin or long-acting nitrates has been prescribed, because adverse hypotensive responses may occur.[12] Modification of the length of the cardiovascular exercise therapy session has been discussed. The patient's THR should remain below the anginal or ischemic threshold (usually 10 to 15 bpm) (Chapter 4).

Diabetes Mellitus

Two types of diabetes must be identified in order to prescribe exercise properly: Type I, or insulin-dependent diabetes (IDDM), is the result of a pancreatic deficiency in insulin production. The type I diabetic is dependent on the regular administration of exogenous insulin, and 10 to 20 percent of the known diabetics in the United States are of this type.[18] In type II, or non-insulin-dependent diabetes (NIDDM), insulin levels may be normal, slightly depressed, or elevated. Usually, decreased cellular sensitivity or responsiveness to exogenous and endogenous insulin is present. Of all known diabetics in this country, 80 to 90 percent are type II. Although this form of diabetes can occur at any age, it is usually diagnosed after age 40 and is associated with obesity.[18] Type II diabetes is typically treated with dietary modification, exercise, oral hypoglycemic medication, and, in some cases, exogenous insulin.[23-25]

Although more research is needed to determine the specific effects of exercise on type I and type II diabetics, existing research indicates that, provided certain guidelines are followed, increased physical activity has several actual and potential benefits to offer the diabetic patient: (1) improvement in insulin sensitivity and potential improvement in glucose tolerance in some individuals, (2) as an adjunct to diet therapy in the promotion of weight loss and the maintenance of body weight,[19] (3) improvement in peripheral hemodynamic function[20] and cardiovascular risk, including the enhancement of work capacity and reduction of body fat, (4) potential reduction in the dosage or need for insulin or oral hypoglycemic agents,[18,21] and (5) enhancement of the quality of life and sense of well-being.

Again, it should be emphasized that more research is needed in regard to the actual benefits and risks and the establishment of specific guidelines for prescribing exercise for both the type I and type II diabetic patient. An exercise program is contraindicated for poorly controlled or uncontrolled diabetic patients (blood glucose greater than 300 mg per dL). Exercise may cause deterioration of metabolic control in such patients.[18]

One of the problems that exercising diabetics may encounter is the hypoglycemic effect of exercise. This effect occurs as a result of the increased mobilization of depot insulin during exercise. This condition may be exacerbated in the type I diabetic if the insulin injection site is in the exercising muscle. Because exercise creates an insulinlike effect, exercising diabetics may have to alter their insulin and carbohydrate intake to avoid hypoglycemic events.[12]

All diabetics (type I and type II) should comply with the following recommendations to assure safe participation in an exercise program:

1. At all times, carry a card or wear a bracelet that identifies the individual as having diabetes mellitus.[2]
2. Exercise with a partner when possible.
3. Be knowledgeable of and alert to the signs and symptoms of hypoglycemia (tachycardia, palpitations, increased sweating, hunger) during and up to several hours following exercise (hypoglycemic episodes may occur from 24 to 48 hours after an exercise session).
4. Have a source of readily absorbable carbohydrate (fruit juice, sugar cubes, glucose tablets, or a solution equivalent to 5 to 20 g of carbohydrate) available during and following exercise to prevent or treat hypoglycemia. (Intramuscular glucagon may be used to treat severe hypoglycemia reactions. The unconscious patient should be given an intravenous injection of glucose.)
5. Avoid the risk of dehydration (which may be a problem when metabolic control is less than satisfactory) by taking extra fluids or by skipping exercise on particularly warm days.
6. Have a careful evaluation of the feet performed by a qualified health professional prior to the initiation of an exercise program. Get instruction regarding the selection of proper footwear and foot protection.

Additional recommendations for the type I (IDDM) patient are necessary.[12,18]

1. Because individuals taking insulin vary considerably in their response to exercise, monitor blood glucose more frequently when beginning an exercise program to determine the response to the type, intensity, and duration of the exercise.
2. Choose an injection site, such as the abdomen, other than the actively exercising muscle.
3. Choose a time to exercise when the blood sugar level is above fasting value, perhaps 1 to 3 hours after a meal, not during peak insulin activity time.
4. It may be necessary to consume extra carbohydrate prior to, during, or following exercise to avoid hypoglycemia episodes.
5. Decreasing the insulin dose prior to an exercise bout may be necessary, but *only as recommended by a physician.*[18] For example, if a patient is well controlled with a single dose of intermediate-acting insulin, the dose may be decreased on days when exercise is planned. Some patients may require a decrease in insulin dosage of 30 to 35 percent. If a patient is using a combination of intermediate- and short-acting insulin, the short-acting dose may be reduced or omitted and the intermediate-acting dose may have to be reduced by up to one third. Under those conditions, a patient may experience hyperglycemia later in the day and require a second injection of short-acting insulin.

Generally speaking, diabetic cardiac patients can participate in the same modes of activity as nondiabetic cardiacs. However, special precautions must be taken when the patient is taking drugs that potentiate exercise-induced hypoglycemia. For example, very high doses of salicylates may alone produce hypoglycemia, and beta-adrenergic blocking agents may prevent the rapid response of the liver, which normally corrects the hypoglycemia.[18]

Type I (IDDM) diabetics should exercise daily, if possible, to assist in the maintenance of a regular pattern of diet and insulin dosage. Because the frequency of exercise is high, the duration may be decreased to 20 to 30 minutes. It is recommended that the intensity of exercise for the type I diabetic be prescribed within the normal range (40 to 85 percent of functional capacity) and on the basis of HR in most cases. The diabetic with autonomic neuropathy, however, may demonstrate chronotropic insufficiency (altered HR response) during exercise. Such patients may also be unable to perceive angina or other symptoms of ischemia. Therefore, they must be carefully monitored, and the RPE methods (Chapter 11) may prove to be helpful in prescribing their exercise intensity.

Type II (NIDDM) diabetic patients should exercise 5 days per week if possible to enhance caloric expenditure. The duration of exercise may be from 40 to 60 minutes in order, again, to assist in weight control. Because the frequency and duration of exercise for type II patients are high, the intensity of the exercise should be maintained in the lower end of the normal range.

Please note that the duration of the exercise sessions given for types I and II diabetic patients represents the maintenance goal for such patients. Diabetic patients, like all cardiac patients, must be carefully and developmentally progressed toward such goals.

The cardiac rehabilitation clinician must be knowledgeable concerning all of the aforementioned recommendations for type I and type II diabetic patients. Specific problems of diabetic patients in various stages of the disease must also be considered. The following examples serve to illustrate the importance of the clinician's need to individualize the exercise prescription for diabetic patients.

Patients with neuropathy have insensitive feet and should avoid exercises that involve running, a potentially traumatizing activity. Cycling and swimming are good alternatives. Recent research indicates that patients with diabetic neuropathic skeletal disease (DNSD) may suffer from fractures of the ankle due to jogging. It has been recommended that jogging not be undertaken by diabetic patients with DNSD or advanced kidney, retinal, or peripheral nerve disease.[22]

Diabetic patients with active proliferative retinopathy, like all cardiacs, should avoid strenuous activities associated with Valsalva-like maneuvers. Such activities cause an undesirable increase in blood pressure. In addition, such patients should avoid participation in activities associated with excessive jarring or jolting of the head.

Exercise for diabetic cardiac patients with hypertension should emphasize rhythmic exercise involving the lower extremities such as walking, jogging (except for patients with DNSD or advanced kidney, retinal, or peripheral nerve disease), or cycling, because intense exercise involving the arms and upper body causes greater increases in blood pressure than exercise involving the major muscle groups of the lower extremities.[18] This recommendation applies to all cardiac patients (Chapters 4 and 11).

The diabetic patient is a special challenge to the cardiac rehabilitation team and must always be observed for symptoms of hypoglycemia and further progression of the disease.

Peripheral Vascular Disease

In patients with claudication, the subjective gradation of pain is a useful technique for evaluating the pain over a period of time and, therefore, measuring slight improvements in exercise tolerance (Table 12–11). This technique also aids in writing the exercise prescription when progressing the patient to higher work levels.

Patients with significant peripheral vascular disease are at a much higher risk of having associated coronary and cerebral vascular disease than those without peripheral impairment.[26] Therefore, an increase in resting systolic BP warrants significant reduction in the THR for the exercise session. Failure of BP to normalize would justify termination of an exercise therapy session. The patient with claudication may initially benefit from intermittent exercise but should be progressed to continuous low-level exercise as soon as it can be tolerated. Exercise therapy sessions should be increased in duration (to a maximum of 60 minutes) at a low level before the intensity is increased. Two exercise periods per day may be beneficial if each session is at least 20 minutes in length. Usually patients can tolerate pain at level 2 during exercise (Table 12–11).

TABLE 12–11 Subjective Gradation of Pain in Patients with
Peripheral Vascular Disease

Grade 4	Excruciating and unbearable pain
Grade 3	Intense pain from which the patient's attention cannot be diverted except by catastrophic events (e.g., fire, explosion)
Grade 2	Moderate discomfort or pain from which the patient's attention can be diverted by a number of common stimuli (e.g., conversation)
Grade 1	Definite discomfort or pain but only of initial or modest level (established but minimal)

Source: From Unger, KM, Moser, K and Hansen, P: Selection of an exercise program for patients with chronic obstructive pulmonary disease. Heart Lung 9:68–76, 1980, with permission.

Restrictive Pulmonary Disease

Restrictive disease creates an inability to adequately increase minute ventilation in response to increasing work load. The result is oxygen desaturation with exercise. This patient population should be referred for pulmonary rehabilitation. The benefits of a pulmonary rehabilitation program can be produced in such patients as well as in those with obstructive pulmonary disease. The use of oximetry can help ensure the safety of exercise intensity in patients with restrictive lung disease. The use of RPE also is important in this group of patients for monitoring exercise intensity.

PULMONARY HYPERTENSION

Patients who present with pulmonary hypertension often have a relatively fixed cardiac output. Therefore, with the onset of exercise, dyspnea, fatigue, and syncope can occur. Exercise must be tailored to low intensity levels and monitored by HR, BP, and oximetry. The benefits of exercise training in this population are, as yet, not encouraging, but judicious use of exercise in these patients is justified. Breathing retraining, energy-saving techniques, pacing, education, and group support are of undeniable benefit to this group.

EXERCISE-INDUCED BRONCHOSPASM

Exercise-induced bronchospasm (EIB) usually occurs 6 to 8 minutes after the onset of continuous exercise in asthmatic patients. The exercising environment is particularly important to patients with EIB. Cold air, low humidity, and pollutants can exacerbate their symptoms. By minimizing the potential hazards, exercise can be accomplished. The appropriate use of warm-up activities is necessary to decrease possible bronchospasm. Bronchodilators administered prior to exercise may help prevent exercise-induced bronchoconstriction. Swimming is the aerobic exercise of choice for asthmatics with EIB because of its controlled environment, availability, and aerobic nature. (For more information on EIB, see Chapter 6.)

Osteoarthritis and Orthopedic Limitations

Any exercise that produces excessive stress on osteoarthritic or injured joints should be avoided. The exercise prescription must emphasize exercises to increase both range of joint motion and strength. Activities that place stress on the weight-bearing joints during inflammatory periods are contraindicated. Intermittent cardiovascular exercise comprised of short bouts of exercise and rest intervals appears to be tolerated better than continuous exercise by orthopedically limited patients.

Obesity

Exercise therapy for the obese patient should be of long duration (maximum of 60 minutes) and low intensity to avoid stressing the weight-bearing joints. The patient thus expends more calories while avoiding the orthopedic problems that may accompany higher-intensity work (Chapter 11).

ENVIRONMENTAL CONSIDERATIONS

Selected patients should be encouraged to exercise at home in addition to the exercise therapy session. It is important to teach such patients how to palpate their own pulses and rate their perceived exertion and to educate them about the effects various environmental factors may have on their ability to exercise. The major concerns are extremes of temperature and humidity. Altitude and air pollution are major factors for patients with pulmonary disease and should be discussed with patients who exercise regularly in areas where the air quality is poor and/or the altitude is high.

Heat

When ambient temperatures range between 40 and 75°F and the humidity is 65 percent or below, conditions are generally recognized as ideal for exercise.[24] In hot weather, however, the body temperature rises faster during exercise and extra precautions must be observed. The harmful effect of higher temperatures is exacerbated by increases in relative humidity. In high heat and humidity, the body struggles to dissipate heat and cool itself. The natural cooling of the body through the evaporation of sweat is ineffective because of the increased humidity. As the core temperature of the body rises, the HR increases (Chapter 4). The volume of blood returning to the heart is reduced by the dilation of the peripheral veins. Therefore, stroke volume, cardiac output, and working capacity are reduced. In this situation, the extra effort demanded by exercise will precipitate ischemic changes and in some cases anginal pain or a more rapid approach to the maximum ventilation. Patients should be instructed on the best time of day to exercise, how to avoid excessive heat and humidity, the appropriate clothing, and the signs and symptoms of heat intolerance.

Cold

Obviously, patients should be informed of the appropriate clothing for cold weather exercise. Low temperatures cause an increase in peripheral resistance at rest and during exercise. The peripheral vasoconstriction associated with cold produces an increase in arterial BP that, when coupled with increased myocardial oxygen demand, causes the patient to reach ischemic threshold more rapidly and consequently may provoke anginal pain.[27]

Cold also affects the pulmonary patient in the form of cold-induced bronchospasm. The cold air that reaches the tracheobronchial tree will cause bronchoconstriction, which makes exercise difficult and unpleasant. Wearing a scarf around the nose and mouth provides a reservoir of warmed air. However, indoor exercise via stationary bicycle, treadmill, or ambulation in a mall may prove to be more advantageous.

Although ischemic responses are related to extremes in temperature and humidity, the same responses have been observed in cardiac patients when there were only moderate changes in temperature.[28] Therefore, all patients should be educated about the dangers associated with exposure to extremes in temperature. It should also be demonstrated to them that in addition to awareness of ambient temperature extremes during exercise, they should try to buffer the effects of temperature extremes in all aspects of daily living, including such situations as bathing and showering, going from air-conditioned buildings or cars out into extreme heat, and vice versa, and drinking very cold or extremely hot beverages.

MOTIVATION AND COMPLIANCE

The goals of outpatient rehabilitation programs are to develop the best possible prescribed therapeutic regimen (including lifestyle modification) for each patient and to enhance compliance with that regimen once it has been established. For the rehabilitation program to be successful, patients must adhere to their programs for months and years following the termination of the formal program. Therefore, all efforts must be made to have the patient understand the factors involved with compliant behavior, and plans must be made to incorporate successful strategies whenever and wherever possible.

Studies indicate that the various techniques utilized by health care professionals to improve patient compliance can be grouped into three broad categories: education, behavior modification, and a combination of the two.[29] Research also indicates that, in terms of therapeutic success, the percent of compliance varies with each category. The lowest compliance rate has been associated with the educational method (50 percent); the highest has been achieved by the behavioral method (82 percent); and an intermediate compliance rate of 75 percent has been demonstrated by combined methods.[30] There are many reasons for the variance. However, to improve patient compliance with exercise therapy, the rehabilitation staff apparently must not only teach patients about their disease, the need for lifestyle change, and exercise requirements but also *motivate* them to continue with their prescribed regimens with behavioral techniques.

Instructors

The key to the success of any program is the competence of the instructional staff.[30] Individuals who work directly with patients must have a thorough and accurate knowledge of exercise physiology, the principles of assessment, exercise prescription, the principles of physical conditioning, and motivational techniques. Many of the techniques used to motivate patients are simple and almost instinctive to individuals who are sincere in their desire to help others achieve goals to which they themselves are dedicated. The instructional staff must provide positive role models for the patients and must always maintain an enthusiastic attitude toward exercise and other lifestyle changes. This type of behavior reinforces patients' attitudes toward the rehabilitative process. They perceive that the changes they are making in their exercise and other habits can and must be a lifetime commitment.

Improving patient compliance involves breaking down barriers to compliance and motivating patient compliance by reinforcing, extrinsically and intrinsically, positive health behaviors. Again, the methods employed to achieve those goals fall into broad categories: educational and behavioral.

EDUCATIONAL TECHNIQUES

Education can be provided in a number of formal and informal situations. The types of educational experience provided by a rehabilitation center will be limited by the

**TABLE 12–12 Weekly Lecture Topics for Cardiac
Rehabilitation Programs**

Risk Factors Associated with Coronary Artery Disease
Anatomy and Physiology of the Heart: What Is a Heart Attack?
Angina: What Is Chest Pain?
Relation of Diet to Heart Disease
Human Sexuality and Heart Disease
Diet and Weight Control
Stress and Stress Management
Cigarette Smoking in Relation to Heart Disease
Drugs Used in the Management of Heart Disease and Their Relationship to Exercise

Source: Adapted from the Cardiac Rehabilitation Program, Northeastern University, Boston, Mass.

staff, facilities, and location of the center. The types of experience that might be provided include patient education manuals written at the appropriate reading level, informal patient education (discussions before, during, and after exercise therapy sessions; bulletin boards), and formal patient education (lectures and individual counseling sessions with or without spouse). Recommended lecture topics for the cardiac and/or pulmonary patient are given in Tables 12–12 and 12–13.

BEHAVIORAL TECHNIQUES

To employ behavioral techniques effectively, an understanding of basic psychological principles is important. These basic principles can be expressed as follows: positive behavioral changes must be reinforced; reinforcement must be delivered immediately following the positive behavioral change; and negative responses should not be emphasized. Here are some examples of how those principles might be applied:

**TABLE 12–13 Weekly Lecture Topics for Pulmonary
Rehabilitation Programs**

Anatomy and Physiology of Respiratory Disease
Chronic Obstructive Pulmonary Disease (COPD)
Pulmonary Hygiene Techniques
Effects of Exercise
Nutrition and Pulmonary Disease
Energy-Saving Techniques
Stress Management and Relaxation
Smoking and Environmental Factors
Medications and Oxygen Therapy
Psychosocial Aspects of COPD
Diagnostic Techniques
General Management of COPD
Community Services
Film: *I Am Joe's Lung*
Signs and Symptoms of Pneumonia

Source: Adapted From the Pulmonary Rehabilitation Program at Massachusetts Respiratory Hospital, Braintree, Mass.

1. Reward measured improvement in percent of body fat, weight loss, vital signs, and functional capacity.
2. Chart or record miles completed, pounds lost, and attendance to break down the patient's goals into smaller goals that guarantee success and then reinforce or reward the patient for achieving each goal. Success breeds success!
3. Give awards, T-shirts, pins, and certificates for attainment of specific goals, such as completion of 50, 100, or 1000 miles.
4. Arrange ceremonies and family nights to help in reinforcing positive attitudes.
5. Reinforce intrinsic motivation through education and role modeling.

Many different skills and factors must be properly combined to make a program successful, but the most powerful motivating force lies in the knowledge, sincerity, enthusiasm, creativity, and dedication of the staff charged with direct patient care.

SUMMARY

Detailed case studies on two patients with cardiovascular disease and two patients with pulmonary disease have been presented to help the clinician better understand the principles relative to THR and RPE and the application of those principles to the daily cardiac and pulmonary exercise therapy session. Examples of readjustments in the exercise prescription based on feedback obtained from the exercise session (such as blood pressure, medication changes, oxygen saturation of the blood) have been included. Those examples will alert the clinician to the necessity for periodic adjustments to the THR or RPE when individual physiological measurements seem to be atypical. Additional modifications of the exercise prescription may be necessary for the patient with cardiopulmonary disease who also has angina pectoris, diabetes mellitus, peripheral vascular disease, asthma, orthopedic limitations, and/or obesity.

Initially, patients should be monitored continuously. Rhythm strips should be obtained during each exercise session for patients with cardiovascular complications. Continuous monitoring can be tapered to intermittent monitoring as the patient progresses. Patients should be instructed about the effects of environmental extremes on HR and BP responses. They should be taught to palpate their own pulses and rate their perceived exertions so they can progress to a home exercise program and do so safely. Suggestions for maintaining patient compliance with the established exercise regimen include educational and behavioral techniques. Of prime importance to the long-term success of any cardiac or pulmonary program are the competency and sincerity of the instructional staff.

REFERENCES

1. Balady, GJ and Weiner, DA: Risk stratification in cardiac rehabilitation. J Cardiopulmonary Rehabil 11:39–45, 1991.
2. Van Camp, SP: Prevention of cardiovascular complications of exercise training. Practical Cardiol 14:31–34, 1988.
3. De Busk, RF, et al.: Identification and treatment of low-risk patients after acute myocardial infarction and coronary artery bypass graft surgery. N Engl J Med 14:161–166, 1986.
4. Leon, AS, et al.: Position paper of the American Association of Cardiovascular and Pulmonary Rehabilitation: Scientific evidence of the value of cardiac rehabilitation services with emphasis on patients following

myocardial infarction. Section I. Exercise conditioning component. J Cardiopulmonary Rehabil 10:79–87, 1990.

5. Hall, LK: Guidelines for cardiac rehabilitation: 1987 to 1990. J Cardiopulmonary Rehabil 11:79–83, 1991.
6. American Association of Cardiovascular and Pulmonary Rehabilitation: Guidelines for Cardiac Rehabilitation Programs. Human Kinetics Publishers, Champaign, IL, 1990.
7. American College of Cardiology. J Am Coll Cardiol 7(2):453, 1986.
8. Reis, A: Position paper of the American Association of Cardiovascular and Pulmonary Rehabilitation: Scientific basis of pulmonary rehabilitation. J Cardiopulmonary Rehabil 10:418–441, 1990.
9. Belman, N and Wasserman, K: Exercise training and testing in patients with chronic obstructive pulmonary disease. Basics Respir Dis 10:1–6, 1981.
10. American Thoracic Society: Evaluation of impairment/disability secondary to pulmonary disorders. Am Rev Respir Dis 133:1205–1209, 1986.
11. Berra, K: Cardiac and pulmonary rehabilitation: Historical and future needs. J Cardiopulmonary Rehabil 11:8–15, 1991.
12. American College of Sports Medicine: Guidelines for Exercise Testing and Prescription. Lea & Febiger, Philadelphia, 1991.
13. Pollock, ML and Froelicher, VF: Position stand of the American College of Sports Medicine. The recommended quantity and quality of exercise for developing and maintaining cardiorespiratory and muscular fitness in healthy adults. J Cardiopulmonary Rehabil 10:235–245, 1990.
14. Dimsdale, JE, et al.: Postexercise period: Plasma catecholamines and exercise. JAMA 251:630–632, 1984.
15. Franklin, BA, et al.: Resistance training in cardiac rehabilitation. J Cardiopulmonary Rehabil 11:99–107, 1991.
16. Wenger, NK: Rehabilitation of the coronary patient: A preview of tomorrow. J Cardiopulmonary Rehabil 11:93–98, 1991.
17. Karvonen, M, Kentala, K and Mustala, D: The effects of training on heart rate: A longitudinal study. Am Med Exp Biol Fenn 35:307, 1957.
18. American Diabetes Association: The Physician's Guide to Type II Diabetes (NIDMM): Diagnosis and Treatment. American Diabetes Association, New York, 1984.
19. National Institutes of Health Consensus Development Conference on Diet and Exercise in Non-Insulin-Dependent Diabetes Mellitus: Draft statement. National Institute of Diabetes, Digestive and Kidney Diseases and the NIH Office of Medical Applications of Research, Bethesda, MD, 1986.
20. Cunningham, LN, et al.: Peripheral hemodynamics and levels of endurance fitness in insulin-dependent diabetic patients. J Cardiopulmonary Rehabil 6:421–429, 1986.
21. La Porte, RE, et al.: Pittsburgh insulin-dependent diabetes mellitus morbidity and mortality study: Physical activity and diabetic complications. Pediatrics 78:1027–1033, 1986.
22. Duda, M: Some diabetics should cycle rather than jog. Phys Sportsmed 14(6):48–50, 1986.
23. Leon, AS: Effects of exercise conditioning on physiologic precursors of coronary heart disease. J Cardiopulmonary Rehabil 11:46–57, 1991.
24. Miller, NH, et al.: Position paper of the American Association of Cardiovascular and Pulmonary Rehabilitation. The efficacy of risk factor intervention and psychosocial aspects of cardiac rehabilitation. J Cardiopulmonary Rehabil 10:198–209, 1990.
25. Staten, MA: Managing diabetes in older adults. Phys Sportsmed 19(3):66–77, 1991.
26. Peterson, LH (ed): Cardiovascular Rehabilitation: A Comprehensive Approach. Macmillan, New York, 1983.
27. de Vries, HA: Physiology of Exercise, ed 4. Wm C Brown Group, Dubuque, IA, 1986.
28. Astrand, P-O: Textbook of Work Physiology, ed 3. McGraw-Hill, New York, 1986.
29. Wiley, MJ: Significant variables associated with compliance in the bio-energetics cardiac rehabilitation population. University of Pittsburgh, 1982. Unpublished master's thesis.
30. Haynes, RB: Strategies for improving compliance: A methodological analysis and review. In Sackett, DL and Haynes, RB (eds): Compliance with Therapeutic Regimens. Johns Hopkins University Press, Baltimore, 1976, pp 69–82.

CHAPTER 13

Risk Factor Modification

There has been a remarkable decline in mortality from cardiovascular and cerebro-vascular disease during the past 30 years.[1-4] During that period, age-adjusted mortality from coronary heart disease (CHD) has decreased approximately 40 percent in the United States. The reasons for the decrease in CHD deaths are not well understood. One can debate that the decrease in mortality is the result of a reduction in the incidence of disease, an improvement in surgical and medical interventions, or a combination of primary and secondary risk factor modification.[5]

The objectives of this chapter are to provide (1) a comprehensive review of each primary risk factor and its association with an increased risk for cardiovascular disease, (2) information regarding the evaluation of each risk factor, and (3) approaches to the management of adverse risk factors (i.e., primary and secondary prevention of CHD).

In the past, risk factors have been classified by the American Heart Association as independent (primary) and secondary.[6,7] The independent risk factors are believed to be directly associated with atherogenesis or to bring about a cardiovascular event. The established independent and modifiable risk factors for CHD are cigarette smoking, hypertension, and hypercholesterolemia. The secondary risk factors believed to worsen the primary factors are also associated with CHD. They are high blood triglycerides, low levels of high-density lipoproteins, diabetes mellitus, obesity, physical inactivity, and certain behavioral characteristics. In more recent years, some investigators have claimed that diabetes, obesity, reduced levels of high-density lipoproteins, and physical inactivity are also independent risk factors for CHD.

It is not the purpose of this section to establish whether a risk factor directly or indirectly influences risk, but to treat the discussion of each risk factor with equal importance. The modifiable risk factors are of greatest interest to the cardiac rehabilitation staff because they are the factors that must be modified if CHD patients are to function as optimally as possible once they leave the formal rehabilitation program and if they are to reduce their risk of recurrent myocardial infarction (Table 13–1).

TABLE 13-1 Rate Your Risk of Heart Attack. Total Your Scores and Rate Your Risk: Less Than 10 = Low Risk; 10 to 19 = Moderate Risk; More Than 19 = High Risk

Risk Factors	4	3	2	1	0	Score
Blood pressure*	Resting blood pressure above 150/95 mm Hg (either number) not under physician care	Resting blood pressure above 150/95 mm Hg (either number) under physician care	Don't know	Resting blood pressure from 140-150/90-95 mm Hg (either number)	Resting blood pressure always less than 140/90 mm Hg (both numbers)	—
Cholesterol*	Above 250 mg/100 mL	250-221 mg/100 mL	220-200 mg/100 mL	Don't know	Below 200 mg/100 mL	—
Smoking*	More than 40 cigarettes daily	40-21 cigarettes daily	20-1 cigarettes daily, cigar or pipe	Stopped smoking	Never smoked	—
Diabetes*	Diabetic with complications	Diabetic taking insulin with no complications	High sugar level controlled by diet or tablets	Don't know	Normal blood sugar	—
Heredity	Two or more blood relatives with heart disease before age 65 years	One blood relative with heart disease before age 65 years	Two or more blood relatives with heart disease after 65 years	One blood relative with heart disease after 65 years	No heart disease in family	—

Age (years)	65–55	54–45	44–35	34–20	Less than 20	
Exercise*		No exercise	Light exercise less than 3 times per week	Vigorous exercise at least 3 times per week	Vigorous exercise every day	___
Stress*		Intense business or personal problems	Daily business or personal problems	Occasional business or personal problems	Rare business or personal problems	___
Weight*		More than 20 lb over ideal weight	20–6 lb over ideal weight	Up to 5 lb over ideal weight	Normal or underweight	___
Drinking* 1 drink = 12 ounces beer 5 ounces wine 1½ ounces liquor		More than 21 drinks per week or drinks frequently	21–15 drinks per week or occasionally	14–8 drinks per week or drinks rarely	7 or fewer drinks per week or never	___
Sex and build			Male, stocky	Male, average or thin build Female, after menopause	Female, still menstruating	___
					TOTAL	___

*This factor can be modified.
Copyright © 1978, St. Catherine Hospital, East Chicago, IN.

MODIFIABLE CORONARY RISK FACTORS

Cigarette Smoking

Smoking has been identified as the number one cause of preventable death in the United States;[11,12] this adverse health habit accounts for one out of every six deaths in the United States.[13] Of the approximately 50 million Americans who smoke regularly, about 390,000 deaths each year can be directly associated with smoking.[14] Over 115,000 of these deaths are due to smoking-related CHDs and 27,500 are due to cerebrovascular disease.[14,15] Smoking is also responsible for over 130,000 deaths related to cancer.[15] In adult men, smoking can account for approximately 90 percent of all deaths from cancer of the lung, trachea, and bronchus. Smoking also accounts for roughly 60,000 deaths annually from chronic obstructive pulmonary disease (COPD), chronic bronchitis, and emphysema[15] (Chapter 14).

In a recent study to assess excess mortality from chronic disease in the United States, nine risk factors were examined singularly for their contribution to deaths from nine different diseases. Of all excess deaths, 33 percent were attributable to cigarette smoking.[16] The numbers and proportions of deaths attributable to risk factors for various chronic diseases are presented in Table 13–2.[16]

The total mortality rate from all causes of death is almost twice as high in heavy smokers as in nonsmokers. Smokers have a 70 percent greater level of CHD risk than nonsmokers. In the heavy smokers group (>2 packs per day) the excessive mortality rate increases to around 200 percent. In the 1979 U.S. Surgeon General's Report, cigarette smoking was equal in importance to the major risk factors of hypertension and hypercholesterolemia.[6] Cigarette smoking has been shown to be a powerful independent risk factor for myocardial infarction (MI) sudden death, peripheral vascular disease, and stroke.[6,17] Overall, approximately 50 percent of CHD deaths are sudden.[19] With sudden death often the first sign of CHD, cigarette smokers present almost a threefold increased risk for sudden cardiac death than nonsmokers. The dose-response relation between the number of cigarettes smoked and CHD risk is significant. Individuals who smoke two or more packs of cigarettes per day have a two-to-three times greater risk of CHD.[17,18] Data relating the number of cigarettes smoked daily to relative risk for CHD by age and sex are presented in Table 13–3.[20]

In a 6-year follow-up on the largest prospective study ever conducted on cigarette smoking,[20] it was reported that almost half of the excess deaths were attributable to smoking. Cigarette smoking is the most important CHD risk factor for both young men and women, and there is greater relative CHD risk in individuals under 50 years of age than in those over 50.[21]

The prevalence of smoking has declined considerably in the United States in the past 25 years, but the decline has been less pronounced in women than in men.[22-24] The prevalence of adult male cigarette smokers declined from 51 percent in 1965 to 34 percent in 1982. On the other hand, during the same period, the decline in adult female smokers has been only from 33 percent in 1965 to 29 percent in 1982.[23] Women are more likely than men to smoke the "low-yield" brands of cigarettes because they believe them to be safer than other kinds of cigarettes,[22] but studies indicate that women who smoke low-yield cigarettes have virtually the same risk of MI as women who smoke the higher-yield brands.

Despite the recent decreases in the number of smokers, nearly one third of all adults in the United States continue to smoke.[24] Cigarette smoking is currently more common among blacks and those of low socioeconomic status.[15,24,25]

TABLE 13-2 Numbers of Deaths and Proportions of Deaths (%) Attributable to Risk Factors for Nine Chronic Diseases*

Risk Factor	Coronary Heart Disease	Stroke	Obstructive Pulmonary Disease	Lung Cancer	Cervical Cancer	Breast Cancer	Colorectal Cancer	Cirrhosis	Diabetes	Total
Total no. deaths	593,111	149,204	71,099	125,511	4,543	40,534	55,811	26,151	37,178	1,103,142
Current/former smoking, %	148,879 (25.1)	35,931 (25.1)	57,791 (81.3)	108,164 (86.2)	1,443 (31.8)				9,703 (26.1)	361,911 (32.8)
Cholesterol level ≥5.20 mmol/L, %	253,194 (42.7)								(23.0)	253,194
Hypertension (systolic blood pressure ≥140 mm Hg), %	171,121 (28.9)	47,431 (31.8)							7,409 (19.9)	225,962 (20.5)
Obesity (≤110/130% of desirable weight), %	190,456 (32.1)	68,483 (45.9)							3,049 (8.2)	261,988 (23.7)
No regular exercise, %	205,254 (34.6)	43,063 (28.9)					8,369 (15.0)			256,686 (23.3)
Alcohol (≥1 oz of ethanol/day)								8,385 (32.1)		8,385 (0.7)
Diabetes, %	77,709 (13.1)	6,993 (4.7)								84,701 (7.7)
Never use mammography %						7,823 (19.3)				7,823 (0.7)
Never use Papanicolaou screening, %					1,658 (36.5)					1,658 (0.2)

*Deaths attributed to risk factors are additive by row (i.e., risk factors), but not by column (i.e., disease).
Source: Adapted from Hahn et al.[16], p. 2657, with permission.

TABLE 13–3 Cigarette Smoking and Relative Risk of CHD
Death in 6 Years by Age, Sex, and Number of Cigarettes
Smoked Daily

Number of Cigarettes Smoked Daily	Relative Risk of CHD Death by Following Ages				
	40–49	50–59	60–69	70–79	40–79*
358,534 Men					
Nonsmoker	1.00	1.00	1.00	1.00	1.00
1–9	1.60	1.59	1.48	1.14	1.45
10–19	2.59	2.13	1.82	1.41	1.99
20–39	3.76	2.40	2.92	2.49	2.39
40+	5.51	2.79	1.79	1.47	2.89
445,875 Women					
Nonsmoker	1.00	1.00	1.00	1.00	1.00
1–9	1.31	1.15	1.04	0.76	1.07
10–19	2.08	2.37	1.79	0.98	1.81
20–39	3.62	2.68	2.08	1.27	2.41
40+	33.1	3.73	2.02	—	3.02

*Unweighted average of relative risks for four age groups: 40–49, 50–59, 60–69, and 70–79. Based on only 5–9 deaths.
Source: Adapted from Arch Environ Health 19:167, 1969. Reprinted with permission of the Helen Dwight Reid Educational Foundation. Published by Heldref Publications, 4000 Albemarle St., NW, Washington, DC 20016. © 1969.

Although there is a continual decline in the number of cigarette smokers in the United States and other Western countries of approximately 1 percent per year, the prevalence in developing countries has increased by 2 percent per year. From 1976 to 1986, half of the global increase in tobacco use has occurred in China.[26]

More recently, studies have shown the negative effects of cigarette smoke on the nonsmoker. The passive, or involuntary, smoker is one who is exposed to the smoke from others. Recent studies have demonstrated that passive smoke increases the nonsmoker's risk of death and heart disease.[27,28] Passive smoking accounts for an estimated 3800 nonsmoker deaths each year from lung cancer.[15]

PATHOPHYSIOLOGIC EFFECTS

Approximately 4000 compounds have been identified in cigarette smoke, including some that are pharmacologically active, toxic, carcinogenic, and antigenic.[18,21] The inhalation of cigarette smoke produces a number of cardiovascular responses in healthy subjects such as increases in both systolic and diastolic blood pressure, heart rate, coronary blood flow, cardiac output, and vasoconstriction of peripheral vessels. Nicotine appears to be the agent producing those increases through stimulation of the sympathetic nervous system, which in turn results in local and systemic catecholamine release. The adverse cardiovascular effects of smoking may also be related to smoking-induced metabolic effects including increases in free fatty acid concentrations, growth hormone, antidiuretic hormone, and blood glucose levels.[21] Carbon monoxide bonds to hemoproteins such as hemoglobin, myoglobin, and cytochrome oxidase. On the average, the cigarette smoker has a fivefold increase in the carboxyhemoglobin level as compared to the nonsmoker. Carboxyhemoglobin is an inactive form of hemoglobin that has no oxygen-carrying capacity. With increases in the carboxyhemoglobin, there is a shift in the hemoglobin dissociation curve resulting in a shift to the left and a reduction in the ability of hemoglobin to deliver oxygen to the tissues. In compensation for the decreased oxygen delivery capacity, smokers maintain a higher hemoglobin level than nonsmokers. Women smokers have a significantly higher mean hemoglobin level than ex-smokers and those who have never smoked.[29] Mean hemoglobin and carboxyhemoglobin levels increased progressively with the number of cigarettes consumed per day. That effect masks the effect of smoking on the detection of anemia.[29]

It appears that cigarette smoking promotes the development of atherosclerosis through repeated injury to the endothelial cells.[21] Carbon dioxide produces hypoxia and increased endothelial permeability. Combined with a possible toxic effect on the endothelial cells by nicotine, this repeated damage to the cells favors an increased lipid deposition in arterial walls. Smokers have an increased platelet aggregation, plasma fibrinogen levels, and decreased clotting times, all of which increase thrombosis development.[21]

When coronary artery disease (CAD) is present, cigarette smoking can cause an imbalance between myocardial oxygen supply and demand primarily through the impairment of oxygen transport and utilization. Pulmonary dysfunction associated with smoking can also produce a tissue hypoxia and possible decrease in coronary blood flow (Chapter 14).

Studies have shown that cigarette smoking increases cardiac automaticity and decreases the ventricular threshold, which results in increased frequency of arrhythmias and sudden death.[21,30,31]

CLINICAL ASSESSMENT OF SMOKING BEHAVIOR

Clinicians in cardiopulmonary rehabilitation have the opportunity and means to modify smoking behavior in their patients. For patients who quit smoking after MI, there is a reduction of reinfarction, sudden cardiac death, and total mortality as compared to patients who continue to smoke.[8,22,32,33] A detailed history of the patient's use of all types of tobacco should be assessed at the time of entry into the program and reviewed every 3 to 6 months. Coronary risk from smoking can be estimated by using Table 13–3. Through self-reporting and clinician-taken medical history, most patients are honest about their habit and will readily admit its deleterious effects.

An assessment of pulmonary function (Chapter 10) that includes measurement of vital capacity and forced expiratory volume in 1 second (FEV_1) should be taken early in life for heavy smokers.[6] Routine annual chest x-rays are recommended only in heavy smokers (Chapter 10).

A number of clinical trials have demonstrated the effectiveness of patient counseling and smoking cessation techniques involving various combinations of counseling, distribution of literature, and nicotine replacement therapy.[14,15,18,34]

Smoking cessation counseling should be offered on a frequent basis to all patients who smoke either cigarettes, cigars, or pipes or use smokeless tobacco. The effectiveness of behavioral interventions varies with age, level of education, years of negative behaviors, and nature of the intervention.[24,35,36]

The major conclusions of a recent report on smoking cessation techniques revealed the following:[8,15,34]

1. Most smokers quit on their own.
2. Interventions using multiple and frequent reinforcements are more successful than those relying on a single intervention technique.
3. The greatest problem in cessation programs is relapse, and preparation for it should be included in the overall smoking cessation strategy.
4. When coupled with other interventions, nicotine gum may facilitate cessation rates.
5. Health care professionals should facilitate multicomponent strategies that incorporate the use of behavioral techniques and scheduled reinforcement.

Assisting the cardiopulmonary patient in the process of smoking cessation should be a high priority for the rehabilitation staff. The patient should be informed in lay terms about the adverse effects of smoking. The information can be contained in a patient education manual or provided as supplemental material for distribution during individual or group counseling. Formal group therapy is not always required to help a patient stop smoking. Many cardiopulmonary patients will have stopped smoking prior to entering a formal exercise rehabilitation program on the advice of their physicians. Therefore, the role of the rehabilitation staff becomes primarily one of reinforcing the patient's compliance with his or her self-motivated behavioral change. Compliance with positive behavior change may be reinforced by reminding the patient of the reason(s) that motivated him or her to stop smoking. The most common reasons are as follows:

1. Concern over the effects on health (particularly fear of recurring coronary events)
2. Desire to set an example for others
3. Recognition of the unpleasant aspects of smoking, for example, nicotine stains, foul-smelling clothing
4. Desire to exercise self-control

Because smoking is one of the most serious of the risk factors associated with CHD, the rehabilitation staff must make a concentrated effort to motivate patients to stop smoking and to educate and encourage patients who have stopped so that the chances of their resuming the habit are significantly reduced.

Hypertension

HYPERTENSION AND CARDIOVASCULAR RISK

Hypertension, defined as a systolic blood pressure greater than or equal to 140 mm Hg and/or a diastolic blood pressure greater than or equal to 90 mm Hg, or individuals already taking antihypertensive medications, occurs in approximately 58 million Americans.[37] The relation of hypertension to CHD is well established.[38,39] Hypertension is a primary risk factor for CAD, congestive heart failure, cerebrovascular disease, and renal disease. Hypertension increases with age in all groups, and it is more common among blacks and those with a positive family history of high blood pressure.[37] It is also more prevalent in the presence of such other well-identified risk factors are as excessive dietary fat intake, obesity, elevated lipids, smoking, diabetes mellitus, excessive alcohol intake, and sedentary lifestyle.[8,37] The incidence of cardiovascular and cerebrovascular disease increases progressively as systolic and diastolic blood pressure increase.

Because of the significantly higher risk present in the "high normal" diastolic blood pressure range (85 to 89 mm Hg), the Joint National Committee on Detection, Evalua-

TABLE 13–4 Blood Pressure Classification Based on Confirmed*
Diastolic and Systolic Pressures in Same Individual
18 Years and Older

Diastolic Blood Pressure (mm Hg)	Systolic Blood Pressure (mm Hg) as Follows:		
	Less Than 140	140–159	160 or Greater
Less than 85	Normal blood pressure	Borderline isolated systolic hypertension	Isolated systolic hypertension
85–89	High normal blood pressure		
90–104		Mild hypertension	
105–114		Moderate hypertension	
115 or greater		Severe hypertension	

*Average of two or more measurements on two more occasions.
Source: Adapted from 1984 Report of the Joint National Committee on Detection, Evaluation, and Treatment of High Blood Pressure. Arch Intern Med 144:1045, 1984, with permission.

tion, and Treatment of High Blood Pressure revised the classification and standards for arterial pressure in 1984.[38] In that report normal blood pressure is defined as a diastolic blood pressure of less than 85 mm Hg and a systolic blood pressure of less than 140 mm Hg. Isolated systolic hypertension (ISH) is defined as systolic blood pressure that is consistently at or above 160 mm Hg with a diastolic blood pressure less than 95 mm Hg. Standards for both diastolic and systolic blood pressure classification for individuals 18 years and older are presented in Table 13–4. The new standards lowered the systolic and diastolic criteria for defining hypertension at 140 mm Hg and/or 90 mm Hg compared to previous standards of 160 mm Hg for systolic pressure and/or 95 mm Hg for diastolic pressure, respectively.

The causes of primary hypertension are not well understood. It has been stated that the majority of all hypertensive cases are of an unknown, or idiopathic, origin.[40]

Hypertension has been shown to be a powerful risk factor, and it rivals the attention that blood lipids play in the development of atherosclerosis. A recent Framingham Study update emphasized that the risk of sudden death more than doubled when blood pressure was mildly elevated.[41] More important was the discovery that isolated systolic hypertension (systolic blood pressure ≥160 mm Hg and diastolic blood pressure <95 mm Hg) was a prognostic factor for major cardiovascular events. Isolated systolic hypertension was the most common form of hypertension; it accounted for 57.4 percent of all hypertensive conditions in men 65 or older and for 65.1 percent in women 65 or older. The risk of cardiovascular death was at least twice as high for persons with ISH as for those with blood pressures consistently below 140/95. During a 24-year follow-up of men aged 45 to 84 in the Framingham Study, the risk of a major cardiovascular event was significantly increased (Fig. 13–1).[41]

EVALUATION OF HIGH BLOOD PRESSURE

Errors in measurement of blood pressure can result from equipment, observer, and/or patient factors. The American Heart Association (AHA) recommends that baseline blood pressure should not be measured immediately after a taxing or stressful situation. Patients should have refrained from smoking, eating, and ingestion of caffeine

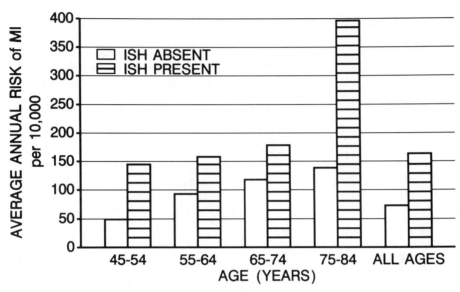

FIGURE 13–1. The presence of isolated systolic hypertension (ISH), defined as systolic blood pressure consistently at or >160 mm Hg with diastolic pressure <95 mm Hg, is an important prognostic factor for major cardiovascular events. Data from 24-year follow-up of men aged 45 to 84 in the Framingham study. (Reprinted with permission. Kannel, WB: CHD risk factor: A Framingham study update. HOSPITAL PRACTICE, Volume 25, issue 7, page 122. Illustration by Albert Miller.)

for at least 30 minutes. The average should be taken of at least two, or more, measurements with the patient seated comfortably with the arm bared, supported, and at heart level. If the first two measurements differ by more than 5 mm Hg, additional readings should be obtained. Hypertension should be confirmed on more than one reading at each of three separate visits.

NONPHARMACOLOGIC TREATMENT OF HYPERTENSION

Once hypertension has been confirmed, a comprehensive history, physical examination, and pathologic assessment should be explored. Because of the possible adverse side effects, cost, and mortality associated with the pharmacologic treatment of hypertension, there is an increasing interest in treating patients with mild, moderate, and severe hypertension by nonpharmacologic or hygienic therapy.[37,42] Several interventions merit review for their contribution in the primary and secondary prevention of CHD.

SODIUM REDUCTION

A blood-pressure-lowering effect of severe dietary sodium restriction (<10 mEq per day) has been recognized for over 40 years.[43] More recent reviews have surveyed the apparent relation between dietary sodium consumption and the prevalence of hypertension. The Intersalt Study examined the relation of electrolyte excretion to blood pressure in over 10,000 people throughout the world.[44,45] Data from this multicenter epidemiologic study revealed a significant correlation between sodium intake and blood pressure. Sodium and the sodium/potassium ratio were significantly related to the blood pressure of the subjects independent of other factors. In the study, a reduction in daily sodium intake of 100 mg was associated with a decrease in systolic pressure of 3.5 mm Hg. Other results in this study revealed that after adjusting for confounding variables, both body mass index and alcohol consumption were positively significant and independently associated with blood pressure.

In recent years, there has been a re-evaluation of the role of sodium in human blood pressure because of two observations. The first is that not all individuals respond to an excessive sodium intake with an increase in blood pressure. Second, not all individuals show a decrease in blood pressure as a result of a reduction in sodium and/or extracellular fluid volume by dietary sodium restriction or diuretic administration.[46] New observations suggest that sodium sensitivity or resistance of blood pressure may be the results of genetics or acquired abnormalities and require further investigation.

The average American diet contains about 5 to 10 g of sodium per day, which is approximately two to three times the recommended amount of 1100 to 3300 mg. Approximately 30 to 50 percent of dietary sodium is in the form of salt added in food preparation or at the table. The remainder of dietary sodium is in the food itself, added as preservative, or added chemicals. It would appear prudent for all individuals, those who are apparently healthy, those with a family history of hypertension, and especially those with documented CHD, to moderate sodium intake in order to reduce the development of hypertension. The reduction of discretionary and nondiscretionary salt and a decrease in sodium-rich foods appears advisable for most patients. Limitations of intake to 1.5 to 2.5 g of sodium (approximately 4 to 6 g of salt) per day produces no serious adverse consequences.[47] Hypertension rarely occurs in populations that have a habitual dietary intake of sodium below 2 g per day.[48] Cardiac patients should be made aware of the sodium content of frequently used prepared food items by analyzing eating patterns and instructing them on the types and amounts of low-sodium foods that should be part of a healthy diet.

WEIGHT REDUCTION

Obesity and hypertension are closely associated.[49-52] Weight gain in young adult life is a patent risk for later development of hypertension.[49] Weight reduction, therefore, is an important nonpharmacologic treatment for hypertension. In 40 to 80 percent of obese hypertensives, weight reduction, even a modest loss, results in sustained decrease in blood pressure to, or toward, normal levels.[51] Weight loss must, however, be maintained in order to benefit from a decrease in blood pressure. In the Framingham Heart Study it was shown that a 1 percent increase or decrease in weight resulted in a 1 percent increase or decrease in blood pressure.[53] The amelioration of hypertension by weight reduction occurs independently of changes in dietary sodium content.[54]

The mechanisms for a decrease in blood pressure associated with weight loss are not fully understood. The effects of weight loss by itself on left ventricular mass have been shown to be decreases in interventricular septal and posterior wall thickness.[55,56] The impact of long-term weight reduction on the incidence of cardiovascular complications in hypertensive overweight patients has not been fully assessed. Weight reduction utilizing a diet low in saturated fat and cholesterol lowers the risk by decreasing important atherogenic risk factors.

ALCOHOL REDUCTION

Elevated blood pressure has been associated with increased alcohol intake in a dose-independent manner.[47,57,58] Although alcohol in moderation (one to two drinks per day) may have a positive effect on lipids, significant increases have been noted in both systolic and diastolic blood pressure in patients consuming more than three drinks per day.[59] Heavy alcohol intake by patients with CHD may impede recovery. It may cause an increase in body weight, triglyceride levels, and uric acid levels and may impair ventricular function and induce atrial and ventricular arrhythmias.

Further complications imposed by medications and their side effects make abstinence from alcohol the prudent choice for most cardiac patients. Patients should be informed about the dangers associated with alcohol consumption. The decision on whether a patient is permitted to consume alcohol is one that must be made in conjunction with the primary physician. Patients should be encouraged to abstain or to select alcoholic beverages containing lower percentages of alcohol per volume, such as light beer or wine. Rehabilitation staff have the ability to assess alcohol use and abuse through use of such instruments as the Michigan Alcohol Screening Test.[61]

PHYSICAL CONDITIONING AND HYPERTENSION

Although still controversial, mounting evidence indicates that regular aerobic exercise does lower blood pressure in hypertensive patients.[62] In 1984, two comprehensive reviews of studies examining exercise conditioning as an antihypertensive therapy in humans reached different conclusions.[63,64] A summary of recent studies that showed a modest but statistically significant decrease in blood pressure following low to moderate levels of aerobic exercise training is presented in Table 13–5.[63]

Because of small numbers of patients and several methodologic and design limitations that could account for the slight reductions of systolic (mean, 9 mm Hg) and diastolic pressure (mean, 7 mm Hg) the studies were found to be inconclusive and "inadequate for the recommendation of exercise conditioning as a replacement for pharmacologic intervention."[63]

In four of five more recent studies on the effect of exercise conditioning on hypertension in humans, however, it was concluded that there were significant decreases in systolic and/or diastolic pressure.[73–77]

BEHAVIORAL MODIFICATION FOR HYPERTENSION

Two behavioral modification methods have been used in the treatment of mild hypertension. Stress reduction/relaxation techniques and biofeedback are often prescribed in conjunction with medical management. In order to be effective, biofeedback must be administered several times per week and for long periods of time before changes are observed.[42] Stress relaxation techniques may be useful as adjunctive treatment in controlling mild hypertension in some patients.[78–80] The influence of intervention on sympathetic activity has been suggested as a possible mechanism for CHD reduction.[79] Although an American Heart Association Task Force concluded that stress alone can elevate blood pressure, it has not been proved to lead to sustained hypertension.[81] At the present time, there is minimal evidence to support the theory that relaxation techniques or biofeedback in and of themselves can serve as effective means of treatment for mild, moderate, or severe hypertension. Control of hypertension should

TABLE 13–5 Effect of Aerobic Exercise Training on Resting Blood Pressure

| Study | No. of Patients | Blood Pressure (mm Hg) | | | | |
| | | Pretraining | | Post-training | | Change (%) Systolic/Diastolic (mm Hg) |
		Systolic	Diastolic	Systolic	Diastolic	
Boyer and Kasch[65]	23	159	105	146	93	−13(8%)/−12(11%)
Choquette and Ferguson[66]	37	136 ± 13	90 ± 7	122 ± 14	82 ± 10	−14(10%)/−9(9%)
Bonanno and Lies[67]	12	148	97	135	83	−13(9%)/−14(14%)
Krotkiewski et al.[68]	27	134 ± 20	87 ± 8	125 ± 20	80 ± 9	−9(7%)/−7(8%)
Roman et al.[69]	12	182 ± 16	113 ± 9	154 ± 7	97 ± 5	−28(15%)/−16(4%)
Kukkonen et al.[70]	12	145 ± 14	99 ± 3	136 ± 10	88 ± 10	−9(6%)/−11(11%)
Hagberg et al.[71]	25	137 ± 5	80 ± 10	129 ± 5	75 ± 10	−8(6%)/−5(6%)
Duncan et al.[72]	44	146 ± 1	94 ± 1	134 ± 1	87 ± 1	−12(8%)/−7(7%)

Source: Adapted from Moir, TW: Nonischemic cardiovascular disease. In Franklin, BA, Gordon, S, and Timmis, GC (eds): Exercise in Modern Medicine. Williams & Wilkins Co, Baltimore © 1989, p. 84, with permission.

initially involve the safest means possible for the CHD patient by using a combination of the nonpharmacologic therapies described above.

OTHER CONCERNS

Recent research has examined the actions of such intracellular ionic abnormalities as elevated levels of cytosolic free calcium in hypertension.[81] High levels of free calcium correlated with elevated blood pressure, which suggests that hypertension is a condition of excess cytosolic free calcium. Conversely, observations of higher levels of free magnesium coincided with lower systolic and diastolic blood pressures. Current studies are examining the role magnesium, calcium, sodium, and pH, or free hydrogen ions, play in hypertension and other metabolic disease syndromes.[81]

Patients must be aware of the exogenous factors that can elevate blood pressure, such as over-the-counter and routinely prescribed medications. Nose drops, sodium-containing antacids, oral contraceptives, postmenopausal estrogens, and nonsteroidal anti-inflammatory drugs should be examined in the treatment of hypertensive CHD patients.[6]

PHARMACOLOGIC TREATMENT OF HYPERTENSION

Pharmacologic treatment of hypertension centers around several available drugs. Diuretics, beta-blockers, calcium antagonists, and angiotensin-converting enzyme (ACE) inhibitors are widely used to treat hypertension. The choice of drug is often related to the severity of hypertension, presence of target organ damage, presence of diabetes mellitus, or other major risk factors for CHD and stroke.[37,42,82-84] The 1988 Report of the Joint National Committee on Detection, Evaluation, and Treatment of High Blood Pressure emphasizes increased flexibility in high blood pressure management to address individual patient needs and medical history, control of other risk factors for cardiovascular disease, and cost of therapy.[37] The primary goal of pharmacologic treatment is to maximize blood pressure control to normal or near normal levels with minimal side effects. The stepped-care approach is outlined in Figure 13-2.

Step 1 is the use of nonpharmacologic approaches that were previously discussed in this chapter. The significance of the 1988 Report was the recommendation for use of nonpharmacologic therapy as the first step in treatment of mildly hypertensive patients. Thiazide diuretics and beta-blockers may have adverse metabolic effects on blood lipid levels, glucose, and uric acid and should be taken into consideration before recommendations for drug therapy are implemented. Thiazide diuretics produce a pattern of elevating total cholesterol, triglycerides, low-density lipoprotein (LDL) cholesterol, and very low density lipoprotein (VLDL) cholesterol. Other adverse side effects are hypokalemia and increased arrhythmias. Careful dietary counseling and supplemental potassium may be required, as well as frequent evaluation of serum potassium levels.[83] Diuretics are often the first-line agents for many hypertensive patients, but they may not be the best choice for exercising patients.

The effects of selective and nonselective beta-blockers in the treatment of hypertension have been well documented. As with thiazide diuretics, beta-blockers, both selective and nonselective, can adversely affect triglycerides and high-density lipoprotein (HDL) cholesterol. The other two classes of first-line antihypertensive agents are calcium channel blockers and ACE inhibitors. Antihypertensive therapy and adverse effects of drug therapy are discussed in Chapter 7.

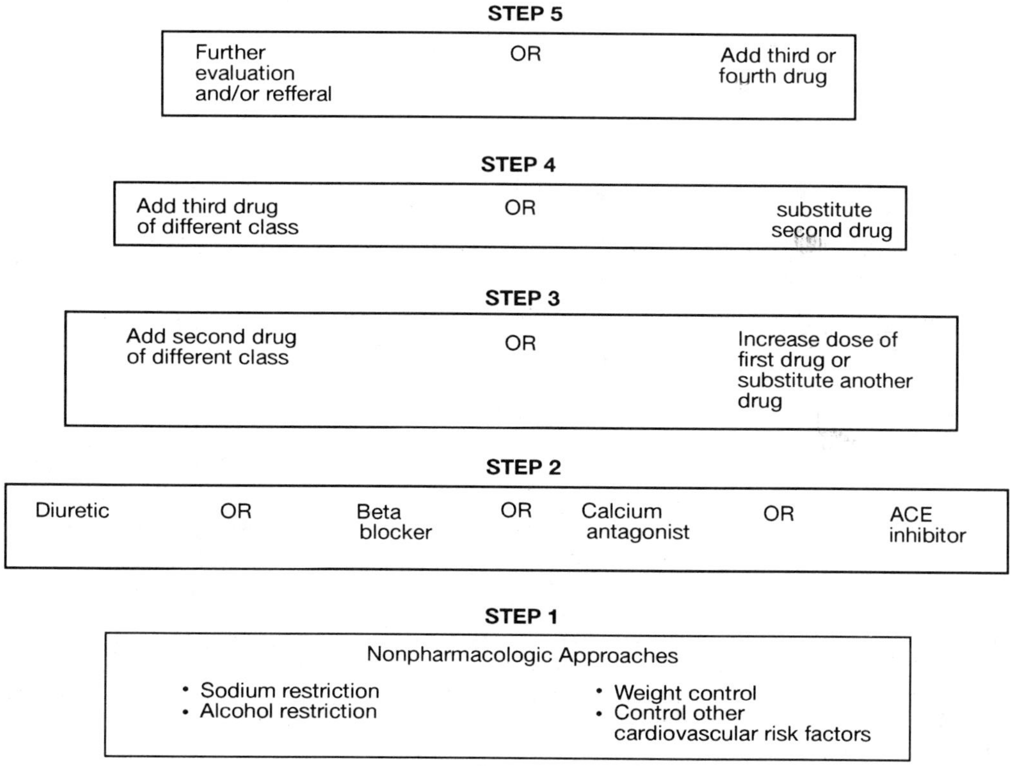

STEP 5

| Further evaluation and/or refferal | OR | Add third or fourth drug |

STEP 4

| Add third drug of different class | OR | substitute second drug |

STEP 3

| Add second drug of different class | OR | Increase dose of first drug or substitute another drug |

STEP 2

| Diuretic | OR | Beta blocker | OR | Calcium antagonist | OR | ACE inhibitor |

STEP 1

Nonpharmacologic Approaches

- Sodium restriction
- Alcohol restriction
- Weight control
- Control other cardiovascular risk factors

FIGURE 13–2. Individualized step-care therapy for hypertension. (From The United States Department of Health and Human Services, NIH Publication #88-1088, Bethesda, MD, 1988, p. 18.)

In summary, cardiac rehabilitation programs provide an opportunity for continued monitoring of blood pressure and supervision of adherence to medications. Hypertension is a major indication for pharmacologic therapy in secondary prevention if such nonpharmacologic measures as regular endurance exercise, sodium restriction, and relaxation techniques are not adequate to control blood pressure.

PLASMA CHOLESTEROL, LIPOPROTEINS, AND TRIGLYCERIDES

There is no longer any doubt about the causative relation linking elevated cholesterol levels to increased rates of premature CHD and to the progression of disease among those with established atherosclerosis.[17,85-87] A number of worldwide retrospective epidemiologic studies have consistently correlated increased serum cholesterol levels with an increased CHD mortality.[88-90]

The Multiple Risk Factor Intervention Trial (MRFIT), a primary-prevention trial, was designed to assess the effect on mortality of intensive, multiple-risk modification in 12,866 high-risk men, aged 35 to 57, from a cohort of 361,662 middle-aged men.[91,92] In that study the relations of serum cholesterol to CHD death were obtained during a 6-year period. The relations of serum cholesterol to age-adjusted 6-year death rate per 1000 men from CHD are presented in Figure 13–3.

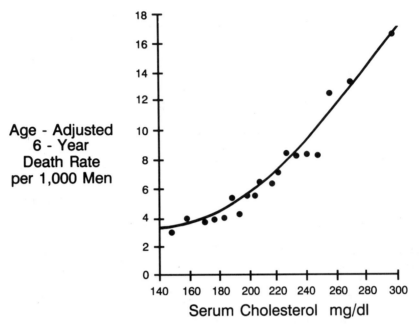

FIGURE 13–3. Relationship of serum cholesterol to age-adjusted 6-year death rate per 1000 men from CHD. Each point represents the median values for 5 percent of the population. Key points are: (1) risk increases steadily, particularly >200 mg/dL, and (2) the magnitude of the increased risk is large—fourfold in the top 10 percent as compared with the bottom 10 percent. (From Martin et al.,[91] p. 933, with permission.)

The results presented in Figure 13–3 show that the risk of CHD mortality increases steadily from serum cholesterol levels as low as 180 mg per dL. The association is continuous throughout the range of cholesterol levels in the study population. At higher levels of serum cholesterol the relation becomes very strong. For men with cholesterol values in the top 10 percent of the population distribution, the risk of CHD mortality is four times as high as the risk in the bottom 10 percent of the population. Even though the study consisted of only men, women are equally susceptible to the effects of lipid-related risk factors for coronary disease.[3,93,94] Plasma cholesterol is a powerful independent risk factor for CHD. In the Framingham Study, individuals whose plasma cholesterol levels were below 175 mg per dL have less than half the risk of MI when compared to those with levels of 250 to 275 mg per dL. In the same study, men aged 31 to 39 years of age with cholesterol levels in excess of 260 mg per dL were twice as likely to die during the 30-year follow-up as men with cholesterol levels below 180 mg per dL.[95]

The association between elevated serum cholesterol levels and an increased risk of CHD is directly related to the LDL cholesterol levels and inversely proportional to HDL levels.[96] In 1985, Doctors Brown and Goldstein were awarded the Nobel Prize for their discovery of a genetic defect or deficiency of LDL receptors on the cell surface proteins.[97] They noted that individuals with a deficiency or absence of LDL receptors are prone to atherosclerosis and premature CHD. They observed that LDL receptors are needed to transfer the body's atherogenic LDL particles to the liver for excretion. Results of dietary studies rich in cholesterol and saturated fatty acids show that the body produced fewer LDL receptors. They concluded that lifestyle-induced deficiencies of LDL receptors result in increased LDL concentration and a greater risk of CHD. The Lipid Research Clinic Coronary Primary Prevention Trial (CPPT) provided evidence that effective primary and secondary prevention can be attained by lowering the LDL-cholesterol level or the total cholesterol/HDL-cholesterol ratio by diet, drugs, or both.[98]

Over a 7-year trial period, more than 3800 hypercholesterolemic, middle-aged men participated in the double-blind trial. The subjects were randomized and treated with either a bile acid sequestrant called cholestyramine or a placebo. Both groups were placed on cholesterol-lowering diets designed to reduce their serum cholesterol levels by about 4 percent. Results of the study showed that subjects in the cholestyramine group had an average reduction in total serum cholesterol of 9 percent greater than those experienced in the placebo group. The cholestyramine group experienced a 19 percent reduction in nonfatal MIs compared to the placebo group. The significance of the results of this study, as well as those of the Framingham Study, is that a 1 percent reduction in an individual's total serum cholesterol level translates into a 2 percent reduction in CHD risk.[93] The 1:2 ratio of lower serum cholesterol to reduce CHD may be even stronger than the two studies suggest.[93,95]

In summary, epidemiologic studies and clinical trials support the conclusion that lowering total and LDL cholesterol levels will reduce the subsequent incidence of CHD events. The studies also indicate that intervention is as effective in secondary prevention as it is in primary prevention.

A basic understanding of the current pharmacological and nonpharmacologic intervention in lipid abnormalities is necessary for the cardiac rehabilitation staff to reinforce behavioral change effectively and provide informal patient education regarding dietary recommendations. Prior to the discussion on interventions for the various dyslipidemias, it is important to briefly review the biochemistry, structure, and function of lipids and lipoproteins.

Biochemistry of Lipids

Cholesterol and phospholipids are essential components of cellular membranes and are necessary for normal bodily functions, including the transport and storage of body

TABLE 13-6 Composition of the Plasma Lipoproteins

Lipoproteins	Protein (%)	Triglycerides (%)	Cholesterol (%)	Phospholipid (%)	Major Apolipoproteins
Chylomicrons	2	84	6	8	A_1, B C_1,C_2,C_3
VLDL	10	50	22	18	B, C_1,C_2,C_3 E
LDL	20	8	50	22	B
HDL	50	7	18	25	A_1, A_2 C_1,C_2,C_3 E

Source: Adapted from Mahley et al.,[100] p. 1277, with permission.

energy and the production of steroid hormones and bile acids. Because lipids are only marginally soluble in an aqueous environment, transportation from their site of origin to their site of use is made possible by the attachment of the lipid molecules to protein molecules known as lipoproteins.[99] Lipoproteins are divided into four major classes based on their size, molecular weight, and density. Each lipoprotein class possesses different proportions of cholesterol, triglycerides, and phospholipids and of the protein components called apolipoproteins. The major classes of lipoproteins are chylomicrons, VLDL, LDL, and HDL. The proportions of cholesterol, triglycerides, protein, and apolipoproteins are shown in Table 13–6.[100]

Chylomicrons

Chylomicrons are synthesized in the intestinal mucosa, and their major lipid component is approximately 85 percent triglyceride, which is derived from dietary fat. When newly ingested triglycerides enter the intestine with the diet, they are hydrolyzed to fatty acids and monoglycerides by pancreatic lipase.[101] Chylomicrons transport the converted dietary lipids into the circulatory system and throughout the body quite rapidly. They deliver most of their fatty acids to the peripheral cells within a few minutes and reach their highest concentration in plasma 2 to 4 hours after a meal. The chylomicron remnants are cleared from the bloodstream by the liver within 10 to 12 hours after ingestion. That is the reason a 14-hour fasting sample is recommended to obtain a reliable triglyceride measurement.

Very Low Density Lipoproteins

VLDLs are triglyceride-rich lipoproteins that are manufactured in the liver. VLDLs transport endogenous triglycerides from the small intestine. The lipid component of VLDLs is about 50 percent triglyceride and 22 percent cholesterol. VLDL breakdown occurs in a series of steps during which triglycerides are removed progressively by tissue lipoprotein lipase. Once the triglycerides are hydrolyzed, the VLDL remnant can follow one of two pathways. The fate of VLDL remnants appears to differ from that of chylomicron remnants. VLDL remnants can be taken up directly by the liver or they can be converted into LDLs. Usually, about 60 to 70 percent of the VLDL remnants are removed by the liver and the remainder are converted to LDL.[101] Thus, VLDL is a precursor of LDL. The mechanism whereby some VLDL remnants are converted to LDL, or the precise independent contribution VLDL has to atherogenesis or CHD risk, remains unknown.[102,103]

Overproduction of VLDL triglycerides can be caused by a genetic dysfunction, an excessive intake of simple carbohydrates or alcohol, non-insulin-dependent diabetes mellitus, estrogen treatment, and obesity.[104] VLDL levels in most cases are estimated by dividing the plasma triglyceride level by five or six.[105,106] This relation does not apply when triglyceride levels exceed 400 mg per dL or in cases of type III or type V hyperlipoproteinemia.[105] It should be noted that acute illness or trauma generally elevates VLDL levels and depresses LDL levels.[107]

Low-Density Lipoproteins

LDLs are the major carriers of cholesterol in plasma. Approximately 60 to 75 percent of the total plasma cholesterol is found in LDL. Consequently, increases in the level of total blood cholesterol are usually the result of increases in LDL-cholesterol. The LDL core consists almost entirely of cholesterol esters. About 75 percent of the serum LDL is cleared by the liver, and the remainder is cleared by the extrahepatic tissues.[108] LDL originates from catabolism of triglyceride-rich lipoproteins, VLDL, and VLDL remnants. Approximately 30 to 40 percent of the VLDL and VLDL remnants are converted to LDL. The rest are removed by the hepatic LDL receptors. LDL delivers cholesterol to tissues via a specific, high-affinity LDL receptor, which controls the uptake of cholesterol by cells as well as intracellular cholesterol synthesis. LDL-receptor activity appears to be a key regulator of LDL cholesterol concentrations.[97] The LDL molecule is small in size and has been shown to pass through the intima to initiate and sustain the process of atherosclerosis. More recent studies have suggested that modified or oxidized LDL is taken up by endothelial cells and smooth muscle cells 3 to 10 times more rapidly than is native LDL and can therefore accelerate endothelial injury and progression of lesions.[102,109] Three basic abnormalities appear to contribute to the development of high serum cholesterol levels.[108] For most people, an increase in cholesterol levels is due to high levels of LDL-cholesterol. The first cause of elevated LDL is a decrease in LDL-receptor activity, which leads to a delayed clearance of LDL and VLDL remnants. This delay in clearance can result in a greater conversion of VLDL remnants to LDL. The second abnormality is an overproduction of LDL caused by an overproduction of apolipoprotein B by the liver (see the section on apolipoproteins) and the decreased uptake of VLDL or VLDL remnants. The final mechanism of hypercholesterolemia is the overloading of LDL molecules with cholesterol esters. A more detailed explanation of the causes of hypercholesterolemia is given elsewhere.[108,110]

Accurate quantification of LDL-cholesterol in the clinical laboratory is difficult. Since all cholesterol in plasma is present on lipoproteins, the concentration of LDL-cholesterol in fasting plasma can be estimated from measurements of total cholesterol, total triglycerides, and HDL-cholesterol. If the triglyceride value is below 400 mg per dL (4.5 mmol per liter), one can divide the triglyceride value by five to estimate the VLDL-cholesterol level.[105] Since total cholesterol is the sum of LDL-cholesterol, HDL-cholesterol, and VLDL-cholesterol, the LDL-cholesterol level can be estimated by the following equation:

$$\text{LDL-cholesterol} = \text{total cholesterol} - \text{HDL-cholesterol} - (\text{triglycerides} \div 5)$$

If the triglyceride level is greater than 400 mg per dL, LDL-cholesterol should not be estimated, but ultracentrifugation of the serum in a specialized laboratory would provide a more accurate LDL-cholesterol level.

The evidence that elevated LDL-cholesterol is a cause of CHD has been well established from epidemiologic, genetic, and animal investigations.[41,91–93,97,98] Moreover, recently completed clinical trials have demonstrated that lowering the LDL-cholesterol ratio by dietary and/or drug interventions can reduce the incidence of CHD.[98,111,112]

High-Density Lipoproteins

HDLs are the smallest particles in the major classes of lipoproteins, and they have the highest density. They are about 50 percent protein, and they contain approximately 18 percent cholesterol and very little triglyceride.[100] HDL is synthesized in both the liver and small intestine. It plays an important role in lipid metabolism by transporting cholesterol from the cells back to the liver, where they are metabolized into bile or bile salts and used in further digestion or excreted from the body via the intestines. This reverse cholesterol transport may be the method whereby HDL protects the body from developing atherosclerosis. Levels of HDL cholesterol vary inversely with total body pools of cholesterol.

The HDL level consists of three subfractions. The plasma level of HDL_2 appears to be the primary cardioprotective and most abundant subfraction of the total HDL-cholesterol.[113] Accurate measurements of HDL subfractions are currently available only in research laboratories. The need to measure HDL subfractions is not suggested because of the high correlation of HDL_2 and total HDL-cholesterol.

Apolipoproteins

Apolipoproteins are the protein subcomponent on the surface of lipoproteins that help deliver the lipoproteins to their sites of metabolism and degradation. They play an important role in maintaining the structure integrity of lipoproteins and the regulation of metabolic enzymes.[100] Nine apolipoproteins have been identified, and almost all are present on the chylomicrons. Quantitative analysis and the role of apolipoproteins in identifying individuals at risk for CHD have received considerable recent attention.[113,114]

TABLE 13-7 Classification and Treatment Decisions Based on LDL-Cholesterol

A. *Classification*

<130 mg/dL	Desirable LDL-cholesterol
130-159 mg/dL	Borderline-high-risk LDL-cholesterol
≥160 mg/dL	High-risk LDL-cholesterol

B. *Dietary Treatment*

	Initiation Level	Minimal Goal
Without CHD or two other risk factors	≥160 mg/dL	<160 mg/dL
With CHD or two other risk factors	≥130 mg/dL	<130 mg/dL

C. *Drug Treatment*

	Initiation Level	Minimal Goal
Without CHD or two other risk factors	≥190 mg/dL	<160 mg/dL
With CHD or two other factors	≥160 mg/dL	<130 mg/dL

Source: Adapted from National Cholesterol Education Program: Report of the Expert Panel on Detection, Evaluation, and Treatment of High Blood Cholesterol in Adults,[132] p. 9, with permission.

The most promising research has focused on apolipoprotein A_1 (apo A_1) and apolipoprotein B (apo B). Apo A_1 and apo A_2 are associated with the chylomicrons and HDL-cholesterol (Table 13–7). Apo B is the major protein constituent of LDL-cholesterol and is a significant component of the chylomicrons and VLDL-cholesterol. Apolipoproteins C_1, C_2, and C_3 are found in the chylomicrons and VLDL-cholesterol. After lipolysis of the VLDL and chylomicrons, the apolipoproteins C's are transferred to the HDL.[114]

Recent evidence has suggested that measurements of apo A_1, apo A_2, and apo B or lipoprotein Lp(a) may provide a stronger indication of CHD risk than concentrations of plasma lipids, HDL-cholesterol, or LDL-cholesterol.[115–117] Currently, the measurement of apolipoproteins is not practical, but in some lipid disorders the measurements can aid in detection of the underlying cause as well as the effects of various interventions.

CLASSIFICATION OF LIPID DISORDERS

Initial classification of lipid disorders begins with the measurement of total serum cholesterol. Recent guidelines were defined by the adult treatment panel of the National Cholesterol Education Program.[118] All adults 20 years of age and older as well as children with a family history of premature CHD and/or a genetic hyperlipidemia should be tested at least once every 5 years. A "desirable level" of serum cholesterol is defined as less than 200 mg per dL. (Table 13–8).[118]

Cholesterol levels between 200 to 239 mg per dL are defined as "borderline-high." Patients with confirmed cholesterol levels in that range without CHD or two other CHD risk factors should be given dietary information and be re-evaluated annually. Borderline-high patients with two other CHD risk factors (including male gender and a family history of premature CHD) or with documented CHD should undergo a 12- to 14-hour

TABLE 13–8 Initial Classification and Recommended Follow-Up Based on Total Cholesterol

A. *Classification*

<200 mg/dL	Desirable blood cholesterol
200–239 mg/dL	Borderline-high blood cholesterol
≥240 mg/dL	High blood cholesterol

B. *Recommended Follow-Up*

Total cholesterol <200 mg/dL	Repeat within 5 years
Total cholesterol 200–239 mg/dL	
Without definite CHD or two other CHD risk factors (one of which can be male sex)	Dietary information and recheck annually
With definite CHD or two other CHD risk factors (one of which can be male sex)	
	Lipoprotein analysis: further action based on LDL-cholesterol level
Total Cholesterol ≥240 mg/dL	

Source: Adapted from National Cholesterol Education Program: Report of the Expert Panel on Detection, Evaluation, and Treatment of High Blood Cholesterol in Adults,[132] p. 8, with permission.

fasting lipoprotein analysis of total cholesterol, HDL-cholesterol, and triglyceride. LDL-cholesterol should be calculated by the method previously mentioned.[105]

Patients with cholesterol levels equal to or greater than 240 mg per dL are classified as having "high" serum cholesterol. The risk of developing CHD in individuals with a high cholesterol at least doubles when compared with levels less than 200 mg per dL.[95] Patients with high total cholesterol levels require a lipoprotein analysis. Once a patient has a lipoprotein analysis, the focus of attention shifts from total cholesterol to the LDL-cholesterol value because of the stronger association of LDL-cholesterol to CHD. This approach allows the clinician to properly identify the lipid disorder and serves as an index for clinical decision making about lipid-lowering therapy.

The "desirable" LDL-cholesterol level is defined as a value less than 130 mg per dL (Table 13–7). Dietary modification is recommended for patients in the 130 to 159 mg per dL borderline-high-risk LDL-cholesterol range as well as those at high-risk LDL-cholesterol in excess of 160 mg per dL. Patients with documented CHD or that present with two other risk factors (including HDL-cholesterol levels less than 35 mg per dL) who have borderline-high or high-risk LDL-cholesterol should have a comprehensive clinical evaluation before initiating cholesterol-lowering intervention. After a minimum of 6 months of intensive dietary intervention and counseling, drug therapy should be initiated for LDL-cholesterol levels greater than 190 mg per dL or 160 mg per dL if two or more risk factors are present.

The clinical evaluation of patients with borderline-high or high-risk LDL-cholesterol may assist in the determination of whether the elevated LDL-cholesterol level is secondary to another disease, a familial or genetic lipid disorder, or an adverse effect of a drug therapy. A more important aim of clinical assessment is to determine the presence or absence of definite CHD and of other heart disease risk factors. The information will aid in decisions on dietary and pharmacologic treatment directed toward lowering LDL-cholesterol. A brief review of the various lipid disorders and their causes will be helpful in assessing risk and determining the appropriate intervention. A more detailed review is given elsewhere.[6,104,107,108,110,118]

SEVERE FORMS OF GENETIC HYPERCHOLESTEROLEMIA

Familial Hypercholesterolemia

Familial hypercholesterolemia (FH) is an autosomal dominant disorder characterized by a defect in the gene encoding for the LDL receptor, which is either absent or nonfunctional. The gene for the LDL receptor is normally inherited from both parents. In very rare incidences, individuals inherit two abnormal genes for LDL receptors and intracellular cholesterol production is out of control. This causes serum cholesterol levels to be in the range of 600 to 1000 mg per dL. The disorder occurs in one in a million people and leads to atherosclerosis by the age of 10 years with survival rarely past 20 years.[110] The heterozygous form of FH occurs in 1 out of 500 people in whom an abnormal gene for the LDL receptor is inherited from only one parent. The affected individual has only one half of the normal number of LDL receptors, and serum cholesterol levels are in the 350 to 450 mg per dL range. Patients with heterozygous FH are prone to premature CHD, usually do not respond adequately to dietary therapy alone, and often require a combination of lipid-lowering medications to bring LDL-cholesterol under control.

Familial Combined Hyperlipidemia

Familial combined hyperlipidemia (FCHL) is another autosomal dominant disorder characterized by multiple patterns of hyperlipidemia phenotypes occurring in a single family. Approximately 1 to 2 percent of the American population appear to have FCHL with about one third of the affected patients having elevated VLDL-cholesterol, one third having increases in LDL-cholesterol alone, and the remainder having either elevated VLDL and LDL or elevated VLDL and chylomicrons. The primary defect appears to be overproduction of apolipoprotein B (apo B). Diagnosis is made by testing first-degree relatives and by finding multiple lipoprotein phenotypes in the same family. Approximately 10 to 15 percent of patients with MI before 60 years of age have familial combined hyperlipidemia.[110]

Severe Primary Hypercholesterolemia

Severe primary hypercholesterolemia is often called polygenic hypercholesterolemia because a definite monogenic inheritance of elevated LDL-cholesterol cannot be demonstrated. The word "polygenic" can be considered to mean that several different defects might cause a monogenic form of moderate hypercholesterolemia. Recently, several metabolic abnormalities, such as mild defects in LDL-receptor function, overproduction of apolipoprotein B-100, and an increased cholesterol absorption, have been identified and are thought to be responsible for polygenic hypercholesterolemia. Patients in this category often do not respond to dietary treatment and require a combination of drugs to lower LDL-cholesterol.

Familial Dysbetalipoproteinemia

Familial dysbetalipoproteinemia (type III hyperlipoproteinemia) is relatively uncommon; it occurs in about 1 in every 5000 people in the United States.[118] An abnormal apolipoprotein E interferes with the normal metabolism of VLDL and chylomicrons and leads to elevated intermediate-density lipoproteins (IDLs) or beta-VLDL. The diagnosis should be suspected when both triglyceride levels and serum cholesterol levels are elevated. Patients with this hyperlipidemia are characterized by the physical findings of palmar tuberous xanthomas and premature CHD and peripheral vascular disease. Frequently these patients are obese, glucose-intolerant, and hyperuricemic.

Familial Hypertriglyceridemia

Familial hypertriglyceridemia (FHTG) is an autosomal dominant disorder characterized by the monogenic inheritance of pure hypertriglyceridemia. In FHTG, serum triglyceride levels are in the range of 300 to 800 mg per dL and serum total cholesterol levels are usually lower than 240 mg per dL. The primary defect is uncertain, but a predominant abnormality may be the overproduction of VLDL-triglycerides by the liver. Some families with FHTG demonstrate a defect in lipolysis of triglyceride-rich lipoproteins that results in either type IV or type V hyperlipidemia.

The diagnosis of FHTG can be made by family screening and finding elevated triglyceride levels in approximately half of first-degree relatives. Patients with FHTG seem to be at lesser risk for CHD than those with familial combined hyperlipidemia.[110,118] Caloric restriction and exercise resulting in maintenance of ideal body weight are strongly recommended for FHTG patients.

Chylomicronemia Syndrome

Chylomicronemia syndrome (formerly type V hyperlipidemia)[119] is due to a combination of defects in lipoprotein metabolism. This hyperchylomicronemia results from defective lipolysis of triglyceride-rich lipoproteins and a defect in triglyceride metabolism from an overproduction of VLDL-triglycerides. Overproduction of VLDL-triglycerides could be either genetic or secondary to excessive alcohol intake, obesity, diabetes mellitus, or chronic renal failure.[110] Abdominal pain, pancreatitis, and eruptive xanthomas are physical findings often associated with this syndrome.

Hypertriglyceridemia

A fasting serum triglyceride level above 500 mg per dL is defined as definite hypertriglyceridemia.[120] Triglyceride levels in the range of 250 to 500 mg per dL are designated as "borderline hypertriglyceridemia." A serum triglyceride level below 250 mg per dL can be considered normal or desirable. The relation between serum triglyceride levels and cardiovascular disease is controversial. In most population studies, serum triglyceride levels were not independently predictive of CHD after being statistically corrected for such associated risk factors as total serum cholesterol, low HDL-cholesterol, cigarette smoking, and obesity.[6] Results from the Framingham Heart Study found that high triglyceride levels are an independent risk factor for CHD in women and possibly also in men.[121] Rather than being a direct cause of atherogenesis, elevated triglyceride levels are usually present with other atherogenic lipoprotein abnormalities that are more directly associated with CHD such as small, dense LDL particles and low levels of HDL-cholesterol.[122] Some patients with borderline or high triglyceride levels and a strong family history of premature cardiovascular disease may have familial combined hyperlipidemia that also increases the risk of CHD. The most common lipoprotein abnormalities produced by hypertriglyceridemia are increased levels of chylomicron remnants and VLDL remnants as well as decreased levels of HDL-cholesterol. The most common lipoprotein abnormalities produced by hypertriglyceridemia are increased levels of chylomicron remnants and VLDL remnants as well as decreased levels of HDL-cholesterol. Changes in lifestyle (weight control, increased physical activity, and alcohol and fat restriction) are the first line of intervention for reducing triglyceride levels. In patients with borderline hypertriglyceridemia, emphasis should be on weight reduction and increased physical activity.

Hypoalphalipoproteinemia

Epidemiologic and research data have shown that concentrations of HDL-cholesterol are inversely related to CHD rates among adult Americans. This inverse relation has been well documented in the Framingham Heart Study.[125,126] An HDL-cholesterol level below 35 mg per dL is defined as abnormal or low. A decrease in HDL levels from 60 to 30 mg per dL is associated with a doubled prevalence of coronary disease.[127]

In men a cholesterol level of 35 mg per dL increases the CHD risk almost 1.5 times the average risk associated with 45 mg per dL. Patients with genetic or primary hypoalphalipoproteinemia frequently have HDL-cholesterol levels in the 20 to 29 mg per dL range. The metabolic abnormalities for these low HDL-cholesterol concentrations are not well understood. Some research has suggested that abnormalities in the metabolism of apolipoproteins (apo) A_1 and A_2 are the primary causes of this dyslipidemia. The secondary causes of reduced serum HDL-cholesterol levels are obesity, physical inactivity, and smoking.[128-130] These negative lifestyle factors depress HDL levels and therefore increase coronary risk. Anabolic steroids and progestational agents also can decrease HDL-cholesterol levels. Beta-blockers and thiazide diuretics, drugs commonly used to treat hypertension, have been found to reduce HDL-cholesterol levels. Hypertriglyceridemia, even in mild forms, is often associated with significantly decreased levels of HDL-cholesterol. For men over age 50 and women at any age, the total cholesterol/HDL-cholesterol ratio is an accurate predictor of CHD risk. The incidence of CHD (based on 4 years of surveillance of participants in the Framingham Study, aged 49 to 82 years) was found to increase when HDL-cholesterol and total plasma cholesterol ratios were high.[131] The strong relation between the incidence of CHD and HDL-C ratio appears to apply to all levels of total cholesterol. The relation applies even to individuals with total cholesterol levels below 200 mg per dL. These findings were also seen for sex-specific rates; as expected, men tend to have higher incidence rates than women. However, the inverse correlation between HDL and CHD is especially strong in women. For every 10 mg per dL change in HDL-cholesterol, CHD risk changed by 50 percent among the Framingham women and by 42 percent among the women of the Lipid Research Clinics follow-up.[93]

EVALUATION OF PATIENT RISK FACTOR MODIFICATION

Regular evaluation of patient compliance with risk factor modification is a standard procedure while the patient is participating in the formal supervised program. However, once the patient leaves the program and is exercising independently at home, compliance to the prescribed plan for risk factor modification and exercise can be assessed through regularly scheduled evaluations. These evaluations are scheduled at intervals determined by the medical status of the patient. After "graduation" from the formal program, the patient should be evaluated at least annually.

Rehabilitation staff should note that in the initial stages of rehabilitation, too much change will defeat the purpose of behavior modification. Patients must not be overwhelmed by the considerable changes that must be made in their lifestyles. Care must be taken to apply developmental principles to the establishment of goals to ensure success in modifying behavior.

Dietary Intervention

Generally, the goals of dietary intervention are to decrease the levels of blood cholesterol and, especially, LDL-cholesterol, since evidence indicates that lowering of

TABLE 13–9 Dietary Therapy of High Blood Cholesterol

Nutrient	Recommended Intake	
	Step-One Diet	Step-Two Diet
Total fat	Less than 30% of total calories	
Saturated fatty acids	Less than 10% of total calories	Less than 7% of total calories
Polyunsaturated fatty acids	Up to 10% of total calories	
Monounsaturated fatty acids	10 to 15% of total calories	
Carbohydrates	50 to 60% of total calories	
Protein	10 to 20% of total calories	
Cholesterol	Less than 300 mg/day	Less than 200 mg/day
Total Calories	To achieve and maintain desirable weight	

Source: From National Cholesterol Education Program,[132] p. 30, with permission.

LDL-cholesterol will decrease the incidence of CHD.[132] In addition, rehabilitation of cardiac patients involves dietary intervention to reduce hypertension or maintain normal blood pressure and to reduce or normalize body weight.

Justification for such intervention is based primarily on the associations among total serum cholesterol, diet, and mortality rates owing to CHD as demonstrated by numerous studies, including long-term epidemiologic investigations such as the Framingham[133] and Chicago[134] studies that followed the progression of the disease in populations that were initially free of CHD.

Treatment for patients with elevated LDL-cholesterol begins with diet therapy. Usually the goal of reduction in LDL-cholesterol (to 160 or 130 mg per dL) can be achieved if the diet therapy management is directed toward lowering total cholesterol levels. This method of dietary management eliminates the additional costs of measuring LDL-cholesterol, since total cholesterol levels of 240 and 200 mg per dL generally correspond to LDL-cholesterol levels of 160 and 130 mg per dL, respectively.[132] (See p. 365).

DIETARY RECOMMENDATIONS

Considerable controversy exists as to the most prudent approach for dietary modifications to manage serum cholesterol levels. The most widely recommended diets are referred to as the Step-One and Step-Two Diets[132] (Table 13–9). Both are designed to reduce the intake of saturated fatty acids and cholesterol and to eliminate intake of excess calories. Diet therapy usually begins with the Step-One Diet (Table 13–10),

TABLE 13–10 Recommended Diet Modifications to Lower Blood Cholesterol: The Step-One Diet

	Choose	Decrease
Fish, chicken, turkey, and lean meats	Fish, poultry without skin, lean cuts of beef, lamb, pork or veal, shellfish	Fatty cuts of beef, lamb, pork; spare ribs, organ meats, regular cold cuts, sausage, hot dogs, bacon, sardines, roe

continued

TABLE 13–10 Recommended Diet Modifications to Lower Blood Cholesterol: The Step-One Diet *Continued*

	Choose	Decrease
Skim and low-fat milk, cheese, yogurt, and dairy substitutes	Skim or 1% fat milk (liquid, powdered, evaporated), buttermilk	Whole milk (14% fat): regular, evaporated, condensed; cream, half and half, 2% milk, imitation milk products, most nondairy creamers, whipped toppings
	Nonfat (0% fat) or low-fat yogurt	Whole-milk yogurt
	Low-fat cottage cheese (1% or 2% fat)	Whole-milk cottage cheese (4% fat)
	Low-fat cheeses, farmer, or pot cheeses (all of these should be labeled no more than 2–6 g fat/ounce)	All natural cheeses (e.g., blue, roquefort, camembert, cheddar, Swiss)
		Low-fat or "light" cream cheese, low-fat or "light" sour cream
		Cream cheeses, sour cream
	Sherbet	Ice cream
	Sorbet	
Eggs	Egg whites (2 whites = 1 whole egg in recipes), cholesterol-free egg substitutes	Egg yolks
Fruits and vegetables	Fresh, frozen, canned, or dried fruits and vegetables	Vegetables prepared in butter, cream, or other sauces
Breads and cereals	Homemade baked goods using unsaturated oils sparingly, angel food cake, low-fat crackers, low-fat cookies	Commercial baked goods: pies, cakes, doughnuts, croissants, pastries, muffins, biscuits, high-fat crackers, high-fat cookies
	Rice, pasta	Egg noodles
	Whole-grain breads and cereals (oatmeal, whole wheat, rye, bran, multigrain, etc.)	Breads in which eggs are major ingredient
Fats and oils	Baking cocoa	Chocolate
	Unsaturated vegetable oils: corn, olive, rapeseed (canola oil), safflower, sesame, soybean, sunflower	Butter, coconut oil, palm oil, palm kernel oil, lard, bacon fat
	Margarine or shortening made from one of the unsaturated oils listed above	
	Diet margarine	
	Mayonaisse, salad dressings made with unsaturated oils listed above	Dressings made with egg yolk
	Low-fat dressings	
	Seeds and nuts	Coconut

Source: From National Cholesterol Education Program: Report of The Expert Panel on Detection, Evaluation, and Treatment of High Blood Cholesterol in Adults,[132] p. 39, with permission.

which recommends a daily fat intake of less than 30 percent of total calories, less than 10 percent of total intake in saturated fatty acids, and less than 300 mg per day of cholesterol. The patient usually remains on this regimen for 3 months. If at the end of that time, the cholesterol levels remain high, the patient is progressed to the Step-Two Diet. The Step-Two Diet further reduces the saturated fatty acid intake to less than 7 percent of total calories and cholesterol to less than 200 mg per day. Patients usually remain on diet therapy for at least 6 months, after which, if cholesterol levels remain high, drug therapy may be considered.

ADDITIONAL DIETARY REGIMENS

Several approaches to dietary modifications have been used to treat various types of hyperlipidemic disorders. Investigation of experimental diets for treatment of all types of hyperlipidemia has yielded specific information about dietary modification. A 10 percent reduction in total serum cholesterol has been reported as a result of therapeutic diet regimens that limit the total dietary cholesterol to 200 mg per day and also limit fat to 30 percent of the total caloric intake, with the ratio of polyunsaturated fat to saturated fat (P/S ratio) 2.0 or greater.[135] Therapeutic diets for hyperlipidemic patients must have a P/S ratio greater than 1.0, and diets with a P/S ratio of 2.0 have been demonstrated to be hypocholesterolemic in effect.[135] In contrast, the average American daily diet contains 500 mg of cholesterol and has a P/S ratio of 0.4.[136] Even greater declines in serum cholesterol (as much as 24 percent) have been reported with therapeutic regimens of 25 mg per day of cholesterol, 10 percent fat (P/S ratio of 1.24), and little protein intake from animal sources.[135] (see Table 13–11).

Further reductions in serum cholesterol can be achieved by increasing the soluble fiber in the diet. This type of fiber is not absorbed by the intestine and is found primarily in plant material. Soluble fiber includes pectins, certain gums, and psyllium. Beta-glucan, a soluble fiber, is found in oat products and beans, and ingestion of 15 to 25 g per day of soluble fiber has been found to lower the plasma cholesterol level by 5 to 15 percent.[132]

Some cardiac rehabilitation centers employ the "Alternative Diet"[135] or some modification of it. This diet has been recommended for initial use in the treatment of all types of hyperlipidemia. Basically, it restricts the daily intake of cholesterol to 100 mg, dietary fat to 20 percent of total calories (high P/S ratio), and meat consumption to 3 to 4 oz per day. It encourages the exclusive use of polyunsaturated fats, complex carbohydrates, and low-cholesterol cheeses.

In comparison, the experimental diet reported by Barnard and associates[137] (Pritikin Longevity Center Diet) restricts the daily intake of cholesterol to 25 mg, dietary fat to 10

TABLE 13–11 A Comparison of the Average American Diet to
the Low-Fat Modified Diet

	Average American Diet	Low-Fat Modified Diet
% fat	42 (P/S ratio 0.4)	30 (P/S ratio 1.0–2.0)
% protein	15 Animal	15 Vegetable and animal
% carbohydrate	42 Simple	55 Complex
	100	100
Cholesterol content	500 mg/day	300 mg/day or less

TABLE 13–12 A Comparison of Diet Plans for CHD Patients

Name of Plan	Cholesterol (mg)	% Fat	P/S Ratio	Meat (oz)	Alcohol	Caffeine	High in Complex Carbohydrates
Alternative	100	20	1.0–2.0	3–4	0–rarely	0	Yes
Pritikin	25	10	1.0–2.0	0–rarely	0	0	Yes
AHA	300 or less	30–35	1.0–2.0	4–6	0–rarely	0	Yes

TABLE 13–13 Quantitative Guidelines for the AHA and Alternative Diet Plans

Food Group	AHA	Alternative
I. Meat Poultry Fish	No more than 2 servings/day One serving = 2–3 oz. meat, fish, poultry	No more than 2 servings/day One serving = 0–2 oz. meat, fish, poultry (If vegetarian, B_{12} supplement may be required)
Legumes Nuts Eggs	1 c. cooked legumes 4 T. peanut butter 3 eggs/week	1 c. cooked legumes No nuts except chestnuts No yolks, 7 whites/week
II. Fruits and Vegetables	4 or more servings/day One serving = ½ c. fruit juice or vegetable juice 1 medium fruit or vegetable ½ c. cooked fruit or vegetable	4 or more servings/day One serving = 1 medium fruit, fresh No fruit juice Avoid canned and processed fruits Use fruit juice and dried fruits as a substitute for sugar in recipes
III. Breads and Cereals	4 or more servings/day One serving = 1 slice bread, french, rye, pumpernickel, pita, containing 1.5 g. fat/slice 1 c. dry cereal ½ c. cooked cereal ½ c. pasta, rice, noodles (no yolk) 1 tortilla, corn 2 graham crackers 1 c. popcorn 1 bagel made without eggs	4 or more servings/day One serving = (same as Lowfat) Use whole grains and unprocessed whole grain products rather than defined products 2 or more different grains/day
IV. Milk Products	2 or more servings/day One serving = Nonfat milk or buttermilk (8 oz.) Lowfat cheese (1 oz.) Lowfat yogurt (8 oz.) ⅓ c. lowfat cottage cheese	2 servings/day One serving = Nonfat milk or buttermilk (8 oz.) Nonfat cheese (2 oz.) Nonfat yogurt (2 oz.) Nonfat milk powder (5 T.) Tofu (2 oz.) Soybeans (2 oz.)
V. Fats	2–4 T. polyunsaturated/day	No processed fats or oils Avoid avocados and olives

percent of total calories (P/S ratio 1.24), and no meat consumption. All protein requirements (13 percent of total calories) are derived from vegetable sources, with the exception of nonfat milk and small amounts of fish or fowl. All remaining calories (77
percent) are consumed in the form of complex carbohydrates. In addition, no caffeine or
alcohol is permitted.[137]

In contrast to the Pritikin Diet are the recommendations of the American Heart
Association.[138] The guidelines for dietary modification recommended by the AHA have
come to be known as the "prudent" diet. The AHA diet restricts the daily intake of
cholesterol to less than 300 mg, dietary fat to 30 to 35 percent of total calories (P/S ratio
1.0), and meat consumption to 4 to 6 oz per day. Table 13–12 summarizes the differences among the three diet plans.

The staff dietitian or nutritionist and the referring physician play the major role in
determining each patient's dietary regimen. However, everyone shares responsibility for
keeping abreast of current trends and research in dietary management of CHD patients.
(See Tables 13–13 and 13–14 for examples of dietary regimens and a summary of
low-fat dietary objectives, respectively.)

DRUG THERAPY

Patients whose LDL-cholesterol remains elevated following at least 6 months of
diet therapy should probably be recommended for drug treatment. Candidates for drug
therapy include those whose LDL-cholesterol remains equal to or greater than 190 mg
per dL and who have no CHD or have two CHD risk factors. Candidates for drug
therapy are also those whose LDL-cholesterol is equal to or greater than 160 mg per dL
and are known to have CHD or two other risk factors (Table 13–15). Individuals whose

TABLE 13–14 Summary of Low-Fat Diet Objectives

1. Reduce the consumption of beef, pork, and lamb.
2. Substitute poultry, fish, and meat substitutes for beef, lamb, and pork.
3. Prepare poultry and seafood without added fat.
4. Increase consumption of meatless meals.
5. Prepare rice, macaroni, and other grains without added fat.
6. Prepare vegetables without added fat.
7. Reduce the consumption of margarine and peanut butter as spreads for breads and rolls. Eliminate butter totally.
8. Use only fat-free salad dressings.
9. Use only skim and low-fat dairy products.
10. Use only low-fat breads and cereals.
11. Avoid commercial baked goods (cakes, pies, cookies).
12. Avoid egg yolks.
13. Avoid foods high in sodium, and do not add salt at the table.
14. Limit the use of sugar in coffee and tea and on cereal.
15. Substitute fruit toppings for jams, preserves, jellies, honey, syrup, and molasses.
16. Use only recommended dessert recipes.
17. Drink decaffeinated coffee and caffeine-free herb teas.
18. Limit alcoholic beverages.

Source: From Frye et al.: A Comprehensive Guide to Cardiac Rehabilitation. The Methodist Hospital, Houston, TX, 1982, with permission.

TABLE 13-15 Risk Status Based on Presence of CHD Risk Factors Other Than LDL-Cholesterol

The patient is considered to have a high-risk status if he or she falls into *one* of the following groups.

Definite CHD: Characteristic Clinical Picture and Objective Laboratory Findings

Definite prior myocardial infarction, *or*
Definite myocardial ischemia, such as angina pectoris

Two Other CHD Risk Factors

Male sex*
Family history of premature CHD (definite myocardial infarction or sudden death before
   age 55 in a parent or sibling)
Cigarette smoking (currently smokes more than 10 cigarettes per day)
Hypertension
Low HDL-cholesterol concentration (below 35 mg/dL confirmed by repeat measurement)
Diabetes mellitus
History of definite cerebrovascular or occlusive peripheral vascular disease
Severe obesity (≥30% overweight)

---

*Male sex is considered a risk factor in this scheme because the rates of CHD are 3 to 4 times higher in men than in women in the middle decades of life and roughly 2 times higher in the elderly. Hence, a man with one other CHD risk factor is considered to have a high-risk status, whereas a woman is not so considered unless she has two other CHD risk factors.

Source: From National Cholesterol Education Program: Report of the Expert Panel on Detection, Evaluation, and Treatment of High Blood Cholesterol in Adults,[132] p. 23, with permission.

LDL-cholesterol exceeds 190 mg per dL are to be considered for drug therapy provided nonpharmacologic intervention through diet, weight control, exercise, and lifestyle modifications (such as quitting smoking and managing stress) have been unsuccessful.

The drugs that are most preferred for lowering LDL-cholesterol are the bile acid sequestrants (cholestyramine and colestipol) and nicotinic acid. In patients who have no concurrent hypertriglyceridemia, the drugs of choice are the bile acid sequestrants. For patients who have concurrent hypertriglyceridemia, the preferred therapy is nicotinic acid.

Newer drugs are currently being used in the treatment of elevated LDL-cholesterol levels, but their side effects, long-term safety, and effectiveness have not been extensively studied. Of the newer medications, the inhibitors of HMG CoA reductase (the rate-limiting enzyme in cholesterol syntheses) are being evaluated, and lovastatin has been approved for marketing. Simvastatin and pravastatin also are inhibitors of HMG CoA reductase, but their use is currently primarily experimental.[132] Among the many medications that are being investigated for use in reducing the risk of CHD are gemfibrozil, probucol, and clofibrate. Gemfibrozil and clofibrate are used for lowering triglyceride levels to reduce the risk of pancreatitis but are not routinely used to lower cholesterol levels and reduce the risk of CHD. Probucol reduces LDL-cholesterol but also has been found to lower the level of LDL-cholesterol. (Table 13-16) A comprehensive discussion of the various medications and drug therapies currently being investigated to decrease the risk of CHD is beyond the scope of this text, and the reader is referred elsewhere. The area of drug therapy will continue to play an important part in the treatment of hyperlipidemia.

TABLE 13–16 Summary of the Major Drugs for Consideration

Drugs	Reduce CHD Risk	Long-Term Safety	Maintaining Adherence	LDL-Cholesterol Lowering, %	Special Precautions
Cholestyramine Colestipol	Yes	Yes	Requires considerable education	15–30	Can alter absorption of other drugs. Can increase triglyceride levels and should not be used in patients with hypertriglyceridemia.
Nicotinic acid	Yes	Yes	Requires considerable education	15–30	Test for hyperuricemia, hyperglycemia, and liver function abnormalities.
Lovastatin*	Not proven	Not established	Relatively easy	25–45	Monitor for liver function abnormalities and possible lens opacities.
Gemfibrozil†	Not proven	Preliminary evidence	Relatively easy	5–15	May increase LDL-cholesterol in hypertriglyceridemic patients. Should not be used in patients with gallbladder disease.
Probucol	Not proven	Not established	Relatively easy	10–15	Lowers HDL-cholesterol; significance of this has not been established. Prolongs QT interval.

*Recently approved by the FDA for marketing.
†Not FDA-approved for routine use in lowering cholesterol. The results of the Helsinki Heart Study should be available soon to define the effect on CHD risk and long-term safety.
Source: From National Cholesterol Education Program: Report of the Expert Panel on Detection, Evaluation, and Treatment of High Blood Cholesterol in Adults,[132] p. 51, with permission.

378

SUMMARY

The primary modifiable risk factors associated with increased incidence of CHD have been identified; they include smoking, hypertension, and high serum cholesterol levels (particularly LDL-cholesterol). They have been discussed in regard to their primary physiologic effects and current trends in the detection, management, and treatment of those factors. In most cases, treatment involves not only medical management but also lifestyle modifications that include exercise, normalizing body weight, dietary changes, and stress management. Increasing evidence supports the continuing need for quality cardiac rehabilitation programs that utilize a multidisciplinary approach as an adjunct to the medical and surgical management of the CHD patient.

REFERENCES

1. Havlik, RJ and Feinleib, M (eds): Proceedings of the conference on the decline in coronary heart disease mortality. US Department of Health, Education, and Welfare, NIH Publication 6 79-1610, Bethesda, MD, 1979.
2. Feinleib, M: The magnitude and nature of the decrease in coronary heart disease mortality rate. Am J Cardiol 54:2C, 1984.
3. Wenger, NK and Schlant, RC: Prevention of coronary atherosclerosis. In Hurst, JW and Schlant, RC (eds): The Heart, Arteries and Veins, ed 7. McGraw-Hill, New York, 1990, p 893.
4. Kueller, L: Risk factor reduction in coronary heart disease: Modern concepts of cardiovascular disease. Am Heart Assoc 53:7, 1984.
5. Sytkowski, PA, Kannel, WB and D'Angostino, RB: Changes in risk factors and the decline in mortality from cardiovascular disease: The Framingham Heart Study. N Engl J Med 322:1635, 1990.
6. Grundy, SM, et al: Cardiovascular and risk factor evaluation of healthy American adults: A statement for physicians by an ad hoc committee appointed by the steering committee, American Heart Association. Circulation 75:1340A, 1987.
7. Grundy, SM: Can modification of risk factors reduce coronary heart disease? In Rahimtoola, SH (ed): Controversies in Coronary Artery Disease. FA Davis, Philadelphia, 1982, p 283.
8. Miller, NH, et al: The efficacy of risk factor intervention and psychosocial aspects of cardiac rehabilitation. J Cardiopulmonary Rehabil 10:198, 1990.
9. Godin, G: The effectiveness of interventions in modifying behavioral risk factors in individuals with coronary heart disease. J Cardiopulmonary Rehabil 9:223, 1989.
10. Hartley, LH, et al: Secondary prevention of coronary artery disease. Task Force 6. Circulation (Suppl)76:I168, 1987.
11. Smoking and health. US Department of Health and Human Services, Publication No PHS 79-50066, Bethesda, MD, 1979.
12. The health consequences of smoking: A report of the Surgeon General. US Department of Health and Human Services, Publication No PHS 82-50179, Rockville, MD, 1982.
13. Smoking-attributable mortality and years of potential life lost: United States, 1984. Centers for Disease Control, MMWR, 36:693, 1984.
14. Reducing the health consequences of smoking: 25 years of progress. A report of the Surgeon General. US Department of Health and Human Services, Publication No DHHS PHS 89-8411, Rockville, MD, 1989.
15. US Preventive Services Task Force: Counseling to prevent tobacco use. In Guide to Clinical Preventive Services: An Assessment of the Effectiveness of 169 Interventions Report of the US Preventive Services Task Force. Williams & Wilkins, Baltimore, 1989, p 289.
16. Hahn, RA, et al: Excess deaths from nine chronic diseases in the United States, 1986. JAMA, 264:2654, 1990.
17. Pooling Project Research Group. Relationship of blood pressure, serum cholesterol, smoking habit, relative weight and ECG abnormalities to incidence of major coronary events: Final report of the Pooling Project. J Chron Dis 31:202, 1978.
18. The health consequences of smoking: Cardiovascular disease. A report of the Surgeon General. US Department of Health and Human Services Publication No DHHS 84-50204, Rockville, MD, 1983.
19. Kannel, WB and Thomas, HE Jr: Sudden coronary death: The Framingham Study. Ann NY Acad Sci 382:3, 1982.

20. Hammond, EC and Garfinkle, L: Coronary heart disease, stroke, and aortic aneurysm: Factors in the etiology. Arch Environ Health 19:167, 1969.
21. Holbrook, JH, et al: Cigarette smoking and cardiovascular disease: A statement for health professionals by a task force appointed by the steering committee of the American Heart Association. Circulation 70:1114A, 1984.
22. Rosenberg, L, Palmer, JR and Shapiro, S: Decline in the risk of myocardial infarction among women who stop smoking. N Engl J Med 322:213, 1990.
23. Remington, PL, et al: Current smoking trends in the United States: The 1981–1983 behavioral risk factor surveys. JAMA 253:2975, 1985.
24. Fiore, MC, et al: Trends in cigarette smoking in the United States: The changing influence of gender and race. JAMA 261:249, 1989.
25. Reducing the health consequences of smoking: 25 years of progress: A report of the Surgeon General. US Department of Health and Human Services Publication No. DHHS 89-8411, Rockville, MD, 1989.
26. Yu, JJ, et al: A comparison of smoking patterns in the People's Republic of China with the United States: An impending health catastrophe in the Middle Kingdom. JAMA 264:1575, 1990.
27. Multiple risk factor intervention trial. Am J Epidemiol 126:783, 1987
28. Helsing, KJ, et al: Heart disease mortality in nonsmokers living with smokers. Am J Epidemiol 127:715, 1988.
29. Nordenberg, D, Yip, R and Binkin, NJ: The effects of cigarette smoking on hemoglobin levels and anemia screening. JAMA 264:1556, 1990.
30. Benowitz, NL: Pharmacologic aspects of cigarette smoking and nicotine addiction. N Engl J Med 319:1318, 1988.
31. Mulcahy, R: Smoking and cardiovascular disease. Cardiology Prac 1:252, 1985.
32. Rosenberg, L, et al: The risk of myocardial infarction after quitting smoking in men under 55 years of age. N Engl J Med 313:1511, 1985.
33. Sparrow, D, Dawber, TR and Colten, T: The influence of cigarette smoking on prognosis after a first myocardial infarction. J Chronic Dis 31:425, 1978.
34. Sohwartz, JL: Review and evaluation of smoking cessation methods: The United States and Canada 1978–1985. Division of Cancer Prevention and Control, National Cancer Institute, NIH Publication No 87-2940, Washington, DC, 1987.
35. The health benefits of smoking cessation: A report of the Surgeon General. US Department of Health and Human Services, Public Health Service, Publication No DHHS 90-8416, Rockville, MD, 1990.
36. Morbidity and mortality weekly report 39:653, 1990. Smokers' belief about the health benefits of smoking cessation, US Committee, 1989. JAMA 264:1933, 1990.
37. 1988 Joint National Committee: The 1988 report of the Joint National Committee on detection, evaluation, and treatment of high blood pressure. Arch Intern Med 148:1023, 1988.
38. US Department of Health and Human Services: The 1984 Report of the Joint National Committee on detection, evaluation, and treatment of high blood pressure. Public Health Service, National Institutes of Health, NIH Publication No 84-1088, Bethesda, MD, 1984.
39. Pooling Project Research Group: Relationship of blood pressure, serum cholesterol, smoking habit, relative weight and ECG abnormalities to incidence of major coronary events: Final report of the Pooling Project. J Chron Dis 31:201, 1987.
40. Kaplan, NM: The control of hypertension: A therapeutic breakthrough. Am Sci 68:537, 1980
41. Kannel, WB: CHD risk factors: A Framingham Study update. Hosp Prac 25:122, 1990.
42. Lucas, CP: Nonpharmacologic and pharmacologic treatment of hypertension. In Hall, LK and Meyer, GC (eds): Cardiac Rehabilitation: Exercise Testing and Prescription, Vol II. Life Enhancement Publications, Champaign, IL, 1988, p 327.
43. Kempner, W: Treatment of kidney disease and hypertensive vascular disease with rice diet. N Carolina Med J 5:125, 1955.
44. Stamler, J, et al: INTERSALT study findings: Public health and medical care implications. Hypertens 14:570, 1989.
45. Sanders, E (ed): Lifestyle factors may affect hypertension, data shows. Nat Med Assoc News, July/Aug: 1, 1990.
46. Weinberger, MH: Salt intake and blood pressure in humans. Contemp Nutr 13:1, 1988.
47. Melby, CL, Lyle, RM and Hyner, GC: Beyond blood pressure screening: A rationale for promoting the primary prevention of hypertension. Am J Health Promotion 3:5, 1988.
48. Inter-Society Commission for Heart Disease Resources: Optimal resources for primary prevention of atherosclerotic diseases. Circulation 70:153A, 1984.
49. Dustan, HP: Obesity and hypertension. Ann Intern Med 103: (part 2):1047, 1985.
50. Messerli, FH: Cardiovascular effects of obesity and hypertension. Lancet 1:1165, 1982.
51. Alexander, JK: Obesity and the cardiovascular system. Hypertension 16:43, 1990.
52. Alexander, JK: The heart and obesity. In JW Hearst (ed): The Heart, ed 7. McGraw-Hill, New York, 1990.
53. Kannel, WB, Brand, N and Skinner, JJ: Overweight and hypertension: The Framingham Study. Ann Intern Med 67:48, 1967.
54. Maxwell, MH, et al: Blood pressure changes in obese hypertensive subjects during rapid weight loss. Arch Intern Med 144:1581, 1984.

55. MacMahon, WS, Wilchen, DEL and MacDonald, GJ: The effect of weight reduction on left ventricular mass: A randomized controlled trial in young, overweight hypertensive patients. N Engl J Med 314:334, 1986.
56. Bray, GA: Obesity and the heart. Mod Concepts Cardiovasc Dis 56:67, 1987.
57. MacMaho, WS: Alcohol consumption and hypertension. Hypertension 9:111, 1987.
58. Saunders, JB, Beevers, DG and Paton, A: Alcohol induced hypertension. Lancet 2:653, 1981.
59. Klasky, AL, et al: Alcohol consumption and blood pressure: Kaiser-Permanente multiphasic health examination data. N Engl J Med 296:1194, 1977.
60. Arkwright, PD, et al: Effects of alcohol and other aspects of lifestyle on blood pressure levels and prevalence of hypertension in a working population. Circulation 66:60, 1982.
61. Selzer, ML: The Michigan Alcoholism Screening Test: The quest for a new diagnostic instrument. Am J Psychiatry 127:1653, 1971.
62. Tanji, VL: Hypertension: How exercise helps. Phys Sportsmed 18(7):77, 1990.
63. Seals, ED and Hagberg, J: The effects of exercise training on human hypertension: A review. Med Sci Sports Exerc 16:207, 1984.
64. Tipton, CM: Exercise, training and hypertension. Exerc Sport Sci Rev 12:245, 1984.
65. Boyer, J and Kasch, F: Exercise therapy in hypertensive men. JAMA 211:166B, 1970.
66. Choquette, G and Ferguson, R: Blood pressure reduction in borderline hypertensives following physical training. Can Med Assoc J 108:699, 1973.
67. Bonanno, J and Lies, J: Effects of physical training on coronary risk factors. Am J Cardiol 33:760, 1984.
68. Krotkiewski, M, et al: Effects of long-term physical training on body fat, metabolism, and blood pressure in obesity. Metabolism 28:650, 1979.
69. Roman, O, et al: Physical training program in arterial hypertension. A long-term prospective follow-up. Cardiology 67:230, 1981.
70. Kukkonen, K, et al: Physical training of middle-aged men with borderline hypertension. Ann Clin Res (Suppl)14:139, 1982.
71. Hagberg, J, et al: Effect of exercise training on the blood pressures and hemodynamics of adolescent hypertensives. Am J Cardiol 52:763, 1983.
72. Duncan, J, et al: The effects of aerobic exercise on plasma catecholamines and blood pressure in patients with mild hypertension. JAMA 254:2609, 1985.
73. Kiyonaga, A, et al: Blood pressure and hormonal responses to aerobic exercise. Hypertension 7:125, 1985.
74. Hagberg, JM and Seals, DR: Exercise training and hypertension. Acta Med Scand (Suppl)711:131, 1986.
75. Nelson, L, et al: Effect of changing levels of physical activity on blood pressure and hemodynamics in essential hypertension. Lancet 2:473, 1986.
76. Harris, KA and Holly, RG: Physiological response to circuit weight training in borderline hypertensive subjects. Med Sci Sports Exerc 19:246, 1987.
77. Gilders, RM, Vaner, C and Dudley, GA: Endurance training and blood pressure in normotensive and hypertensive adults. Med Sci Sports Exerc 21(6):629, 1989.
78. Herd, JA, et al: Psychophysiologic factor in hypertension. Circulation 76(1, Pt 2):I89, 1987.
79. Patel, C, et al: Trial of relaxation in reducing coronary risk: Four year follow-up. BMJ 290:1103, 1985.
80. Sutherland, JE: The link between stress and illness: Do our coping methods influence our health? Postgrad Med 89(1): 1991.
81. Resnick, LM: Ionic hypothesis: The link between hypertension, obesity, insulin resistance, and left ventricular hypertrophy. Prac Cardiol 16(12):36, 1990.
82. Julius, S, et al: The association of borderline hypertension with target organ changes and higher coronary risk: Teromusen blood pressure study. JAMA 264:354, 1990.
83. Ames, RP: Antihypertensive therapy and risk factors for coronary heart disease. Pract Cardiol 15(10):49, 1989.
84. Tanji, JL: Hypertension. Part 2. The role of medication. Phys Sports Med 18(8):87, 1990.
85. Gordon, T, et al: Predicting coronary heart disease in middle-aged and older persons: The Framingham Study. JAMA 238:497, 1977.
86. Neaton, JD, et al: Total and cardiovascular mortality in relation to cigarette smoking, serum cholesterol concentration, and diastolic blood pressure among black and white males followed up for five years (MRFIT). Am Heart J 108:759, 1984.
87. Schlant, RC, et al: The natural history of coronary heart disease: Prognostic factors after recovery from myocardial infarction in 2,789 men. The 5-year findings of the Coronary Drug Project. Circulation 66:401, 1982.
88. Keys, A (ed): Coronary heart disease in seven counties. Circulation (Suppl)41:I2, 1970.
89. Kannel, WB, et al: Serum cholesterol, lipoproteins, and the risk of coronary heart disease. The Framingham Study. Ann Intern Med 74:1, 1971.
90. Goldbourt, U, Holtzman, E and Neufeld, HN: Total and high density lipoprotein cholesterol in the serum and risk of mortality: Evidence of a threshold effect. Br Med J 290:1239, 1985.
91. Martin, MJ, et al: Serum cholesterol, blood pressure, and mortality: Implications from a cohort of 361, 662 men. Lancet 2:933, 1986.

92. Multiple Risk Factor Intervention Trial Research Group: Multiple risk factor intervention trial: Risk factor changes and mortality results. JAMA 248:1465, 1982.
93. American Heart Association Task Force on Cholesterol Issues: The cholesterol facts: A summary of the evidence relating to dietary fats, serum cholesterol, and coronary heart disease. A joint statement by the American Heart Association and the National Heart, Lung, and Blood Institute. Circulation 81:1721, 1990.
94. Godsland, IF, et al: Sex, plasma lipoproteins and atherosclerosis: Prevailing assumptions and outstanding questions. Am Heart J 114:1467, 1987.
95. Anderson, KM, Castelli, WP and Levy, D: Cholesterol and mortality: 30 years of follow-up from the Framingham Study. JAMA 257:2176, 1987.
96. Kannel, WB: Contributions of the Framingham Study to the conquest of coronary artery disease. Am J Cardiol 162:1109, 1988.
97. Brown, MS and Goldstein, JL: A receptor mediated pathway for cholesterol homeostasis. Science 232:34, 1986.
98. The Lipid Research Clinics Program. The Lipid Research Clinics Coronary Primary Prevention Trial results. I. Reduction in the incidence of coronary heart disease. II. The relationship of reduction in incidence of coronary heart disease to cholesterol lowering. JAMA 251:351, 365, 1984.
99. Fredrickson, DS, Levy, RI and Lees, RS: Fat transport in lipoproteins: An integrated approach to mechanisms and disorders. N Engl J Med 276:34, 1967.
100. Mahley, RW, et al: Plasma lipoproteins: Apolipoprotein structure and function. J Lipid Res 25:1277, 1984.
101. Grundy, SM: Metabolism of triglyceride-rich lipoproteins. In Cholesterol and Coronary Disease: Reducing the Risk. Science and Medicine, New York, 1988, p 4.
102. Steinberg, D and Witztom, JL: Lipoproteins and atherogenesis: Current concepts. JAMA 264:3047, 1990.
103. Havel, RJ: Role of triglyceride-rich lipoproteins in progression of atherogenesis. Circulation 81:694, 1990.
104. Grundy, SM: Hypertriglyceridemia: Pathophysiology and relation to coronary heart disease. In Cholesterol and Coronary Disease: Reducing the Risk. Science and Medicine, New York, 1988, p 2.
105. Friedewald, WT, Levy, RI and Fredrickson, DS: Estimation of the concentration of low-density lipoprotein cholesterol in plasma, without use of the preparative ultracentrifuge. Clin Chem 18:499, 1972.
106. DeLong, DM, et al: A comparison of methods for the estimation of plasma low- and very low-density lipoprotein cholesterol. The Lipid Research Clinics Prevalence Study. JAMA 256:2372, 1986.
107. Glueck, CJ: Classification and diagnosis of hyperlipoproteinemia. In Rifkind, BM and Levy, RI (eds): Hyperlipidemia: Diagnosis and Therapy. Grune & Stratton, New York, 1977, p 17.
108. Grundy, SM and Vega, GL: Causes of high blood cholesterol. Circulation 81:412, 1990.
109. Steinberg, D, et al: Beyond cholesterol: Modifications of low-density lipoprotein that increase its atherogenicity. N Engl J Med 320:915, 1989.
110. Grundy, SM: Classification of Lipid Disorders. Gower Medical Publishing, New York, 1990, pp 2, 3.
111. Canner, PL, et al: Fifteen-year mortality in Coronary Drug Project patients: Long-term benefit with niacin. J Am Coll Cardiol 8:1245, 1986.
112. Blankenhorn, DM, et al: Beneficial effects of combined colestipol-niacin therapy on coronary atherosclerosis and coronary venous bypass grafts. JAMA 257:3233, 1987.
113. Miller, NE, et al: Relation of angiographically defined coronary artery disease to plasma lipoprotein subfractions and apolipoproteins. BMJ 282:1741, 1981.
114. Huff, MW, et al: Metabolism of apolipoproteins C-11, C-111, and B in hypertriglyceridemic men: Changes after heparin-induced lipolysis. Arteriosclerosis 8:471, 1988.
115. Brunzell, JD, et al: Apoproteins B and A-1 and coronary artery disease in humans. Arteriosclerosis 4:79, 1984.
116. Kottke, BA, et al: Apolipoproteins and coronary artery disease. Mayo Clin Proc 61:313, 1986.
117. Scanu, AM and Fless, GM: Lipoprotein (a): Heterogeneity and biological relevance. J Clin Invest 85:1709, 1990.
118. The Expert Panel: Report of the National Cholesterol Education Program Expert Panel on Detection, Evaluation and Treatment of High Blood Cholesterol in Adults. Arch Intern Med 148:36, 1988.
119. Dunn, FL: New guidelines for the diagnosis and treatment of hyperlipidemia. Roche Biomedical Laboratories p 4, 1988. Clinical monograph.
120. Consensus Development Conference: Treatment of hypertriglyceridemia. JAMA 251:1196, 1984.
121. Castelli, WP: The triglyceride issue: A view from Framingham. Am Heart J 112:432, 1986.
122. Grundy, SM: Cholesterol and coronary heart disease: Future directions. JAMA 264:3053, 1990.
123. Treatment of hypertriglycerides. NIH Consensus Development Conference summary. Arteriosclerosis 4:296, 1984.
124. Tools for patient management: A basic outline of triglyceride disorders. In Cholesterol and Coronary Disease: Reducing the Risks. Science and Medicine, New York, 1988, p 9.
125. Castelli, WP, et al: HDL cholesterol and other lipids in coronary heart disease: The cooperative Lipoprotein Phenotyping Study. Circulation 55:767, 1977.
126. Gordon, T, et al: Lipoproteins, cardiovascular disease and death: The Framingham Study. Arch Intern Med 141:1128, 1981.

127. Abbott, RD, et al: High density lipoprotein cholesterol, total cholesterol screening, and myocardial infarction: The Framingham Study. Arteriosclerosis 8:207, 1988.
128. Wolf, RN and Grundy, SM: Influence of weight reduction on plasma lipoproteins in obese patients. Arteriosclerosis 3:160, 1983.
129. Phillips, NR, Havel, RJ and Kane, JP: Levels and interrelationships of serum and lipoprotein cholesterol and triglycerides: Association with adiposity and the consumption of ethanol, tobacco, and beverages containing caffeine. Arteriosclerosis 1:13, 1981.
130. Kannel, WB: Update on the role of cigarette smoking in coronary artery disease. Am Heart J 101:319, 1981.
131. Castelli, WP, et al: Incidence of coronary heart disease and lipoprotein cholesterol levels: The Framingham Study. JAMA 256:2835, 1986.
132. National Cholesterol Education Program: Report of the Expert Panel on Detection, Evaluation, and Treatment of High Blood Cholesterol in Adults. US Department of Health and Human Services, National Heart, Lung, and Blood Institute, National Institutes of Health, Publication No 89-2925, Bethesda, MD, 1989.
133. Dawber, TR: The Framingham Study: The Epidemiology of Atherosclerotic Disease. Harvard University Press, Cambridge, MA, 1980.
134. Truett, J, Cornfield, J and Kannel, W: A multivariate analysis of the risk of coronary disease. J Chronic Dis 20:511–524, 1967.
135. Connor, WE and Connor, SL: Dietary treatment of hyperlipidemia. In Rifkind, BM and Shekelle, RB (eds): Hyperlipidemia: Diagnosis and Therapy. Grune & Stratton, New York, 1977.
136. Levy, RI, et al: Nutrition, lipids, and coronary heart disease: A global view. In Levy, RI, et al (eds): Nutrition in Health and Disease. Raven Press, New York, 1979.
137. Barnard, JR, et al: Effects of an intensive exercise and nutrition program on patients with coronary artery disease: Five year follow-up. J Cardiac Rehabil 3:183–190, 1983.
138. American Heart Association: Heartbook: A Guide to Prevention and Treatment of Cardiovascular Diseases. Dutton, New York, 1980.

CHAPTER 14

Additional Components of Pulmonary Rehabilitation

Although aerobic exercise training is an integrant of pulmonary rehabilitation, the pulmonary patient requires additional information to optimize his or her exercise capabilities and to improve the quality of life. The topics presented below are often termed "adjuncts" to pulmonary rehabilitation, but the inference that they are somehow of secondary importance is inaccurate. The following discussion covers the essential elements of a pulmonary rehabilitation program: secretion removal techniques, ventilatory muscle training and breathing reeducation, energy-saving techniques, and smoking cessation.

SECRETION REMOVAL TECHNIQUES

Secretion retention can occur when there is an increase in the amount of secretions produced by the goblet cells and mucous glands that line the tracheobronchial tree (bronchiectasis, chronic bronchitis, and asthma), a change in the composition of the secretions (cystic fibrosis), or a decrease in the action of the cilia within the tracheobronchial tree (immotile cilia or smoking). In any case, the resultant increase in secretions can interfere with ventilation and the diffusion of oxygen and carbon dioxide. An assessment of the pulmonary system will identify the areas of secretion retention (Chapter 10). An individualized program of secretion removal techniques directed to the areas of involvement can optimize a patient's ventilation and therefore gas exchange capabilities.

Patients with secretion retention may improve their performance of an exercise regimen if the proper secretion removal techniques are provided prior to the exercise session. The following discussion includes the techniques of postural drainage, percussion, shaking, vibration, and airway clearance as they pertain to the patient population who might participate in an outpatient pulmonary rehabilitation program. There is no intent to cover all patients who are acutely ill with pulmonary dysfunctions.

Postural Drainage

Positioning a patient in such a way that the bronchus of the involved lung segment is perpendicular to the ground is the basis for postural drainage. By utilizing gravity, the positioning assists the mucociliary transport system in removing excessive secretions from the tracheobronchial tree. Lorin and Denning[1] found that secretion clearance improved in patients with cystic fibrosis when postural drainage coupled with coughing was compared to coughing alone. Postural drainage can be employed by itself as a treatment program. Each appropriate postural drainage position is maintained for at least 5 minutes and may last up to 20 minutes if large amounts of secretions are present. An appropriate method of airway clearance, for example, cough, should be encouraged during and after each postural drainage position. Postural drainage can also be used in conjunction with other manual techniques (described in this chapter) as part of a treatment program.

Standard postural drainage positions are pictured in Figure 14-1. Although they are the optimal positions for gravity drainage of specific lung segments, they may not be realistic for some patients. The standard position for postural drainage could make a patient's respiratory status, or a concomitant problem, worse. Modification of the standard positions may prevent any untoward effects and still enhance secretion removal. The following list of precautions should be considered prior to instituting postural drainage with patients enrolled in an outpatient pulmonary rehabilitation program. They are relative precautions rather than absolute contraindications.

A. Precautions for the use of the Trendelenberg position (bed in a tipped, head-down position)
  1. Circulatory: pulmonary edema, congestive heart failure, hypertension
  2. Abdominal: obesity, abdominal distention, hiatal hernia, nausea, recent food consumption
  3. Shortness of breath made worse with the Trendelenberg position
B. Precautions for the use of the side-lying position
  1. Vascular: axillo-femoral bypass graft
  2. Musculoskeletal: arthritis, recent rib fracture, shoulder bursitis, tendonitis making positioning uncomfortable

This list is not meant to be all-inclusive, but it does provide the reader with a range of dysfunction that should be considered prior to instituting postural drainage.

Percussion

Percussion (or clapping) is a force rhythmically applied with the therapist's cupped hands to the patient's chest wall (Fig. 14-2). The percussion technique is applied to a specific area on the thorax that corresponds to an underlying involved lung segment. The appropriate site for the application of the percussion technique is shown in Figure 14-1. The technique is typically administered from 2 to 5 minutes (or to patient tolerance) to each involved lung segment, although there have been reports in the literature of the utilization of from 30 seconds to 20 minutes of percussion.[2,3] Percussion is thought to release the pulmonary secretions from the wall of the airways and into the lumen of the airway.[4] Unfortunately, this process seems to be nondirectional; that is, the

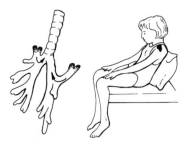

UPPER LOBES Apical Segments

Bed or drainage table flat.

Patient leans back on pillow at 30° angle against therapist.

Therapist claps with markedly cupped hand over area between clavicle and top of scapula on each side.

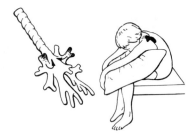

UPPER LOBES Posterior Segments

Bed or drainage table flat.

Patient leans over folder pillow at 30° angle.

Therapist stands behind and claps over upper back on both sides.

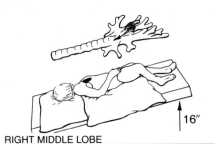

16″

RIGHT MIDDLE LOBE

Foot of table or bed elevated 16 inches.

Patient lies head down on left side and rotates ¼ turn backward. Pillow may be placed behind from shoulder to hip. Knees should be flexed.

Therapist claps over right nipple area. In females with breast development or tenderness, use cupped hand with heel of hand under armpit and fingers extending forward beneath the breast.

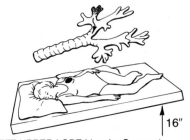

16″

LEFT UPPER LOBE Lingular Segments

Foot of table or bed elevated 16 inches.

Patient lies head down on right side and rotates ¼ turn backward. Pillow may be placed behind from shoulder to hip. Knees should be flexed.

Therapist claps with moderately cupped hand over left nipple area. In females with breast development or tenderness, use cupped hand with heel of hand under armpit and fingers extending forward beneath the breast.

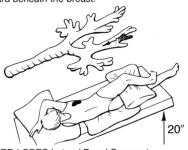

20″

LOWER LOBES Lateral Basal Segments

Foot of table or bed elevated 20 inches.

Patient lies on abdomen, head down, then rotates ¼ turn upward. Upper leg is flexed over a pillow for support.

Therapist claps over uppermost portion of lower ribs. (Position shown is for drainage of right lateral basal segment. To drain the left lateral basal segment, patient should lie on his right side in the same posture).

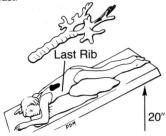

Last Rib

20″

LOWER LOBES Posterior Basal Segments

Foot of table or bed elevated 20 inches.

Patient lies on abdomen, head down, with pillow under hips. Therapist claps over lower ribs close to spine on each side.

FIGURE 14–1. Postural drainage.

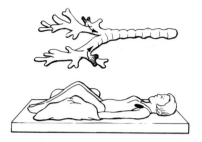

UPPER LOBES Anterior Segments

Bed or drainage table flat.

Patient lies on back with pillow under knees.

Therapist claps between clavicle and nipple on each side.

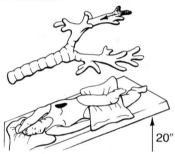

LOWER LOBES Anterior Basal Segments

Foot of table or bed elevated 20 inches.

Patient lies on side, head down, pillow under knees.

Therapist claps with slightly cupped hand over lower ribs. (Position shown is for drainage of left anterior basal segment. To drain the right anterior basal segment, patient should lie on his left side in same posture).

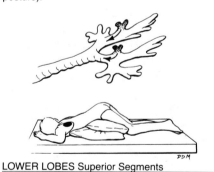

LOWER LOBES Superior Segments

Bed or table flat.

Patient lies on abdomen with two pillows under hips.

Therapist claps over middle of back at tip of scapula on either side of spine.

FIGURE 14–1. *Continued.* (From Rothstein, JM, Roy, SH, and Wolf SL: The Rehabilitation Specialist's Handbook. FA Davis, Philadelphia, pp. 624–625, with permission.)

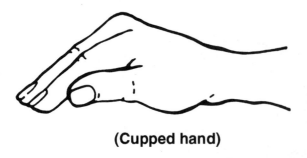

(Cupped hand)

FIGURE 14–2. Cupped hand for the percussion technique. (From the National Cystic Fibrosis Foundation, Courtesy of Bettina C. Hilman, MD, with permission.)

secretions may be moved closer to the glottis or deeper into the pulmonary parenchyma. By coupling percussion with the appropriate postural drainage position for a specific lung segment, the probability of secretion removal is enhanced.[5–7] Since percussion is a force directed to the thorax, there are conditions that must be evaluated prior to its use.

A. Precautions for the use of percussion
   1. Circulatory: hemoptysis, coagulation disorders (increased partial thromboplastin time (PTT) or prothrombin time (PT), decreased platelet count below 50,000, and medications that interfere with coagulation.
   2. Musculoskeletal: fractured ribs, flail chest, degenerative bone disease

Again, the list is by no means all-inclusive. It does provide some general guidelines that deserve consideration when percussion is part of the therapeutic regimen. It should also be noted that some modification of this technique to enhance patient tolerance can occur.

Shaking

Shaking is used to hasten the removal of secretions via the mucociliary transport system. Following a deep inhalation, a bouncing maneuver is applied to the rib cage throughout the expiratory phase of breathing. This maneuver, the shaking, is applied to a specific area on the thorax that corresponds to the underlying involved lung segment (Fig. 14–3). It is commonly used following percussion in the appropriate postural drainage position.[8,9] Five to seven deep inhalations, each followed by shaking on exhalation, are adequate to promote secretion clearance without risking possible hyperventilation. Since the technique is a force applied to the thorax, the same precautions as noted in the application of percussion are needed.

Vibration

The sustained co-contraction of the therapist's upper extremities produces a vibration that is transmitted from the therapist's hands to the patient's thorax during the expiratory phase of respiration. Vibration can also be produced by a mechanical device and be transmitted to the patient's chest wall. It, again, is applied to a specific area on the thorax that corresponds to an underlying involved lung segment. Vibration is used to enhance the mucociliary transport system. Since little to no pressure is placed to the

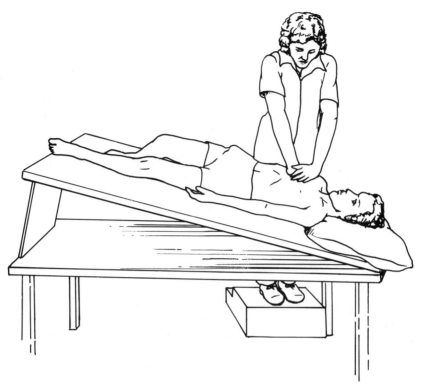

FIGURE 14–3. Shaking being performed over the involved right anterior segment, upper lobe. (From the National Cystic Fibrosis Foundation, Courtesy of Bettina C. Hilman, MD, with permission.)

thorax during the vibration technique, there are no contraindications to its use. Vibration is often used when percussion and shaking are contraindicated. Postural drainage positions, if appropriate, can be coupled with vibration to optimize effectiveness.

Airway Clearance

Once the secretions have been mobilized with postural drainage, percussion, and shaking or vibration, removing them from the airways is necessary. Coughing is the most common and easiest means of clearing the airway. There are many variations of the cough maneuver. For the patient enrolled in a pulmonary rehabilitation program, the cough, huff, and forced expiratory technique (FET) are most often used.

COUGH

A cough is the simplest way in which to clear secretions from the upper airways. It is produced by a coordinated effort made up of the following steps: Inhale deeply, close the glottis, create an increased intrathoracic pressure by contracting the abdominal muscles ("bearing down"), and then release the glottis and expel the air while continually contracting the abdominal muscles.[10] Expiratory flow rates during a cough can be as high as 70 mph. The upright sitting position has been found to produce the highest expiratory flow rates and is therefore thought to be the most effective position for coughing.[11]

HUFF

A huff uses many of the same coordinated steps as the cough with the omission of a closed glottis. The patient is asked to take a deep inhalation and rapidly contract the abdominal muscles for a series of forced expirations through an "open" airway. It is as if the patient were saying "Ha, ha, ha." High intrathoracic pressure generated during the compression phase of coughing can close off small airways in some patients with chronic obstructive pulmonary disease (COPD). By trapping the air behind the closed airway, the cough becomes ineffective. A huff has been shown to stabilize collapsible airway walls, making expiration and secretion removal more effective in this patient population.[12]

FORCED EXPIRATORY TECHNIQUE

The performance of the FET is characterized by breathing control and huffing from mid to low lung volumes. The patient is first taught breathing from the lower chest (diaphragmatic breathing). He or she is then asked to inhale a normal amount of air (tidal inhalation) and, from that point, to contract the abdominal muscles to produce a forced exhalation.

The sequence of performing this technique is summarized as follows:[13]

1. Breathing control
2. Thoracic expansion exercises (with or without percussion and shaking)
3. Breathing control
4. One or two huffs from mid to low lung volumes
5. Breathing control

FET is thought to milk the more peripheral airways of their secretions and make overall lung clearance more effective.[14] It has been effective in patients with COPD, asthma, and cystic fibrosis.

In summary, the combination of postural drainage, percussion, shaking, vibration, and airway clearance directed to specific areas of secretion retention can remove excessive pulmonary secretions, improve ventilation, and subsequently improve gas exchange. Patients with secretion retention who participate in a pulmonary rehabilitation program might benefit from a session of secretion removal techniques prior to the exercise session.

VENTILATORY MUSCLE TRAINING AND BREATHING REEDUCATION

The inability to increase ventilation sufficiently is often the limiting factor in activities and exercise tolerance of patients with pulmonary dysfunction. Optimizing the ventilatory function can decrease the work of breathing and improve the ability to perform work. Ventilatory muscle training has been utilized to improve the strength and endurance of the muscles of ventilation and thereby increase the efficiency of breathing.

Breathing reeducation teaches a more efficient pattern of ventilation, which decreases the work of breathing.

Ventilatory Muscle Training

The ventilatory muscles can be physiologically trained similarly to all other skeletal muscles. Traditionally, skeletal muscles are trained by either loading them against a high resistance for strengthening or by high-frequency repetition for enhancing endurance. In general, they have the capacity for specificity of training. Whereas general aerobic exercise alone can improve the strength and endurance of the ventilatory muscles[15], specific training regimes for those muscles have been suggested.[16] Leith and Bradley[17] report a 55 percent increase in the strength and a 19 percent increase in the endurance of the ventilatory muscles following a 5-week training program.

There are specific devices, inspiratory muscle trainers (IMTs), that load the inspiratory muscles via graded aperture openings. The patient breathes in through the narrowed opening, which loads the inspiratory muscles and thereby trains the muscles of inspiration.[18] Exhalation is unresisted in most IMT devices. Exercise programs that provide both strength and endurance training of the inspiratory muscles can be formulated. Training sessions are recommended at a frequency of one to two times per day and a duration of 15 to 30 minutes.[18,19] By changing the size of the aperture opening, the intensity of training can be modulated.

An appropriate exercise intensity can be determined in either of two ways. First, the maximum static inspiratory mouth pressure (MSIP) from functional residual capacity is determined. Inspiratory muscle strengthening programs then utilize an aperture opening that provides a resistance between 30 and 40 percent of MSIP.[20] A second way to determine exercise intensity is to select the smallest aperture (opening) the patient can tolerate for a 10-minute exercise period.[18] Endurance training would use a lower percent of MSIP, or the aperture opening, that would allow a longer exercise duration.

The objective of this type of training is to decrease the oxygen consumption of the inspiratory muscles during ventilation, and thereby improve exercise capacity.[21] By training the inspiratory muscles, patients may also be more able to resist ventilatory muscle fatigue. This is advantageous during exercise sessions as well as during exacerbations of their respiratory disease.

Breathing Reeducation

DIAPHRAGMATIC BREATHING

Teaching a more efficient pattern of breathing, although not a physiological training technique, can alter the work of breathing. By encouraging the use of the diaphragm, the principal and most efficient muscle of inspiration, the oxygen cost of breathing, can be decreased. Instructing a patient in diaphragmatic breathing exercises begins by placing him or her in the comfortable semi-Fowler's (reclined sitting) position. The patient's own hand is placed over the costochondral angle. "Sniffing" is then used to facilitate the contraction of the diaphragm, allowing the patient to palpate the muscle and ensuring proper hand placement. Allowing the hand to rise during inspiration and fall during expiration encourages a relaxed and efficient pattern of ventilation. It is most desirable to inspire nasally, thus ensuring a slow, even inspiration. Exhalation orally provides for the least resistance to air flow.

Decreasing the use of accessory muscles also decreases the work of breathing. Biofeedback can emphasize the proper use of the diaphragm and inhibit the use of accessory muscles during the ventilatory cycle.

Even though a good breathing pattern is often taught in a semirecumbent comfortable position, a progression must be established.[20] The continued use of that same breathing pattern during sitting, standing, walking, and stair climbing is necessary to make breathing reeducation useful in the overall rehabilitation of the patient with pulmonary disease.

PURSED LIP BREATHING

Pursed lip breathing, when used by patients with COPD, has been shown to decrease respiratory rates and increase tidal volumes.[21] It may delay or prevent airway collapse and allow for better gas exchange,[22] and it should be done during a passive, not a forced, exhalation. By the use of the technique, minute ventilation is maintained while the work of breathing is decreased. Though many patients have learned to purse lip breathe without any instruction, the therapist can ensure that the activity is carried out correctly and that it is maintained during exercise.

Both techniques of ventilatory muscle training and breathing reeducation strive to decrease the work of breathing. By incorporating them in the exercise session, a more effective exercise program can be performed.

ENERGY-SAVING TECHNIQUES

Patients with pulmonary dysfunction may become dyspneic while performing varying levels of activities of daily living (ADLs). The activities that produce dyspnea are thereafter often avoided. The result may be a dependence on others, with both physical and emotional consequences. During the initial evaluation, the therapist must determine which ADLs are problematic. The individual's goals for the rehabilitation program should reflect the difficulties and offer resolution of the problems. Instruction in the use of energy-saving techniques (ESTs) should be part of the patient's treatment plan. Regaining the ADLs can renew a patient's independence and sense of well-being.

ESTs should be employed when the usual performance of an activity would precipitate dyspnea. An EST combines the techniques of assistive and adaptive equipment, activity planning and preparation, pacing, and efficient breathing patterns. Together, the techniques lower the energy expenditure and the oxygen consumption of an activity.

Assistive and Adaptive Equipment

The use of assistive and adaptive equipment alone can allow a patient to perform an activity. A patient with pulmonary disease who has moderate obesity over the abdomen may become dyspneic while putting on shoes and socks. That task can be accomplished without dyspnea by using a stocking-aid and long-handled shoehorn. A patient with moderate to severe dyspnea will often find it very difficult to shower, since the activity requires long periods of standing, bending, upper extremity work, and frequency of breath holding. The patient may be able to shower by using a shower bench, soap on a rope, a hand-held shower nozzle, a long-handled brush, and a terry cloth bathrobe. Even a microwave oven, because it requires less cooking time and little attention during cooking, may allow a patient to better prepare more nutritious meals more frequently with decreased levels of dyspnea. These are only a few examples of how assistive and adaptive equipment can be used in pulmonary rehabilitation.

Activity Planning and Preparation

Activity planning and preparation is another key component of energy-saving techniques. The scheduling, organizing, and prioritizing of tasks can make a difference in the functional abilities of patients with pulmonary disease.[23] Many bouts of dyspnea can be avoided by efficient scheduling of activities. Activities that most significantly increase the demands on the cardiopulmonary system should be spaced throughout the day, week, and month to allow for maximum rest and recovery time between them. They should also be scheduled around availability of friends and relatives to assist in the more demanding work. Many patients with pulmonary disease find the mornings most difficult. By performing as many activities as possible the evening before and organizing the tasks ahead, the mornings can be made less demanding. Meal preparation is another important activity that often is not performed adequately because of dyspnea. Even when the meal is prepared, the patient may have become too fatigued to eat. Proper organization from the start of the meal preparation can minimize the demands of the activity. Proper planning ensures that only one trip to the refrigerator or cupboard is necessary. Commonly used meal ingredients and utensils should be very accessible to the preparation site. Meals can be prepared while seated instead of standing. By carefully planning and preparing for an activity, it can be completed without dyspnea and fatigue. Note that such activities as cooking should be performed with good ventilation and oxygen precautions when applicable.

Pacing

Pacing is another integral component of ESTs and pulmonary rehabilitation. It is so simple in nature that the patient is somehow expected to know and use the concept intuitively. That is often not the case, however, and pacing has to be taught. Pacing can be defined as the performance of an activity within the limits or boundaries of the patient's breathing capacity. Often that means the activity must be broken down into components so that it is performed at a tempo that does not exceed the patient's breathing limitations. For example, stair climbing is performed only on exhalation and by taking one or two steps at a time. The patient is asked to remain on that step until there is full recovery. The next two or three steps are ascended, again on exhalation, followed by a rest period until recovery. The sequence is continued until the full flight of stairs is accomplished without dyspnea. (Pursed lip breathing and recovery breathing should also be employed with pacing when necessary.)

Often a patient may complain the activity took too long to perform or that he or she felt foolish walking that way. To the patient, pacing is viewed as slowing down. It is often helpful to prove to the patient that the pacing technique may actually save time. First, ask the patient to climb a flight of stairs his or her own way. A person with COPD typically climbs the stairs in the following manner: an upward look at the awesome task ahead, ascent of the first few steps, some shortness of breath, and then an increase in the speed of ascent to assure that the top will be reached. By the time the patient reaches the top, he or she is visibly dyspneic, and it may take him or her minutes to regain control of respirations. Time the activity from the onset of stair climbing until breathing is recovered at the top of the stairs. Now repeat the task with pacing. With pacing, the task will undoubtedly take less time and the patient will remain comfortable throughout. As to looking foolish, how foolish did the patient appear to be at the top of the stairs in the first climb while gasping for air? The patient should also expect that the activity will look much more polished with practice.

The goal of pacing is to complete an activity safely and without dyspnea. Pacing can and should be part of every activity that would otherwise cause dyspnea. By breaking activities down into component parts and interspersing rest periods between components, the total activity can be completed without dyspnea and fatigue.

Pacing should be employed in such tasks as ADLs, ambulating, stair climbing, and lifting. It is not a technique to be used during the aerobic portion of a pulmonary rehabilitation program. During exercise, some shortness of breath should and will occur.

SMOKING CESSATION

Smoking is the leading cause of chronic bronchitis and emphysema as well as a contributing cause of many other disease processes.[24] Therefore, a special focus on the effects of smoking and smoking cessation should be included in pulmonary rehabilitation programs. According to the 1987 position statement of the American Thoracic Society, smoking cessation should be of highest priority in the comprehensive care of patients with COPD.[25]

With regard to smoking, there are four categories of patients: those who never smoked, those who used to smoke, those who are currently smoking but would like to quit, and, finally, those who are currently smoking and wish to continue smoking. For the two groups of nonsmokers, the hazards of primary smoke and passive ambient smoke need presentation. The effects of smoking and the benefits of being smokeless must be reinforced.[26]

The currently smoking patient demands careful consideration. A patient who has the desire to quit smoking, regardless of personal success, needs assistance to break the behavior pattern most effectively. There are many smoking cessation techniques; examples are cold turkey, behavior modification,[27] rapid smoking,[28] diversion therapy,[29] and nicotine gum[30] (Table 14–1). No single method can claim a higher long-term success rate than another. A comprehensive treatment approach incorporating many different smoking cessation strategies has a higher abstention rate than any single specific technique.[31–33] It is the role of the clinician to guide the patient toward smoking cessation, not necessarily to provide the service. The American Lung Association and the American Cancer Society are good sources of available smoking cessation centers. That the clinician be a sympathetic and encouraging professional during the process of smoking cessation is very important.

A patient who has no intention of quitting smoking should be dealt with quite differently. The patient must fully understand the consequences of smoking and how the habit is altering the degree of illness. If the patient still plans to smoke, the benefits of continuing in a pulmonary rehabilitation program are questionable. There may be

TABLE 14–1 Types of Smoking Cessation Techniques

Propaganda
    Mass media messages
    Posters
    Brochures
	Therapy programs
	    Smoking cessation clinics
	    Group therapy
	    Individual counseling
	    Psychotherapy
	    Hypnosis

Drugs
    Lobeline
    Dextroamphetamine
    Imipramine
    Nicotine gum
	Behavior modification
	    Self-monitoring
	    Stimulus control
	    Contingency management
	    Self-management
	    Desensitization

Aversion–satiation
    Rapid smoke
    Imagination
    Smoky air in face or mouth
    Electric shock
	Role-playing
	    Self-punishment
	    Values clarification
	    Sensory deprivation
	    Gradual reduction
	    Problem solving

Cognitive approach
    Information
    Books
    Articles
    Physician's order
	Others
	    Prayer
	    Meditation
	    Relaxation

Affective approach
    Fear
	Exercise
	    Acupuncture

Source: From Peters, J, and Lim, V: Smoking cessation techniques. In Hodgkin, J et al. (eds): Pulmonary Rehabilitation: Guidelines to Success. Butterworth Publishers, Boston, 1984, p. 94. Used by permission of J. Hodgkin, MD.

little or no motivation for being well, for being responsible for one's own care, or for complying with the demands of pulmonary rehabilitation.

Nutrition

Patients with chronic lung disease may require more calories per day than their peers who do not have lung disease. Even with the use of pancreatic enzyme replacements, patients with cystic fibrosis require up to 50 percent more calories per day than the average person.[37] However, eating certain foods and large meals is difficult for many patients with pulmonary disease. The preparation of food, the need to breath-hold during swallowing, the side effects of medication regimens, and the limitations of diaphragmatic excursion as a result of a full stomach can make eating uncomfortable and unpleasant. As a result, patients may lose their appetites and lose weight; they could become malnourished. Strength, endurance, and the ability to ward off infection also are affected. Small meals and readily available snacks that are high in carbohydrates may provide better nutrition, patient comfort, and compliance. Nutritional counseling to identify individual dietary needs is often necessary for overall wellness.

SUMMARY

In summary, pulmonary rehabilitation is more than an exercise therapy session. A comprehensive care plan that will "return the patient to the highest possible functional capacity allowed by his pulmonary handicap and overall life situation"[33] is the goal of pulmonary rehabilitation. Additional components of the exercise sessions, secretion removal techniques, ventilatory muscle training and breathing reeducation, energy-saving techniques, smoking cessation, and nutritional requirements are imperative to meet that goal, and they have been presented in this discussion.

REFERENCES

1. Lorin, M and Denning, C: Evaluation of postural drainage for measurement of sputum volume and consistency. Am J Phys Med 50(5):215–219, 1971.
2. Murphy, M, Concannon, D and Fitzgerald, M: Chest percussion: Help or hindrance to postural drainage? Irish Med J 76:189–190, 1983.
3. Zidulka, A, et al: Clapping or percussion causes atelectasis in dogs and influences gas exchange. J Appl Physiol 66(6):2833–2838, 1989.
4. Kigin, C: Advances in chest physical therapy. In Current Advances in Respiratory Care. American College of Chest Physicians, Park Ridge, 1984.
5. Chopra, S, et al: Effects of hydration and physical therapy on tracheal transport velocity. Am Rev Respir Dis 115:1009–1014, 1977.
6. Denton, P: Bronchial secretions in cystic fibrosis. Am Rev Respir Dis 86:41–46, 1962.
7. Mazzocco, M, et al: Physiologic effects of chest percussion and postural drainage in patients with bronchiectasis. Chest 88:360–363, 1985.
8. Frownfelter, D: Chest Physical Therapy and Pulmonary Rehabilitation: An Interdisciplinary Approach, ed 2. Year Book Medical Publishers, Chicago, 1987.
9. Zack, M and Oberwaldner, B: Chest physiotherapy: The mechanical approach to antiinfective therapy in cystic fibrosis. Infection 15(5):381–384, 1987.
10. Starr, J: Lesson 8, In Touch Series. American Physical Therapy Association, Alexandria, VA, 1990.
11. Starr, J: The effect of position and trial on the effectiveness of cough in the postoperative patient. Boston University, 1980. Unpublished thesis.
12. Hietpas, B, Roth, R and Jensen, W: Huff coughing and airway patency. Respir Care 24(8):710–713, 1979.
13. Pryor, JA: Respiratory Care. Churchill Livingstone, New York, 1991, pp 80–82.
14. Sutton, P, et al: Assessment of the forced expiratory technique: Postural drainage and directed coughing in chest physiotherapy. Eur J Respir Dis 64:62–68, 1983.
15. Keens, T, et al: Ventilatory muscle endurance training in normal subjects and patients with cystic fibrosis. Am Rev Respir Dis 116:853–860, 1977.
16. Kim, M: Respiratory muscle training: Implications for patient care. Heart Lung 13:333–340, 1984.
17. Leith, D and Bradley, M: Ventilatory muscle strength and endurance training. J Appl Physiol 41:508–516, 1976.
18. Sonne, L and David, J: Increased exercise performance in patients with severe COPD following inspiratory resistive training. Chest 81:436–439, 1982.
19. Chen, H, Dukes, R and Martin, B: Inspiratory muscle training in patients with chronic obstructive pulmonary disease. Am Rev Respir Dis 131:251–255, 1985.
20. Darbee, J and Cerney, F: Exercise testing and exercise conditioning for children with lung dysfunction. In S Irwin and J Tecklin: Cardiopulmonary Physical Therapy, ed 2. CV Mosby, Philadelphia, 1990, pp 469–470.
21. Belman, M and Mittman, C: Ventilatory muscle training improves exercise capacity in chronic obstructive pulmonary disease patients. Am Rev Respir Dis 121:273–280, 1980.
22. Adkins, H: Improvement of breathing ability in children with respiratory muscle paralysis. Phys Ther 48:577–581, 1968.
23. Thoman, R, Stoker, G and Ross, J: The efficacy of pursed-lips breathing in patients with chronic obstructive pulmonary disease. Am Rev Respir Dis 93:100–106, 1966.
24. Kigin, C: Breathing exercises for the medical patient: The art and the science. Phys Ther 70(11):700–706, 1990.
25. Shanfield, K and Hammond, M: Activities of daily living. In Hodgkin, K, Zorn, E, and Connors, G (eds): Pulmonary Rehabilitation: Guidelines to Success. Butterworth Publishers, Boston, 1984, pp 171–193.
26. Burki, N: Pulmonary Diseases. Medical Examination Publishing, Garden City, NY, 1982, p 271.

27. American Thoracic Society: Standards for the diagnosis and care of patients with chronic obstructive pulmonary disease (COPD) and asthma. Am Rev Respir Dis 136(1):225–244, 1987.
28. Fielding, J: Smoking effects and control: Part I. N Engl J Med 313(8):491–498, 1985.
29. Guilford, J: Group treatment versus individual initiative in the cessation of smoking. J Appl Psychol 56(2):162–167, 1972.
30. Relinger, J, et al: Utilization of adverse rapid smoking in groups: Efficacy of treatment and maintenance procedures. J Consult Clin Psychol 45(2):245–249, 1977.
31. Harris, M and Rothberg, C: A self-control approach to reducing smoking. Psychol Rep 31:165–166, 1972.
32. Russell, M, Raw, M and Jarvis, M: Clinical use of nicotine chewing gum. BMJ 280(6231):1599–1602, 1980.
33. Horn, D and Waingrow, S: Some dimensions of a model for smoking behavior change. Am J Public Health (Suppl 56)12:21–26, 1966.
34. Peters, J and Lim, V: Smoking cessation techniques. In Hodgkin, J, Zorn, E, and Connors, G (eds): Pulmonary Rehabilitation: Guidelines to Success. Butterworth Publishers, Boston, 1984, pp 91–120.
35. Lando, J: Successful treatment of smokers with a broad spectrum behavior approach. J Consult Clin Psychol 45(3):361–366, 1977.
36. Petty, T: Pulmonary rehabilitation: Basics of RD. American Thoracic Society, New York, 1975.
37. Tecklin, J: Pediatric Physical Therapy. JB Lippincott, Philadelphia, 1989, p 165.

APPENDIX A

Patient Program Application Forms

Dear

Enclosed are the preliminary application forms that we discussed via telephone. Please complete the enclosed forms as indicated (x).

_____ Medical and Personal History Form

_____ Dietary Profile Form

_____ Insurance Information Form

_____ Medical Release Authorization Form

These forms must be completed by you and returned to _____ before your therapy can be initiated. Referral forms will be forwarded to your personal physician, cardiologist, and/or other medical specialist for specific medical information that we require.

Upon receiving your forms and the physician referral forms, we will contact you to schedule an orientation/observation session. Instructions for the session are enclosed in this mailing. When you are contacted to schedule your orientation/observation session, record the date and time of your appointment on this form.

_____ offers complete rehabilitative services. Whether you are a patient (cardiac, diabetic, arthritic, post-surgical, etc.) requiring a prescribed rehabilitation program, or a person seeking help in beginning an exercise and/or weight-control program, the staff works as a team to design and supervise an individualized program for you. Our staff of physicians, exercise and medical physiologists, registered nurses, physical therapists, nutritionists, and other health professionals work together to promote health through lifestyle modification and applied education.

The specific needs of each individual are considered; therefore, the appropriate treatment, as well as the cost of treatment will vary among patients. Your medical/health insurance will pay for the major portion of your treatment; however, the percentage of reimbursement is dependent upon individual insurance policies. Transportation costs incurred during treatment are also tax-deductible.

Please do not hesitate to contact me if you have any questions regarding our services or the completion of the enclosed forms.

Sincerely,

Director

PLEASE COMPLETE AND RETURN TO:

Medical and Personal History Forms: <u>PLEASE PRINT</u>

NAME: _____ AGE ____ SEX ____ BIRTHDATE ____ / ____ / ____

I. Conditions which you have had/or currently have:

	Yes	No	Unknown	Date Occurred
Allergies	—	—	____	_____
Specify			_____	_____
Congenital heart defect	—	—	____	_____
Rheumatic fever	—	—	____	_____
Heart murmur	—	—	____	_____
Vascular diseases:	—	—	____	_____
Coronary artery disease	—	—	____	_____
Artery diseases, other	—	—	____	_____
Varicose veins	—	—	____	_____
Leg cramps (claudication)	—	—	____	_____
Phlebitis	—	—	____	_____
Heart attack(s)	—	—	____	_____
High blood pressure	—	—	____	_____
Hyperlipidemia (elevated cholesterol, triglycerides)	—	—	____	_____
Obesity (MORE THAN 20 lb above ideal weight)	—	—	____	_____
Diabetes	—	—	____	_____
Gout	—	—	____	_____
Hernia(s)	—	—	____	_____
Epilepsy	—	—	____	_____
Arthritis	—	—	____	_____
Specify (knees, elbows, spine, etc.)			_____	_____
Injuries to:				
Back	—	—	____	_____
Muscles	—	—	____	_____
Bones	—	—	____	_____
Joints	—	—	____	_____
Lung disease	—	—	____	_____
Kidney disease	—	—	____	_____
Liver disease	—	—	____	_____
Psychological/emotional problems	—	—	____	_____

II. Operations: Date Occurred

1. _____ _____
2. _____ _____
3. _____ _____
4. _____ _____
5. _____ _____

III. Other medical problems:

_____
_____
_____

IV. Current medications & dosages:
      MEDICATIONS   DOSAGES

_____   _____
_____   _____
_____   _____
_____   _____
_____   _____
_____   _____

V. Risk Factors:
  A. Family History: Have any of your relatives had?

	Yes	No	Unknown
Heart attacks	—	—	_____
Specify relative			_____
High blood pressure	—	—	_____
Specify relative			_____
Hyperlipidemia	—	—	_____
Specify relative			_____
Heart operations	—	—	_____
Specify relative			_____
Diabetes	—	—	_____
Specify relative			_____
Other diseases			_____

  B. Smoking: Did you smoke in the past? _____ Age when you started smoking _____ Do you smoke now? _____ If you have stopped smoking, when did you and why? _____
_____

     Currently smoking: cigarettes   cigars   pipe   (please circle)
     Number per day? _____.

  C. Diet: Present weight _____ lb   Weight 1 year ago _____ lb
     Weight at age 21 _____ lb
     Are you dieting presently? _____ Why? _____
     What type of diet? _____

  D. Employment/Occupation:
     Current employment status:
     Full time _____   Retired _____   Unemployed _____
     Part time _____   Disabled _____
     Occupation _____ Number of years _____
     Employer _____
     Do you plan to return to this job or continue in the occupation? _____
     Physical activity required in occupation:

(continued)

	Almost All	(½)+	(½)	−(½)	Almost None
Time spent sitting	————	——	—	——	—————
Time spent walking	————	——	—	——	—————
Time spent standing	————	——	—	——	—————
Time spent standing/sitting with arm work	————	——	—	——	—————

Lifting or carrying heavy objects: Seldom   Sometimes   Often
(please circle one)
Approximate weight range ——— to ——— lb

Transportation to and from work: (please circle one of the following)
car   bus   railroad   ferry   subway   walking

If walking to work: (please circle one)
Less than 1 block   1–2 blocks   3–4 blocks   5–9 blocks
10–19 blocks   1 mile   2 miles+

Working hours per week: (please circle one)
Less than 25   25–35   36–40   41–50   51+

E. Physical Activity:
In addition to your occupation, do you exercise on a regular basis? ——————
If so, list your activities:

ACTIVITY	NUMBER OF TIMES PER WEEK
——————————————	——————————————
——————————————	——————————————
——————————————	——————————————

Have you previously participated in an exercise class or program? ——————
If so, describe the activities you performed: ——————————————
————————————————————————————

F. Stress:

Are you:	Yes	No
Frustrated when waiting in line, often in a hurry to complete work or keep appointments, easily angered, irritable?	——	——
Impatient when waiting, occasionally hurried, or occasionally moody?	——	——
Comfortable when waiting, seldom rushed, and easygoing?	——	——

PLEASE COMPLETE AND RETURN TO:

Name _____

Dietary Information Form

1. Are you on a specialized diet at this time? _____ yes _____ no
2. If so what type of diet? (e.g., low salt, low fat, number of calories, etc.)
   _____
3. Who recommended this diet? _____
4. Have you recently gained or lost weight? _____ yes _____ no
5. If yes, how much gained? _____ lost? _____
6. Describe your use of salt. _____
7. Check all of the following commercially prepared foods which you use:
   _____ Canned, dehydrated, or frozen soups or stews
   _____ Canned or frozen casseroles
   _____ Frozen dinners
   _____ Pretzels, chips, or snack crackers
   _____ Fast-food chain foods
8. Do you eat meals out frequently (3 times per week or more)? _____
9. Name any foods you *cannot* eat. _____
10. What foods would be particularly hard for you to give up? _____
    _____

Daily Dietary Habits

List foods and beverages commonly consumed. Include ALCOHOL, sugar, milk, or cream
used in beverages, butter or margarine used, and dressing used on salads.

Breakfast:

Lunch:

Dinner:

Snacks:

Food preference: <u>Check</u> the foods that you eat almost every day. <u>Circle</u> the foods that you
                  eat at least once a week.

Milk and Dairy Products:
— whole milk   — 2% milk   — skim milk   — buttermilk
— evap. milk   — cream   — cheese   — prc. cheese and spreads
— cottage cheese   — yogurt   — ice cream   — low-fat cottage cheese

Vegetables:
— green and yellow beans   — carrots   — lettuce and salad greens
— beets   — corn   — broccoli, brussel sprouts
— sweet potatoes   — peas   — lima beans
— squash   — potatoes   — cabbage
— tomatoes   — baked beans

Fruits and Juices:
— citrus fruits   — citrus juice   — pineapple   — pineapple juice
— apples   — peaches   — bananas   — apple juice
— grapes   — grape juice   — cherries
— berries   — prune juice   — plums

Breads/Cereals/Pasta:
— cereal, dry, unsweet.   — cereal, dry, sweet.   — cereal, cooked
— muffins   — bread   — rice
— biscuits   — crackers   — rolls
— macaroni   — spaghetti   — noodles

Meat/Fish/Poultry/Eggs:
— eggs   — beef   — poultry   — fish
— liver   — pork   — bacon   — shellfish
— cold cuts   — dried beans   — frankfurters   — peanut butter

Fats/Oils/Snacks:
— salad dressing   — pastries   — peanuts and other nuts
— margarine   — cookies   — potato chips and other chips
— butter   — candy   — popcorn
— oil   — pie   — cake

PLEASE COMPLETE AND RETURN TO:

Insurance Information Form

Patient's Name _____ Date _____ / ___ / ____
  (Last, First, MI)
Address _____ Phone: Home _____
_____ Work _____
  Zip Code
Patient's Date of Birth _____
Insurance Company _____
Address _____
Telephone Number _____
Insured's Name _____ Insured's Date of Birth _____
  Last, First, MI   SS# ____-____-____
Insured's Employer _____   Occupation _____
Insured's relationship to patient ___ self ___ spouse___ child ___ other
Insurance ID Number _____
Group Name or Number _____
Are you covered by any other plans which provide medical benefits or
services? ___ yes ___ no
If "yes," list all other insurance companies or service plans providing coverage:
Company Name _____ Insured's Name _____
Company Address _____ ID Number _____
_____ Group Name or Number _____
  Zip Code
Referring Physician: _____
Most recent diagnosis/symptoms   Date illness/injury
1. _____   _____
2. _____   _____
3. _____   _____
4. _____   _____
Date of first treatment _____
I certify that the above information is correct to the best of my knowledge.
_____
  SIGNATURE

PLEASE COMPLETE AND RETURN TO:

Medical Records Release Authorization

TO: _____

_____

(Physician's Address)

I HEREBY AUTHORIZE AND REQUEST YOU TO RELEASE TO:

Records and/or pertinent information in your possession concerning my illness/treatment.

Name _____ Date _____ / / _____

Address _____

Signature: _____

(If relative, state relationship)

Witness: _____

Instructions for Orientation/Observation Sessions

Name _____
Appointment   _____   _____   _____
                   Month   Date   Time

Clothing
     Bring soft-soled shoes, e.g., tennis or walking shoes, socks, cotton shorts and a cotton shirt; and wear no unnecessary jewelry. (If you are more comfortable in slacks, feel free to wear them.)

          DO NOT WEAR A NYLON SHIRT.

Day of the Orientation/Observation Session:
     1. Do not eat for at least two hours preceding the session.
     2. Do not vary your medications (regular).
     3. Do not ingest coffee, tea, coke, or other stimulants.
     4. Do not engage in excessive physical activity.
     5. Do not ingest alcohol or other depressants.
     6. Do not smoke for at least two hours preceding the session.

     The procedures will take approximately one hour and are not particularly stressful or uncomfortable to most people. You should try to remain as relaxed as possible during all of the procedures.

APPENDIX B

Referring Physician Forms

To _____ M.D.

We have been contacted by _____
concerning participation in one of our rehabilitation programs.

The enclosed form must be completed and returned to us prior to the initiation of therapy. Your recommendations concerning your patient's participation in the program will be adhered to completely. Please do not hesitate to contact us should you have any questions regarding your patient's therapy.

Thank you for your time and consideration.

PLEASE COMPLETE AND RETURN TO:

Referring Physician Form

Patient's Name _____ Age _____
Etiology: _____
Diagnosis(es): _____
Medications: _____
Blood Analysis: Date _____ CBC: Hgb __ HCT __ WBC __ Diff __
                              Lipids: Trig __ Chol __ HDL __ LDL __ HDL/Chol __
Urinalysis: Date _____   Alb _____   Glucose _____   Micro _____
Other Tests (please attach findings) _____
Treadmill Report (if applicable):

   Date of test   __/__/__   Protocol   _____

   Resting heart rate _____   Resting BP _____/_____

   MAX heart rate   _____ bpm   MAX BP   _____/_____

   Maximum METs _____
12-Lead ECG Interpretation/Comments (Rhythm/abnormalities): _____
_____
_____

STAT and PRN Orders
   1. Nitroglycerin 1/150 gr. SL PRN for chest pain.
   2. Lidocaine 50 mg. bolus IVP for PVCs 6–7/min. or V-bigeminy or V-tachycardia.
   3. Atropine 0.6 mg. IVP q 2–3 hrs. PRN for heart rate 40/min.
   4. Oxygen Intranasal 2–6 liters/min. PRN.
   5. Hang 250 D_5W and run at KVO rate.
   6. Defibrillate for ventricular fibrillation:
    Start at: 200–300 joules delivered energy; if no results 360 joules delivered energy;
   7. Additional (specify): _____
_____
_____
_____

                              _____, M.D.
                                        Signature
                         Date __/__/__

Physician Re-Referral Form

Patient's Name _____ Date _____ / ___ / _____
Address _____ Telephone _____
Date of conducted laboratory evaluation or exercise session episode _____
_____
_____
_____

YOU RECOMMEND:
_____ 1. Discontinue participation in the cardiac rehabilitation program.
_____ 2. Temporarily discontinue participation in the cardiac rehabilitation program
        while further investigation procedures are conducted. Probable date of renewed
        participation _____.
_____ 3. Continue participation in the cardiac rehabilitation program while further in-
        vestigative procedures are conducted. Probable date of completion of investiga-
        tive procedures _____.
_____ 4. Continue participation in the cardiac rehabilitation program. No further inves-
        tigative procedures to be conducted.

Physician's Name _____ Date _____ / ___ / _____

Physician's Signature _____

Informed Consent Forms

Graded Exercise Tolerance Test Informed Consent

I, the undersigned, authorize the _____ Diagnostic Laboratory to administer and conduct the Exercise Tolerance Test. This test is designed to measure my fitness for work and/or sport; to determine the presence or absence of clinically significant heart disease; and/or to evaluate the effectiveness of my current therapy.

I understand that the test will require that I either walk on a motor-driven treadmill or pedal a bicycle ergometer. During the performance of physical activity, my electrocardiogram will be monitored and my blood pressure will be measured at periodic intervals and recorded. Exercise will be progressively increased until I attain a predetermined endpoint corresponding to a moderate work level, or become distressed in any way, or develop an abnormal response the administrator of the test considers significant, whichever of the above occurs first.

Every effort will be made to conduct the test in such a way as to minimize discomfort and risk. However, I understand that in performing diagnostic tests on individuals with pre-existing medical problems (diagnosed or undiagnosed) that there are potential risks associated with such tests. In particular, an exercise tolerance test may elicit episodes of transient light-headedness, fainting, chest discomfort, or leg cramps, and very rarely heart attack or death may occur. I further understand that emergency equipment, drugs, and trained personnel are available to provide usual and customary care in unusual situations that may arise including: basic and advanced life support and transportation of a patient by ambulance to the nearest hospital.

Questions: _____

_____

Reply: _____

_____

_____ __/__/__ _____ __/__/__
       Witness   Date   Signature of Patient   Date

Informed Consent/Release

1. Explanation of Program

    You will be participating in a rehabilitation program that will include physical exercise, nutritional counseling, and patient education and may include stress management/relaxation therapy. The intensity and type of exercise you will perform will be based on your cardiovascular response to an initial graded exercise tolerance test that will be performed at the _____ clinic or by your personal physician within one month prior to beginning your exercise therapy. You may also be given other tests as needed to estimate body composition, desirable weight, lung function, various physiological parameters, personality traits, and stress levels. You will be given instructions regarding the amount and kind of regular exercise you should do. Exercise treatment visits will be available on a regularly scheduled basis. Your exercise prescription may be adjusted by the staff depending on your progress. You will be given the opportunity for re-evaluation at regularly scheduled intervals after beginning the rehabilitation program. Other re-evaluations may be recommended as needed. Progress reports will be sent to your personal physician on a regular basis.

2. Monitoring

    Your blood pressure will be monitored regularly as part of your program. You will be taught to monitor your own pulse rate before, during, and after each exercise session. In addition, ECG monitoring will be performed as a routine part of your program and according to individual needs.

3. Risks and Discomforts

    In rehabilitating individuals with pre-existing medical problems (diagnosed or undiagnosed), there exists the possibility of certain physiological changes occurring during the exercise treatment visits. These changes include abnormal blood pressures, fainting, and irregular heart beats, and in rare instances a heart attack or death may occur. We emphasize that every effort will be made to minimize the danger associated with the aforementioned changes by review of referring physician information, preliminary examination, and through observations of your exercise sessions. Emergency equipment, drugs, and trained personnel are available to provide basic life support at times when unusual situations arise. A registered nurse, physician, or emergency medical technician are available to provide advanced life support within a reasonable period of time. If required, patients may be transported by ambulance to the nearest hospital.

4. Benefits to be Expected

    Participation in the rehabilitation program may not benefit you directly in any way. The results obtained may help in evaluating the types of activities in which you might engage safely in your daily life. No assurance can be given that the rehabilitation program will increase your functional capacity, although widespread research and experience indicates that improvement is usually achieved.

5. Responsibility of the Participant

To gain expected benefits you must give priority to <u>regular attendance and adherence to prescribed amounts of intensity, duration, frequency, and type of activity</u>.

   To assure the safest exercise environment:

DO NOT:
   A. Withhold any information pertinent to symptoms from the professional staff.
   B. Exceed target heart rate.
   C. Exercise when you do not feel well.
   D. Exercise within 2 hours after eating.
   E. Exercise after drinking alcoholic beverages.
   F. Expose yourself to extremes in temperature; e.g., hot shower after exercising, saunas, steam baths, and similar extreme temperatures, as well as iced or hot drinks.
   G. Undertake isometric or straining exercise.

DO:
   A. Report any unusual symptom you experience before, during, or after exercise.
   B. Before leaving the site, check out with a member of the staff.

6. Use of Medical Records

   The information obtained during evaluation performed at the clinic and/or while I am a participant in the rehabilitation program will be treated as privileged and confidential. It is not to be released or revealed to any person except my referring physician without my written consent. The information obtained, however, may be used for statistical analysis or scientific purpose with my right to privacy retained.

7. Inquiries

   Any questions about the rehabilitation program are welcome. If you have doubts or questions, please ask us for further explanation.

8. Freedom of Consent

   Your permission to engage in this rehabilitation program is voluntary. You are free to deny consent if you so desire, both now and at any point in the program.

   I acknowledge that I have read this form in its entirety or it has been read to me and that I understand the rehabilitation program in which I will be engaged. I accept the rules and regulations set forth. I consent to participate in the _____ rehabilitation program.

Questions: _____

Response: _____

9. Release

   I have read the foregoing and I understand it. Any questions that have occurred to me have been answered to my satisfaction. Therefore, for guidance and supervision in exercise therapy, life-style change counseling, and/or diet therapy, I hereby for myself, my heirs, Executors and Administrators, waive and release any and all rights and claims for damages I may now and hereafter have against the staff of the _____ Rehabilitation Program, its Agents, Representatives or Assigns and Consultants.

_____	_____	_____
Signature of Patient	Signature of Director	Signature of Witness
Date _____	Date _____	Date _____

Emergency Procedures, Medications, and Basic Emergency Equipment

Standing Emergency Orders

The following emergency procedures have been adapted to make the procedures more practical to the real environment of the prehospital setting and are presented as guidelines only. Keep in mind that the prehospital setting is very different from the hospital setting in terms of the advanced surgical procedures used in the care of cardiac and other trauma patients. Also, it should be noted that there is more than one acceptable way to manage most situations. Clinicians must get advice from the medical director as to how emergency situations might best be handled in specific areas of the country.

General Procedures

The following orders delegate authority to the nurse to initiate emergency and resuscitative treatment in the absence of a physician. All patients participating in rehabilitation programs provided by _____ shall be covered under these orders — with or without a written order by the physician.

The following is the basic outline of all procedures and medications covered by this policy:

A. Initial response to emergency
   1. Evacuation of the exercise area. When an emergency situation arises, the staff shall immediately order evacuation of the exercise area. Patients should exit to the hallway area and proceed to cool-down. Patients should remain outside the exercise area until the endangered patient has been safely transported out of the building.
   2. Notify the _____ ambulance authority. Use the emergency message posted by the phone.
   3. Notify the physician in charge.
B. CPR, PRN: All nursing personnel must be certified in basic life support (BLS) as

described by the AHA or Red Cross. Certification must be current and evidence of certification must be on file at each clinic.

C. Defibrillation: For ventricular fibrillation (VF) and
                      ventricular tachycardia (VT)

   Start at 200 joules; if no change in cardiac rhythm, 200 – 300 joules; if no change, 200 – 300 joules; if no change, 360 joules, maximal output.

D. Initiating IV therapy: All patients in a life-threatening situation must have a route whereby IV therapy can be administered if necessary. The nurse may start an IV of 250 ml D5/W, KVO, using an angiocath.

E. ECG: In an emergency or a justifiably abnormal situation, e.g., patient experiencing persistent chest pain, obtain an ECG and monitor continuously PRN.

F. Oxygen: Give intranasal O_2, PRN 2 L/min rate. To increase flow rate, notify physician.

Procedures for Specific Situations Including the Administration of Medications

A. Hypotension: Systolic BP <90 mmHg
                   Symptomatic
                   HR >60 bpm
   1. Elevate feet
   2. Notify physician
   3. Obtain ECG

B. Fainting:
   1. Lay flat; elevate feet
   2. Use ammonia ampules
   3. Give O_2 PRN
   4. Notify physician
   5. Obtain ECG

C. Bradyarrhythmias: Ventricular rate <60 bpm
                        Symptomatic
   1. Notify ambulance and physician
   2. Assure adequate airway and ventilation; O_2 PRN
   3. IV therapy
   4. If HR <50 bpm, give atropine: 0.5 or 0.6 mg IV bolus
   5. Obtain ECG

   If circulatory collapse and loss of consciousness occur, proceed to BLS measures appropriate to shock and/or other dysrhythmia.

D. Asystole: Carotid pulse = 0; Respiration rate <2/min
   1. Begin BLS, notify ambulance and physician
   2. Obtain ECG and give O_2
   3. Continue BLS until spontaneous respiration and circulation are established (presence of carotid pulse)
   4. If no response:
      a. IV therapy
      b. Give epinephrine: 5 – 10 ml of a 1 : 10,000 solution IV
      c. Give sodium bicarbonate: 1 mEq/kg IV Bolus

5. If a change in cardiac rhythm occurs, proceed to appropriate cardiac dysrhythmia protocol.

6. If asystole persists:
   give calcium chloride: 5 ml of a 10% solution IV

7. If asystole persists:
   give atropine: 0.5 mg IV bolus

8. Continue the following sequence if asystole persists:
   a. Epinephrine: 0.5 mg (5 ml) q 5 min IV bolus
   b. Sodium bicarbonate: ½ mEq/kg q 10 min IV
   c. Calcium chloride: 0.5 mg 10% (5 ml) IV bolus q 10 min. Do not mix calcium chloride with sodium bicarb.
   d. Atropine: 0.5 mg IV bolus q 5 min to maximum 2 mg

9. If a change in rhythm occurs, proceed to appropriate dysrhythmia protocol

10. Obtain ECG

E. Symptomatic PVCs: New onset of PVCs, PVCs >6/min, R on T phenomenon, change in mental status with symptomatic PVCs, salvos

   1. Notify physician
   2. Assure adequate airway and ventilation, O_2 PRN
   3. IV therapy
   4. Obtain ECG strips, 12-lead if possible
   5. Give lidocaine: 50–100 mg IV bolus, int. dose (1 mg/kg)
   6. Begin lidocaine drip, premixed 2g/500ml D5/W at 2–3 mg/min (30 ml/hr) (30 mcgtts/min)
   7. Additional 50 mg bolus (0.5 mg/kg) may be given q 5 min if necessary to total of 225 mg
   8. Increase infusion by 1 mg/min with additional bolus to a maximum of 4 mg/min (60 ml/hr) (60 mcgtts/min)
   9. Watch for signs of toxic RXN—slurred speech, altered consciousness, muscle twitches, seizures
   10. If change in rhythm occurs, follow appropriate cardiac rhythm sequence

F. Symptomatic PVCs: Ventricular rate <60 bpm
                     Patient symptomatic
                     Systolic BP <90 mmHg

   1. Notify physician and ambulance
   2. Assure adequate airway and ventilation
   3. Give atropine: 0.5 mg IV bolus, repeat q 5 min to total dosage of 2 mg
   4. If ineffective in increasing hr to >60 bpm and overriding PVCs, start isuprel drip. Mix 1 mg in 250 ml D5/W (4 mcg/ml): titrate between 2–20 mcg/min to maintain hr 60–100 BPM and override PVCs

G. Ventricular Tachycardia: Patient conscious and symptomatic

   1. Notify ambulance and physician
   2. Provide adequate airway and ventilation and give O_2 PRN
   3. IV therapy
   4. Obtain ECG strips and 12-lead if possible
   5. Give lidocaine: 50–100 mg IV bolus int. dose (1 mg/kg)
   6. Begin lidocaine drip premixed 2 g/500 ml D5/W (Start at 2 mg/min, 30 ml/hr)

7. Additional 50 mg bolus (0.5 mg/kg) may be given q 5 min if necessary to a total of 225 mg
8. Increase infusion by 1 mg/min with additional bolus to a maximum of 4 mg/min
9. Watch for CNS signs of toxic RXN — slurred speech, altered consciousness, muscle twitching, seizures
10. If change in rhythm occurs, follow appropriate cardiac rhythm sequence

H. Ventricular Tachycardia: Patient unconscious p̄ max lidocaine infusion
1. Witnessed and monitored: give precordial thump
2. Begin BLS and continue until spontaneous respiration and circulation are established
3. Give lidocaine 50–100 mg IV bolus (1 mg/kg)
4. Defibrillate: 200–300 joules
5. If change in rhythm occurs, follow appropriate cardiac rhythm sequence and:
6. Begin lidocaine infusion: 2 g/500 ml D5/W (0.4%) at 2 mg/min (30 ml/hr) (30 mcgtts/min)
7. Repeat step 5
8. If ineffective:
   a. Give sodium bicarbonate 1 mEq/kg IV
   b. Give lidocaine 0.5 mg IV bolus
   c. Increase lidocaine infusion to max 4 mg/min (60 ml/hr) (60 mcgtts/min)
   d. Cardiovert with 200–300 joules

If no change in cardiac rhythm occurs p̄ max of 10 min lidocaine infusion, follow sequence for recurrent ventricular tachycardia

I. Recurrent Ventricular Tachycardia: Patient unconscious p max lidocaine infusion
1. Continue BLS until spontaneous respiration and circulation are established
2. Discontinue lidocaine infusion

J. Ventricular Fibrillation:
1. Notify ambulance and physician
2. Obtain ECG strips, 12-lead if possible
3. If onset of VF witnessed, give precordial thump
4. If ineffective or if patient is found in VF, begin CPR and defibrillate immediately: 200–300 joules
5. If change in cardiac rhythm occurs, follow appropriate cardiac sequence
6. If first defibrillation is unsuccessful, deliver second countershock of 360 joules immediately
7. Repeat step 5
8. If ineffective:
   a. Give epinephrine: 0.5 mg (5 ml of 1 : 10,000) IV bolus
   b. Give sodium bicarbonate: 1 mEq/kg IV
   c. Continue CPR for 2 min
   d. Defibrillate with 360 joules
9. Repeat step 5
10. If ineffective, or if VF recurs after successful defibrillation,
    a. Give lidocaine 50–100 mg IV bolus and start infusion of 2–3 mg/min
    b. Continue CPR for 2 min
    c. Defibrillate with 360 joules

11. Repeat step 5
12. Repeat steps 10b and 10c
13. Repeat step 5
14. If no change in cardiac rhythm:
    a. Continue CPR for 2 min
    b. Defibrillate with 360 joules
15. Repeat step 5
16. If no change in cardiac rhythm:
    a. Continue CPR
    b. Give sodium bicarbonate (½ mEq/kg) if 10 min have elapsed
    c. Defibrillate with 360 joules
17. Repeat step 5
18. If no change in cardiac rhythm occurs:
    a. Continue CPR
    b. Give epinephrine: 0.5–1 mg (5–10 ml of 1 : 10,000) IV bolus q 5 min
    c. Give sodium bicarbonate: ½ mEq/kg q 10 min

K. Supraventricular Tachycardia: Patient symptomatic; i.e., change in mental status, Systolic BP <90 mmHg

1. Notify physician
2. Assure adequate airway, ventilation and O_2 PRN
3. Obtain ECG
4. Instruct patient to perform Valsalva maneuver
5. Perform carotid massage (under direct physician supervision only)
6. IV therapy

Medications

1. Atropine Sulfate: 0.1 mg/ml in 10 ml syringe
   Dosage: 0.5 mg–1.0 mg = 5–10 ml
   Repeat at 5 min intervals to achieve desired HR generally, do not exceed 2 mg

2. Calcium Chloride: 10% solution, 100 mg/ml in 10 ml syringe
   Dosage: 500 mg = 5 ml
   May repeat dose q 10 min PRN

3. Dopamine: 200 mg in 5 ml ampule
   Dosage: 200 mg in 250 ml D5/W = 800 mcg/ml
   Infusion: 2–10 mcg/kg/min

4. Epinephrine: 1 : 10,000 solution, 0.1 mg/ml in 10 ml syringe
   Dosage: 0.5 mg–1.0 mg = 5–10 ml IV
          Repeat dose q 5 min PRN in cardiac arrest
   Infusion: 1 mg in D5/W (4 mcg/ml in 250 ml; 2 mcg/ml in 500 ml)
          Rate: 1 mcg/min for maintenance of BP

5. Isoproterenol (Isuprel): 0.2 mg/ml in 5 ml ampule
   Dosage: 1 mg in D5/W (4 mcg/ml in 250 ml; 2 mcg/ml in 500 ml)
   Infusion: 2–20 mcg/min; titrate; beware of PVCs

6. Lidocaine: 1% (10 mg/ml; 100 mg/10 ml) and 2% (20 mg/ml; 100 mg/5 ml) for IV bolus
   for infusion after bolus: 4% (40 mg/ml; 1 g/25 ml)
   Dosage: 1%: 75 mg = 7.50 ml
            2%: 75 mg = 3.75 ml
            2 g/500 ml D5/W or 1 g/250 ml D5/W premixed = 4 mg/ml
   Infusion: 1–4 mg/min
   For breakthrough ventricular ectopy, additional 50 mg bolus q 5 min to suppress ectopy—total 225 mg; increase drip: 4 mg/min

7. Procainamide: 100 mg/ml in 10 ml ampule for IV bolus
                 500 mg/ml in 2 ml ampules for infusion p bolus
   Dosage: 20 mg/min until:
       a. Dysrhythmia suppressed
       b. Hypotension ensues
       c. QRS widens by 50%
       d. Total of 1 g given
   1 g/250 ml D5/W = mg/ml; infusion: 1–4 mg/min
   Monitor ECG and BP. Give cautiously in patients with acute MI.

8. Sodium Bicarbonate: 1 mEq/ml in 50 ml = 50 mEq
   Dosage: 1 mEq/kg or 75 ml initial dose for average-sized adult
   Repeat according to pH. If not available, use ½ initial dose q 10 min

9. Dextrose: 5% in water premixed 250 ml bag

All Orders and Medication Instructions Approved

_____ M.D. _____
Medical Director   Date
_____ Clinic

Basic Emergency Equipment
    Portable Cart
    Defibrillator
    IV lines, needles, syringes
    Ambu bags
    Airways and O_2 tank
    ECG equipment
    Stethoscope
    Sphygmomanometer

APPENDIX E

Flexibility Exercises

Stretching I

Discontinue any exercise that causes you pain or discomfort.
Don't hold your breath—breathe slowly and deeply.
Stretch slowly and gently—no bouncing.
Try not to strain. Relax while you stretch.

1. Wall Stretch

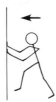

Stand facing wall with feet a shoulder-width apart. Take one step forward with right leg, bending knee. Keep back heel on floor. Place hands a shoulder-width apart on the wall for support. Hold. Repeat with other leg.

2. Stand and Reach

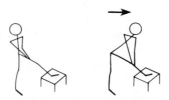

Using a bench or stool, place one foot up on bench, keeping leg straight. Slowly extend arms down leg. Hold. Repeat with other leg.

3. Standing Foot Hold

Stand with left hand on chair or wall for support. Bend right leg and grasp foot with right hand. Gently pull foot toward body. Repeat with other leg.

4. Groin Stretch

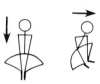

Sit on mat with feet together. Place hands on ankles. Gently pull them in close to hips. Slowly bend forward, keeping back straight. Relax. Repeat.

5. Straddle

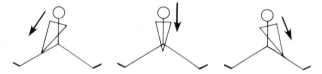

Sit on mat with legs apart extended straight out. Extend arms out, reaching toward right foot. Return to center. Reach toward left foot. Return to center and reach forward. Relax. Keep back straight.

6. Spinal Twist

Sitting on mat, extend right leg to front, and place left foot on mat on other side of right knee. Reach over left leg with right arm. Use left hand behind you for balance. Turn upper body to left, looking over left shoulder. Repeat to other side.

7. Curl Stretch

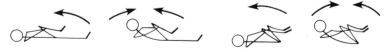

Lie on back on mat with legs extended. Bring right knee up to chest. Hold hands just below knee. As you stretch slowly, bring head up toward knee. Relax. Repeat with other knee. Relax. Bring both knees up and slowly curl head up. Relax.

8. Neck Limber

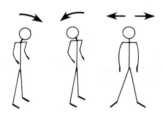

Seated or standing, pull head down toward chest and hold for 10 seconds. Return to starting position and then pull head back and hold for 10 seconds. Repeat for left and right side and as many angles in between as you wish.

9. Arm Circle

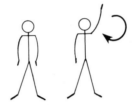

Seated or standing, begin with right arm, depressing shoulder down toward floor with arm extended. Continue to raise arm slowly up toward ceiling and around toward back. Keep arm extended and stretch throughout movement. Repeat with other arm.

Name _____

Flexibility and Muscular Strength and Endurance Data Sheet

Kinetic Activities

| Date | Flexibility Exercises | | | | | | | Muscular Strength and Endurance | | | | | | |
	Calf	Hamstring	Quads	Groin	Trunk	Shoulder	Neck	1	2	3	4	5	6	BP

APPENDIX **F**

Coronary Outpatient Exercise Guidelines

Coronary Outpatient Exercise Guidelines

Level	Approx. No. of Weeks after Event	Calisthenics No. of Repetitions	Medically Supervised			Unsupervised (85% of Supervised)	
			Bicycle Ergometer	Arm Ergometer	Treadmill or Walk-Jog	Bicycle Ergometer	Walk
Phase II (Therapeutic)							
1	3–4	6	8 min (×2) 35% MET-ET or 50 r/min at 150 KPM	8 min (×2) 30% MET-ET or 100 T at 150 KPM	12 min* 50% MET-ET† or 22-min time	8 min (×2) 50 r/min at 130 KPM	12 min* 25-min mile
2	3–4	7	8 min (×2) 40% MET-ET or 50 r/min at 225 KPM	8 min (×2) 35% MET-ET or 125 T at 225 KPM	12 min* 60% MET-ET† or 22-min mile	8 min (×2) 50 r/min at 190 KPM	12 min* 25-min mile
3	3–4	8	8 min (×2) 45% MET-ET or 50 r/min at 300 KPM	8 min (×2) 45% MET-ET or 125 T at 300 KPM	12 min* 70% MET-ET† or 20-min mile	8 min (×2) 60 r/min at 225 KPM	12 min* 22-min mile
4	5	10	12 min 45% MET-ET or 60 r/min at 300 KPM	8 min (×2) 45% MET-ET or 150 T at 300 KPM	12 min* 75% MET-ET† or 18-min mile	12 min 60 r/min at 225 KPM	12 min* 20-min mile
5	5	10	15 min 45% MET-ET or 70 r/min at 300 KPM	8 min (×2) 45% MET-ET or 150 T at 300 KPM	12 min* 75% MET-ET† or 18-min mile	15 min 70 r/min at 225 KPM	12 min* 20-min mile
6	5	10	15 min 45% MET-ET or 70 r/min at 300 KPM	8 min (×2) 45% MET-ET or 150 T at 300 KPM	12 min* 75% MET-ET† or 18-min mile	15 min 70 r/min at 255 KPM	12 min* 20-min mile
7‡	6	12	15 min 60 r/min at 300 KPM or 3.7 MET	175 T at 300 KPM or 4.5 MET	1.5 min§ 3.9 MET, 16-min mile walk; or 6.0 MET, 14-min mile walk; or 8.6 MET, 12-min mile jog; or 10.2 MET, 10-min mile jog	15 min 60 r/min at 255 KPM or 3.1 MET	1.5 min 3.9 MET or 16-min mile walk

425

Coronary Outpatient Exercise Guidelines—*continued*

Level	Approx. No. of Weeks after Event	Calisthenics No. of Repetitions	Medically Supervised			Unsupervised *(85% of Supervised)*	
			Bicycle Ergometer	Arm Ergometer	Treadmill or Walk-Jog	Bicycle Ergometer	Walk
Phase II (Therapeutic)							
8‡	7	18	15 min 60 r/min at 450 KPM or 4.9 MET	200 T at 375 KPM or 5.5 MET	2.0 min§ 3.9 MET, 16-min mile walk; or 6.0 MET, 14-min mile walk; or 8.6 MET, 12-min mile jog; or 10.2 MET, 10-min mile jog	15 min 60 r/min at 380 KPM or 4.2 MET	2.0 min 3.9 MET or 16-min mile walk
9‡	9	18	15 min 60 r/min at 450 KPM or 4.9 MET	200 T at 450 KPM or 6.4 MET	2.25 min§ 6.0 MET, 14-min mile walk; or 8.6 MET, 12-min mile jog; or 10.2 MET, 10-min mile jog; or 11.0 MET, 9-min mile jog	15 min 60 r/min at 380 KPM or 4.2 MET	2.25 min 3.9 MET or 16-min mile walk
10‡	11	18	15 min 60 r/min at 600 KPM or 6.1 MET	250 T at 450 KPM or 6.4 MET	2.5 min§ 6.0 MET, 14-min mile walk; or 8.6 MET, 12-min mile jog; or 10.2 MET, 10-min mile jog; or 11.0 MET, 9-min mile jog	15 min 60 r/min at 500 KPM or 5.2 MET	2.5 min 6.0 MET or 14-min mile walk

11‡	12	18	15 min 60 r/min at 600 KPM or 6.1 MET	250 T at 450 KPM or 6.4 MET	2.75 min§ 6.0 MET, 14-min mile walk; or 8.6 MET, 12-min mile jog; or 10.2 MET, 10-min mile jog; or 11.0 MET, 9-min mile jog	15 m 60 r/min at 500 KPM or 5.2 MET	2.75 min 6.0 MET or 14-min mile walk
12‡	13	18	15 min 60 r/min at 600 KPM or 6.1 MET	250 T at 450 KPM or 6.4 MET	3.00 min§ 6.0 MET, 14-min mile walk; or 8.6 MET, 12-min mile jog; or 10.2 MET, 10-min mile jog; or 11.0 MET, 9-min mile jog	15 min 60 r/min at 500 KPM or 5.2 MET	3.00 min 6.0 MET or 14-min mile walk

Phase III (Maintenance)

13‡	14 on	18	15 min 60 r/min at 600 KPM or 6.1 MET	250 T at 450 KPM or 6.4 MET	3.00 min 9–12-min mile or 11.0–8.6 MET jog-walk	15 min 60 r/min at 500 KPM or 5.2 MET	3.00 min 6.0 MET or 14-min mile walk

Levels 1–6 typically accomplished in a 2-week period. Telemetry ECG monitoring may aid in heart rate and rhythm evaluation during this period. Supervised programs, 3 sessions weekly. Unsupervised programs 3–4 sessions weekly. MET-ET = MET level on treadmill test. KPM = bicycle resistance in kilo and meters. T = turns of 60–75 revolutions per minute (r/min). Event = myocardial infarction, coronary bypass surgery, or coronary angioplasty.

*Plus an additional 1-min warm-up and 1-min cool-down.
†As designated on exercise treadmill (calibrated).
‡Levels 7–13, rowing machine may be used for 3–5 min, progressing from slight to moderate resistance.
§Select pace on an individual basis considering activity level in previous weeks and patient's cardiovascular status.
Source: From Fletcher, GF and Cantwell, JD: Exercise and Coronary Heart Disease, ed 2, 1977, p. 175. Courtesy of Charles C Thomas, Publisher, Springfield, Illinois.

APPENDIX G

Dietary Goals for the United States*

1. To avoid overweight, consume only as much energy (calories) as is expended; if overweight, decrease energy intake and increase energy expenditure.

2. Increase the consumption of complex carbohydrates and "naturally occurring" sugars from about 28 percent to about 48 percent of energy intake.

3. Reduce the consumption of refined and other processed sugars by about 45 percent to account for about 10 percent of total energy intake.

4. Reduce overall fat consumption from approximately 40 percent to about 30 percent of energy intake.

5. Reduce saturated-fat consumption to account for about 10 percent of total energy intake and balance that with polyunsaturated and monounsaturated fats, which should account for about 10 percent of energy intake each.

6. Reduce cholesterol consumption to about 300 mg per day.

7. Limit the intake of sodium by reducing the intake of salt (sodium chloride) to about 5 g per day (2 g sodium).

*From Select Committee on Nutrition and Human Needs, U.S. Senate: Dietary Goals for the United States, ed 2. December 1977.

428

Index

An "f" following a page number indicates a figure; a "t" following a page number indicates a table.

Centriacinar emphysema, 103
Cephalosporin, 142
Cerebrovascular disease(s)
    hypertension and, 354
    smoking and, 350
CF. *See* Cystic fibrosis
Chair step test protocol, 238t
CHD. *See* Coronary heart disease
Chemoreceptor(s)
    control of heart beat and, 27–28
    regulation of respiration and, 53, 55–56
Chest lead(s)
    modified V₅, 161, 161f, 229
    reference sites for, 159f
Chest pain
    nitrates and, 115, 118
    streptokinase and, 132–133
Chest roentgenogram(s) (CXR)
    chronic lung diseases and, 100, 102, 105,
        107–108, 111–112
    pulmonary assessment and, 254, 261, 281
    smoking and, 353
CHF. *See* Congestive heart failure
Cold, exercise therapy and, 342–343
Cholesterol. *See also* High-density lipoproteins;
        Low-density
lipoproteins; Plasma cholesterol; Very low density
        lipoproteins
    aerobic exercise and, 70
    classification and recommended follow-up for,
        367t
    coronary artery disease and, 130
    dietary intervention and, 371–372, 372t–373t,
        374, 376
    drugs to lower, 130t
    genetic hypercholesterolemia and, 368–371
    goals for the United States, 428
    hypertension and, 360
    lipid disorders and, 367–368
    relationship to age-adjusted coronary heart
        disease death rate, 362f
Chronic diseases, deaths attributable to risk
        factors for, 351t
Chronic heart failure, 92
Chronic lung disease(s), 98–113
    pharmacologic management of, 118, 133–142
Chronic obstructive pulmonary disease (COPD),
        98–101
    arterial blood gas analysis and, 60–61
    exercise testing and, 7–8, 278
    forced expiratory flow and, 265
    huff and, 390
    oxygen therapy and, 294
    pulmonary impairment and, 282
    pulmonary rehabilitation and, 392–394
    right ventricular failure and, 93
    smoking and, 350, 394
Chylomicron(s), 364, 366–367
    genetic hypercholesterolemia and, 369–370
Chylomicronemia syndrome, 370
Cigarette smoking. *See* Smoking
Circulation
    aerobic exercise and, 64, 68, 71
    collateral, 80, 82–83, 108
    congestive heart failure and, 91

coronary
    atherosclerosis and, 79, 84
    myocardial infarction and, 87
    heart and, 13–32, 92–93
    systemic adjustments to, 64–65
CK. *See* Creatine kinase
Class I antiarrhythmic(s), 126–128, 186
Class II antiarrhythmic(s), 128–129
Class III antiarrhythmic(s), 129
Class IV antiarrhythmic(s), 129–130
Claudication, 340
Clot lysis system, 132
CO₂. *See* Carbon dioxide
Community exercise programs, 7
Compensated heart failure, 92–93
Complete heart block, 185–186, 186f
Compliance with rehabilitation program
    chronic obstructive pulmonary disease and,
        9–10
    exercise therapy and, 343–345
    nutrition and, 395
    risk factor modification evaluation and, 371
    smoking and, 354
Conducting airways, 39–43
    lower conducting airways, 42f
    upper conducting airways, 41f
Conduction, 18–19. *See also* Impulse conduction
    antiarrhythmics and, 122, 126
    arrhythmias and, 170–173
    atrial impulse, 20f
    atrioventricular blocks and, 183–185
    cardiac catheterization and, 83
    cardiac glycosides and, 121
    drugs, 195–196
    electrocardiogram and, 152–155, 167, 267
    electrophysiologic studies and, 193
    heart blocks and, 182, 186–187
    myocardial fibers and, 21–22
    myocardial infarction and, 84, 88
    pacemakers and, 188–189, 191
    pathways of, 21f
    sinus tachycardia and, 170
    sudden cardiac death and, 91
    ventricular, 21f
Confidentiality, medical records and, 222
Congenital heart disease, 91, 93
Congestive heart failure (CHF)
    atrial arrhythmias and, 174
    coronary artery disease and, 89, 91–92
        antiarrhythmics and, 127–128, 130
    exercise and, 195, 293
    heart blocks and, 186
    hypertension and, 354
    pharmacologic management of, 118, 120–121,
        127–128, 130
Connective tissue, 100–101
Contraction
    atrioventricular node, 177
    bundle branch blocks, 187
    coronary artery disease and, 115, 118–121,
        126–127
    electrocardiogram and, 152–154, 156, 194
    heart failure and, 88–89, 91–94
    pacemakers and, 190
    premature nodal, 177

Q

U

Uncompensated heart failure, 92–93
Unstable angina, 82
Urine analysis, 217, 220–221
Urokinase, 83, 132–133

V

Vagal stimulation, 174, 177
Valsalva maneuver
    atrial arrhythmias and, 173, 177
    diabetes and, 340
    exercise prescription and, 293
Valve replacement(s), 278
Variant angina, 82–83
Vasoconstriction
    chronic bronchitis and, 102
    cold and, 342
    coronary artery disease and, 118
    emphysema and, 104
    perfusion and, 52
    regulation of peripheral resistance and, 30
Vasodilation
    aerobic exercise and, 68
    myocardial infarction and, 88
    perfusion and, 52
    verapamil and, 120
Vasodilators, 93, 132. *See also* Nitrates
VC. *See* Vital capacity
VDS. *See* Dead space volume
VE. *See* Minute volume
VEmax. *See* Maximum minute ventilation
Venous return (preload), 92
Venous stasis, 89
Venous thrombi, 89
Ventilation
    acid-base balance and, 56
    aerobic exercise and, 65, 68
    arterial blood gas analysis and, 57–58
    chronic obstructive pulmonary disease and, 99, 133
    forced expiratory technique and, 390
    partial pressures of, 50t
    perfusion relationship and, 53, 54f, 102–104, 107, 109–110
    pulmonary assessment and, 255–256, 264–267, 270
    pursed lip breathing and, 392
    respiration regulation and, 54–55, 55f, 56
    secretions and, 384
Ventilatory muscle training, 390–391
Ventricular arrhythmia(s)
    alcohol reduction and, 358
    atrioventricular blocks and, 184
    automatic implantable cardioverter-defibrillator and, 193
    bigeminy, 180f
    drugs, electrocardiogram and, 195–196
    electrocardiogram and, 178–182
    exercise therapy and, 311
    normal sinus rhythm with unifocal premature contraction, 179f
    premature contractions, 179f

progression of, 182f
    tachycardia, 181f
Ventricular conduction, 21f
Ventricular failure, 93–94, 95f
Ventricular fibrillation (VF)
    automatic implantable cardioverter-defibrillator and, 193
    electrocardiogram and, 181–182, 182f
    emergency procedures for, 417
    myocardial infarction and, 88
    sudden cardiac death and, 91
Ventricular function
    coronary artery bypass graft and, 145
    exercise prescription and, 280–281
    myocardial infarction and, 84
Ventricular tachycardia(s) (VT), 193
    electrocardiogram and, 180–181, 181f
    emergency procedures for, 416–417
Ventriculogram, 144
Verapamil
    atrial arrhythmias and, 173–174, 176–177
    coronary artery disease and, 120, 129–130
Very-low-density lipoprotein(s) (VLDL), 360, 367, 369–370
Vertebrae, 34–35, 37
VF. *See* Ventricular fibrillation
Vibration, 388–389
Visual disturbances, 122, 128
Vital capacity (VC), 46–48
    asthma and, 107
    pulmonary assessment and, 261–263
    restrictive lung disease and, 111
    smoking and, 353
Vital signs, 255–256
VLDL. *See* Very-low-density lipoprotein(s)
VO2max. *See* Maximal amount of oxygen
VT. *See* Tidal volume
VT. *See* Ventricular tachycardia

W

Walk test, 268–269
Walking
    chronic obstructive pulmonary disease and, 7–8
    exercise prescription and, 290–291
    pulmonary rehabilitation and, 392
Wandering atrial pacemaker(s), 171, 171f
Warm-up period(s)
    exercise and, 290, 294, 311, 341
    stress testing and, 233–234
Waves, complexes, and intervals, 154–164. *See also* names of individual waves and intervals, e.g., T wave, P-R interval
Water retention, 89, 91–92, 94
Wheezing, 102, 105, 107, 254, 260
Weight
    diet and, 372
    hypertension and, 357
    loss of, 70–71, 370, 395
    percent body fat and, 292
    physical measurement of, 223, 251
    pulmonary assessment and, 256